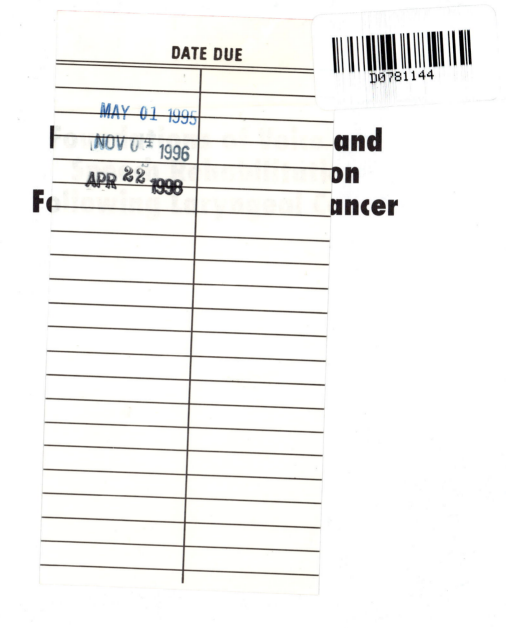

DATE DUE

MAY 01 1995
NOV 04 1996
APR 22 1998

Foundations of Voice and Speech Rehabilitation Following Laryngeal Cancer

Philip C. Doyle, Ph.D., CCC-SLP, SLP(C)

Associate Professor
Department of Communicative Disorders
University of Western Ontario
London, Ontario, Canada

SINGULAR PUBLISHING GROUP, INC.
San Diego, California

Singular Publishing Group, Inc.
4284 41st Street
San Diego, California 92105-1197

©1994 by Singular Publishing Group, Inc.

Typeset in 10/12 Palatino by ExecuStaff
Printed in the United States of America by BookCrafters

Library of Congress Cataloging-in-Publication Data

Doyle, Philip C.
    Foundations of voice and speech rehabilitation following laryngeal cancer / by Philip C. Doyle.
       p.   cm.
    Includes bibliographical references and index.
    ISBN 1-56593-109-2
    1. Larynx—Cancer—Patients—Rehabilitation.   2. Speech therapy.
  3. Voice disorders—Patients—Rehabilitation.   I. Title.
    [DNLM: 1. Speech, Alaryngeal.   2. Laryngeal Neoplasms—
  rehabilitation.   3. Speech Therapy—methods.   WV 540 1994]
  RC280.T5D69   1994
  616.99'42206—dc20
  DNLM/DLC
  for Library of Congress   94-7648
                                                                CIP

Contents

Foreword

In 1980 the American Cancer Society estimated that approximately 10,500 new cases of laryngeal cancer would be diagnosed each year in the United States. A decade later they revised their estimate upward to 13,000 new cases each year. General aging of the population is likely to accelerate this trend, and modern medicine will improve the 5-year survival rate, yielding increasing numbers of laryngectomized patients. The occurrence of laryngeal cancer can be devastating to the patient and his or her family and poses difficult challenges to the health care professionals who must manage the situation.

Fortunately, Dr. Doyle has written a lucid, comprehensive text that will contribute significantly to the knowledge of laryngectomee communication rehabilitation. He has served as a clinician, teacher, and researcher and imparts a broad perspective to the clinical endeavor. Dr. Doyle presents a consistent philosophy throughout the text that yields principles and goals

of patient management. The guiding principles evolve into practical *what* and *how to* methodology. Relevant information has been clearly summarized in tables for clinicians and students and an extensive literature review offers direction for further study. Most importantly, a strong sense of humanity permeates the text to remind us that cancer patients confront many daunting issues that impact on their quality of life.

The text has been organized in a practical, logical sequence for patient care. Each chapter is subdivided into sections for quick reference of information and also summarized. Chapters 1 and 2 present an introduction to the incidence and causation of laryngeal cancer. Chapter 3, "Diagnosis and Treatment of Laryngeal Cancer: An Overview for the Speech-Language Pathologist," provides a valuable, practical guide to the medical diagnosis and management of laryngeal cancer. This presentation will assist the speech-language pathologist to interpret information communicated by other health care professionals and evaluate the possible impact on the patient. The potential contribution of the lymphatic system to cancer metastasis, tumor grading, and clinical staging are discussed. Conservative surgical approaches and the impact on voice are described in addition to total laryngectomy. The roles of radiation treatment and chemotherapy complete this chapter.

Chapter 4 introduces communication rehabilitation of the laryngectomee by defining the role of the speech-language pathologist. An effective clinical process begins with the establishment of a positive relationship between the clinician and patient, but the professional is reminded that the patient's fear of cancer may interfere with communication between them. The speech-language pathologist's role is multifaceted and encompasses providing, interpreting, and facilitating information. Dr. Doyle quite properly chooses to conclude a discussion of the professional's role by presenting 12 attitudes of health care workers that can be detrimental to the rehabilitation process. Chapter 5, "Voice and Speech Treatment Following Partial Laryngectomy," presents traditional therapy techniques for managing vocal pitch, loudness, and quality appropriate for each postsurgical method.

The speech-language pathologist's role and a positive response to detrimental attitudes is extended to Chapters 6 and 7 which address pre- and postoperative communication counseling, respectively. These chapters are complete and present broad issues and review *what* information to present and *how* to present it. Multidisciplinary roles are clearly delineated, and the patient's and spouse's psychological state is to be considered, including recognizing that comprehension may be reduced due to the stress. The advantages and potential problems of visitations to the patient by laryngectomized individuals are discussed. Chapter 8, "Alaryngeal Voice and Speech Options," suggests a

patient-centered, clear philosophy that, if given adequate information, the laryngectomee ultimately chooses his or her own method of alaryngeal communication. Effective communication and psychological well-being are the goals. In recognition of individual differences, potential advantages and disadvantages of each method are presented.

Pre- and postoperative communication counseling is followed by chapters devoted to each individual method of alaryngeal communication. Chapter 9, "Esophageal Function," describes the voicing mechanism and surgery's impact on esophageal and tracheoesophageal voice. The subsequent chapter, "Esophageal Speech," addresses clinical management issues including further discussion of the pharyngoesophageal segment as it relates to voice production and possible speech difficulties. Specific methods of facilitating esophageal insufflation are described and a systematic program of extending esophageal voice to functional speech is presented. An eloquent plea for communication as the ultimate goal is presented in Chapter 11, "Artificial Laryngeal Speech." Controversial issues are discussed and essentially resolved by redirecting the focus to patient needs rather than clinician bias. The different types of artificial larynges are described, and a clear program of rehabilitation is presented. Chapter 12 is a thorough presentation of tracheoesophageal speech. Clinical management issues are discussed in a logical sequence that includes patient selection criteria. The surgical puncture technique is described, and the general speech success rate is reviewed. Dr. Doyle guides the reader through prosthesis fitting, voice assessment, and problem-solving procedures. A complete rehabilitation program is outlined including cleaning and inserting the prosthesis, methodology for voice production, and utilization of the tracheostoma breathing valve. Finally, functional comparisons of the alaryngeal methods of communication are presented in Chapter 13, "Comparative Performance by Esophageal, Artificial Laryngeal, and Tracheoesophageal Speakers."

It is appropriate that Dr. Doyle has chosen to devote the final three chapters to a major theme of his text, namely, to consider the total impact of a laryngectomy on individuals' lives. He reminds us in Chapter 14, "Long-Term Counseling of the Patient," that a laryngectomy creates myriad problems that can require considerable time to resolve. A team of professionals must assist the patient to adjust to physical and psychological changes in order to return to an essentially normal life. It is also suggested that the patient could benefit from participation in a laryngectomy support group. In Chapter 15, Dr. Doyle has written an especially sensitive and thoughtful treatise on the potential effects of laryngeal cancer and its treatment on the quality of the patient's life. Patients and their loved ones must consider the best method of controlling the cancer and confront the likelihood of its recurrence. Physical disfigurement and loss of normal verbal communication can create social isolation. Patients do not live in a vacuum, and health care professionals must understand that communication is the primary means for initiating, maintaining, and terminating relationships with other people. The impact of communication loss confirms that it is not just the continuation of life, but also the quality of one's life that is important. An individual must experience a life that is worth living and has meaning for him- or herself and others. The final chapter weaves these themes into a discussion of how we can better serve the patient. To consider the patient as a person, not just a communication disorder, indicates that multidisciplinary care is essential. Dr. Doyle implores us to consider laryngectomy rehabilitation guided by one primary goal: to assist the patient to return to as normal a life as possible.

This text is written by a master clinician for clinicians. Dr. Doyle has provided a compassionate and comprehensive examination of the rehabilitation process for individuals with laryngeal cancer. He has made a significant contribution to the professional growth of speech-language pathologists and, ultimately, the care of patients.

Charles G. Reed, Ph.D.
Chief, Audiology & Speech
Pathology Service
Department of Veterans
Affairs Medical Center
San Francisco, California

Preface

When the speech-language pathologist encounters a patient who has undergone laryngectomy, the classic textbooks by Diedrich and Youngstrom (1966), Snidecor (1978), and Gardner (1971) remain essential and primary sources of information to the clinician. These sources were a rich and invaluable resource during the preparation of the present text. In many instances, these sources remain steadfast in their clinical utility and application. However, much has changed in the management and rehabilitation of patients following laryngeal cancer over the past two decades. To understand these changes the topic must be viewed in a broader, more comprehensive fashion than has existed previously.

I will always remember a rather lengthy discussion I had with Dr. Jack Snidecor in 1979 while I was a graduate student at the University of California, Santa Barbara. This meeting was arranged by Dr. Ted Hanley following my expression of interest in the area of alaryngeal speech rehabilitation. Dr. Snidecor knew that significant advances in alaryngeal speech rehabilitation were on the horizon and that the complexion of clinical care would change in the years ahead. Fifteen years later, I continue to reflect on Dr. Snidecor's clarity of thought and the influence of that warm October afternoon conversation on the present work.

The initial motivation to pursue writing the present text had its conception in several different, yet overlapping concerns. It was my desire to meet several challenges; foremost among these concerns was the desire to produce a comprehensive and contemporary source of information on speech and voice rehabilitation following laryngeal cancer. Second, I wanted to produce a resource that could lead to better patient care. To produce such a resource, issues other than those typically found in the communicative disorders literature would need to be addressed concurrently. A deliberate attempt was made to offer an expanded view of laryngeal cancer not only as a disease process, but of the concomitant influence of the condition on the individual's recovery and well-being. Hence, the practicing speech-language pathologist or student may develop a better appreciation of what a laryngectomy entails and its consequences; this may, therefore, permit an enhanced understanding of what the speech-language pathologist will observe clinically.

In preparing a text on the topic of voice and speech following laryngeal cancer, the prevailing focus clearly centers on the rehabilitation of verbal communication. But other factors that influence the patient must also be acknowledged, particularly those that influence recovery and the overall success of rehabilitation. One particular element that continually surfaced during the developmental stages of the writing process was the effects of a malignancy that extend beyond those of the disease. Cancer appears to affect not only those who have the disease, but those with whom they come in contact. It seems cancer is not only feared but shunned by society.

In one of the last interviews before his death from prostate cancer in December 1993, the musician Frank Zappa stated that the diagnosis of cancer carries substantial emotional upheaval for the individual patient. Specifically, Zappa stated "The minute somebody tells you that you have cancer, your life changes dramatically, whether you beat it or you don't. It's like you have a . . . brand put on you." The social penalties associated with any form or site of cancer appear to be significant. This is no less true for those diagnosed with laryngeal malignancy. When coupled with the loss of verbal communication, the effects may be devastating.

Attempts to meet these broad objectives certainly offered a considerable challenge given the rather cumbersome body of literature which addresses laryngeal cancer. There are literally thousands of references related to the generic topic of laryngeal cancer; these references originate from a variety of disciplines and perspectives. This information is distributed across the medical, social, and behavioral sciences. The generous body of available information offers both distinct advantages and disadvantages to the speech-language pathologist who works with individuals treated for laryngeal cancer.

The advantages are found primarily in the fact that patients with laryngeal cancer are of interest to members of multiple professions. Accordingly, this diversity provides a unique and valuable framework for understanding the more complex and multidimensional nature of laryngeal cancer. Speech-language pathologists *cannot* function in an insular fashion if high quality care is to be provided to patients and members of their family. Offering different perspectives on the problem provides the reader with an opportunity to view both some of the "trees," as well as a few acres of the "forest." Yet disadvantages also stem directly from this diversity. Namely, the extensive variety of sources from which information about people with laryngeal cancer can be gleaned is quite simply overwhelming. Researching and addressing the topic of laryngeal cancer from a variety of viewpoints and perspectives does, however, begin to offer a more "holistic" and perhaps progressive view of the patient and what lies ahead following a diagnosis of laryngeal cancer. Successful rehabilitation following laryngeal cancer is comprised of more than one's verbal skill.

Comprehensive knowledge about laryngeal cancer as a disease process, the rationale for and methods underlying specific medical treatments, and the breadth of its sequelae across physical, psychological, and social boundaries are limited from a speech-language pathology point of view. That is, while the importance of many "nonspeech" issues are certainly acknowledged in our literature, they are less prevalent compared to basic speech issues.

This text includes information from many sources beyond those found in the communication disorders and sciences literature which may be of direct value to the clinician, and perhaps most importantly, to the patients we serve. Many sources utilized in the present text may not always be readily accessible to the speech-language pathologist. The primary information presented was obtained from germinal papers, as well as from sources that the speech-language pathologist may not typically delve into, but which may be of clinical value. The need for information that transcends the sterile and technical aspects of the patient's postlaryngectomy status is often lost or overlooked, but it is definitely an essential component of treatment efforts if rehabilitative success is to be achieved. Efforts at determining what would be included and what would be excluded was indeed the most difficult challenge encountered during preparation of the text. Clear shortcomings nevertheless remain. Some information has been omitted either by choice or perhaps by frank omission. This in no manner reflects on their quality, but rather, simply bears witness to the fact that all things cannot be included in a single source without offering the potential reader a complimentary abdominal truss and a handtruck. Hopefully, the information that is included will provide a more complete view of both laryngeal cancer as a disease, in addition to its impact on the patient as a person.

The other, although not necessarily secondary, motivating factor for undertaking this project was the people who experience the problem. This dimension of laryngectomy rehabilitation has always provided the most significant source of interest and inspiration to me. Cancer is not a disease one wishes to think about even though most of us are highly likely to have to confront this disease entity in some form, either directly or indirectly, during our lifetime. Few individuals can state that they have not experienced the effects of cancer in an at least an indirect manner; most can speak of some experience with a loved one, friend, colleague, or acquaintance.

Few individuals have the opportunity to meet so many people of such diverse backgrounds. I consider myself fortunate to have this opportunity. Individuals who have been "branded" by one of the most feared diseases of mankind often exhibit substantial grace, composure, and resourcefulness in spite of the situation they face. I continue to be amazed at the shear courage that many of these people exhibit at such a difficult time. One might even view their response as heroic. The generosity of spirit that many of these patients exhibit to others is often overwhelming.

Through my contact with patients I have been able to meet a truly remarkable group of people that I would not have otherwise come to know. I continue to remember each and every patient, but both my professional and personal life have been influenced the most by one particular patient, Mattathias N. Smith. Matt was one of the most remarkable human beings I will ever know. When the call beckoned for Matt to move on, I am certain that his sojourn ended with a warm greeting by angels. Matt's courage in confronting his illness and his continuing joy of life will always be remembered. He taught me much about living. Matt and the others I have worked with ultimately provided the most compelling reason for undertaking the task of preparing this text. I hope that it will be of help to both patients and clinicians in the future.

Acknowledgments

Needless to say, many people freely gave of their time, knowledge, opinions, and support during this entire endeavor. I was able to repeatedly call on a group of individuals to read chapters, or sections thereof, along the way or to argue over inclusions and omissions, suggest tables or figures, or check specific tidbits of information. This was frequently done on very short notice. My sincere appreciation is extended to Herbert A. Leeper, Gerald Martin, William Ryan, Rob Haaf, Candace Myers, Charles Reed, Eric Blom, Elizabeth Skarakis-Doyle, J.B. Orange, Joy Armson, Joe Kalinowski, Mark Taylor, Siobhan Wooten, and Jeff Lear.

I would like to single out several of these folks as they went "above and beyond" what I requested of them. My sincere appreciation is extended to my friend and colleague Andy Leeper who continually offered his comments and suggestions on numerous chapters along the way. To Gerry Martin I am indebted for his clear thinking and guidance along the way and for his careful review of information presented in Chapter 3 "through the eye's of a head and neck surgeon." Candace Myers provided detailed feedback on issues related to counseling and offered many valuable suggestions which were at times incorporated throughout the entire text. Betsy Skarakis-Doyle offered unique perspectives and editorial advice on topics found within several chapters, but most particularly in relation to issues of quality of life.

To my mentor Chuck Reed, I am once again grateful for his willingness to share his vast knowledge in the area over the years. I now have a better appreciation of why he so often asked me "What else?" Everyone should be fortunate to have a teacher like Chuck, but not everyone is as lucky as I.

I would also like to extend a special thank you to Carl E. Silver, M.D., of the Montefiori Medical Center in New York for his gracious consent to reprint figures from his excellent book *Cancer of the Larynx* in Chapter 3. Dr. Silver's figures are probably the finest in the literature, and his willingness to share this information with the speech-language pathology community is sincerely appreciated. Tom Rush provided the expertise to computerize the graphic images from Dr. Silver's text. Rob Haaf helped determine what additional figures should be included and provided ample opportunity for humorous distraction during the process.

A specific thanks is due to Pam McAndrew who helped piece together a thoroughly unruly and rough manuscript during her evenings and weekends. Donna Costello helped generate many of the tables included in the text and stood at the ready by the copying machine when copies were needed. Carol Anne Stephenson was a vigilant intermediary to the overnight courier.

My appreciation is offered to Jeff Danhauer for encouraging me to pursue this project and for once again believing that I could offer something of value to the profession. Thanks are due to the staff at Singular Publishing—particularly to Marie Linvill and Sadanand Singh, and Randy Stevens for their patience when I confronted roadblocks during this process.

I must also acknowledge as a group many former graduate students who have helped me to look at things in different ways. To several of my recent or current graduate students—Karen Grabowski, Jeff Lear, Charlene O'Neill, Carolyn Chalmers, Natalie Huckle, Leslie Sigmund-Styba, and Frances Reimer—who deserved more of my time, I am most appreciative of your tolerance over the last year.

I would also like to acknowledge the continuous *nonsupport* of work in the general area of alaryngeal voice and speech rehabilitation by both federal and provincial granting agencies in Canada.

Last, but certainly never least, my love and appreciation is extended to my wife Betsy and our children Kate and Peter who tolerated a phantom spouse and father during this whole ordeal. While I cannot recoup the time lost, I am once again home for all of you!

Dedication

To the loving memory of my Mother
Elinore Vagim Doyle
Noren gu hantibig erarou
and
To my Father
Charles Doyle
Go mbeidh sadghal fada agat

Cancer of the Larynx: An Overview of the Problem

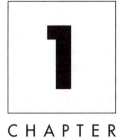

In the first sentence of his classic textbook *Speech Rehabilitation of the Laryngectomized*, Snidecor (1978) noted that laryngeal cancer has plagued humans for thousands of years. Unfortunately, until the middle of the 20th century the typical course of laryngeal cancer was its progression until death. Since the work of Sands (1865) and Billroth (1873) significant changes in both the understanding of laryngeal cancer and its medical management have ensued (Silver, 1981). Over the past 40 years many advances in approaches to medical management of laryngeal cancer have emerged and subsequent increases in long-term survival have been observed (Bailey, 1985a).

Although the individual who undergoes treatment for laryngeal cancer is never completely free of fear in regard to cancer death, significant improvements in 5-year survival rates have been observed over the past 25 years (American Cancer Society, 1990, 1993; Mendez, Maves, & Panje, 1985; Silverberg, 1983; Wynder, 1975). Since the 1950s the primary emphasis of medical management has transcended radical ablative surgery as an all-inclusive approach to treatment of laryngeal cancer. That is, less radical, partial surgical approaches (conservation laryngeal surgery) have been used with increased frequency over the past 40 years (Biller, 1987). Further, the use of radiation treatment (Goffinet, Fee, & Goode, 1984; Hendrickson, 1985; Kirchner, 1985), as well as laser surgery as a primary method of management for early glottic cancers (Casiano, Cooper, Lundy, & Chandler, 1991; Koufman, 1986; Shapshay, Hybels, & Bohigian, 1990) may now be more common. It is within this contemporary period of development that clinical interest in laryngeal cancer has been extended beyond the more traditional and often singular considerations of identification and diagnosis of disease. This has permitted the patient rather than the disease to become a more prominent focus of comprehensive rehabilitation efforts.

The purpose of this chapter is to provide a brief overview of literature on laryngeal cancer with a particular emphasis on the evaluation of contemporary issues that impact treatment and rehabilitation efforts. These issues pertain not only to primary medical management, but to rehabilitation in the postsurgical period. Much of this information is provided in the context of its relationship to verbal communication. Subsequent chapters are structured so as to provide the reader with an enhanced appreciation of what has transpired in years past and what is now currently accepted in relation to medical management and postsurgical voice and speech rehabilitation. Additionally, in this chapter an attempt is made to address several generic areas of concern that would appear to have a significant influence on the successful long-term rehabilitation of the individual. Finally, it is hoped that an appreciation of current limitations in the care of those diagnosed with laryngeal cancer can be provided. This information is believed to be of benefit to speech-language pathologists and other professionals who serve this clinical population.

Treatment of Laryngeal Cancer: Changing Perspectives Over Many Years

Bailey (1985a) suggested that the 120 years that have transpired since seminal reports on surgical treatment of laryngeal cancer first appeared[1] (mid-1800s) could be segmented into three distinct 40-year periods of philosophical evaluation and change. According to Bailey (1985a), each of these three periods of development were characterized by innovative although frequently controversial ideas regarding the disease and its medical treatment. Specifically, Bailey (1985a, p. 258) termed the first 40-year period (approximately 1860–1900) one of "reluctant acceptance of the concept of conservation surgery." The second period which emerged in the early part of the 20th century (1900–1940) was described by Bailey as the period of "popularization and basic development." The most recent period (1950–1980) was dominated by what Bailey termed "rapid development in medical science." This domination in the most recent period has clearly continued into the 1990s. From a rehabilitative viewpoint, the most dramatic changes in postsurgical voice and speech have taken place over the past 40 years.

Bailey's (1985a) division of this 120-year period clearly reflected philosophies that influenced how extensive surgical treatment would be. Prior to more comprehensive understanding of laryngeal lymphatics (Pressman, 1956) total laryngectomy was the surgical method of choice in all but small glottic tumors (Bailey, 1985a). Therefore, primary medical treatment before the 1950s usually centered on *which* approach to the *surgical treatment* of laryngeal cancer would be pursued. However, as more information on tumor spread and invasion was obtained, additional and more selective procedures were developed. The general philosophical underpinnings which characterized each period of development in laryngology (Bailey, 1985a) is not uncommon to "cancer" as a generic category of disease. That is, approaches to the medical management of all forms of cancer have also been influenced by reluctance, popularization, and development as it relates to the understanding of the induction, spread, and management of the malignancy.

Within each 40-year period outlined by Bailey (1985a) specific elements of

---

[1]Although some treatment options such as the tracheotomy had certainly been reported prior to the 19th century (see Silver, 1981), these techniques were indeed palliative in nature.

development and refinement in medical diagnosis and treatment were evident. However, the emergence and acceptance of issues that extended beyond diagnosis and surgical treatment are generally phenomena associated with the most recent period. Over time, this increased awareness of factors other than the disease itself clearly has stimulated change in the prevailing attitude-of-the-day and philosophy toward the treatment of laryngeal cancer. With laryngeal cancer, the broadening awareness of interrelated issues has resulted in a multidisciplinary approach to rehabilitation and the acknowledgment that rehabilitation is optimized using such a framework (UICC, 1980).

Laryngectomy: Development of a Comprehensive Rehabilitation Strategy

Arguably, the greatest advances in diagnosis, definition, and management of laryngeal cancer have occurred within the last 40-year period (Bailey, 1985a). It is during this period that an increased awareness of physical, psychological, and social problems that emerge postsurgically has moved to the forefront of clinical concerns for those who serve patients with laryngeal cancer (Gates, Ryan, Cantu, & Hearne, 1982; Gates, Ryan, Cooper, Lawlis, et al., 1982; Goldstein & Price, 1987; Mathieson, Stam, & Scott, 1990; Ryan, Gates, Cantu, & Hearne, 1982, and others). Although this awareness has expanded considerably, a clear understanding of the relationship and interdependency of such factors (i.e., physical, psychological, etc.) as a critical rehabilitative issue is at times lacking. Successful rehabilitation following treatment for laryngeal cancer unquestionably requires at least a basic understanding of many issues that extend beyond those spe-

cific to surgical treatment and voice and speech rehabilitation.

Changing Trends in Understanding Laryngeal Cancer

Although it appears that an increase in the overall occurrence of malignancies has been observed over the past several decades (American Cancer Society, 1990, 1993; Byrne, Kessler, & Devesa, 1992; UICC, 1987), this is believed to be a phenomenon primarily related to the general aging of the population (Endicott et al., 1989; UICC, 1987). Unfortunately, as individuals live longer their chance of experiencing a malignancy also increases (Endicott et al., 1989). Substantial improvement in the diagnosis of early malignant neoplasms in a variety of bodily systems has also occurred in the recent 40-year period as a result of technological advances. This has subsequently led to generally improved long-term survival rates for many different types of cancer including that of laryngeal cancer (American Cancer Society, 1990).

In some instances increases in life expectancy, as well as improvements in diagnostic technology have likely influenced the apparent increase of laryngeal cancer that has been observed. It is clear, however, that the distribution of head and neck cancers, in general, and laryngeal cancer specifically, is changing. This is most evident in the apparently increased incidence of head and neck cancer in younger individuals and women (American Cancer Society, 1993; Carniol & Fried, 1982; DeRienzo, Greenberg, & Fraire, 1991). Thus, speech-language pathologists will not only be likely to encounter an increasing number of patients, but an increased number of patients at both the younger and older ends of the age continuum. This may offer new challenges to the clinician beyond those that have traditionally been noted in the rehabilitative process.

The literature on laryngeal cancer has most frequently addressed information related to identification, diagnosis, treatment, and eventual postoperative outcome (i.e., cancer survival), as well as the functional sequelae associated with the management of laryngeal cancer. These data clearly suggest that smoking and alcohol consumption are often strongly correlated to malignancies of the aerodigestive system (Gray, Coldman, & MacDonald, 1992; Muscat & Wynder, 1992). Further, the incidence of laryngeal cancer has historically been male dominated. However, these patterns may be changing particularly in regard to the age of onset and shifts in gender ratios (Robin et al., 1989). This information suggests that new perspectives in rehabilitation may be necessary in future years.

Developing a Framework for Postsurgical Rehabilitation of Patients with Laryngeal Cancer

When the literature is evaluated carefully, multiple perspectives from a wide range of disciplines including medicine, nursing, speech sciences, speech-language pathology, and epidemiology are quite evident. Information in the literature on laryngeal cancer also covers an extremely wide breadth of topics given the complex nature of laryngeal cancer and the consequences of treatment. This includes issues pertaining directly to identification and diagnosis of early as well as more advanced and widespread laryngeal malignancies, the progression of the cancer, in addition to changing methods and attitudes toward treatment of individuals with laryngeal cancer. Although this body of literature serves to provide a framework from which laryngeal cancer as a process may be viewed, common strands are often diffi-

cult to extract from this work. In fact, substantial controversies continue to exist. This is most notable in relation to medical/surgical management of laryngeal cancers. Due to differences in the approach to medical/surgical management of particular sites of laryngeal cancer, considerable variation exists in postsurgical anatomy and physiology. Thus, data on postoperative functional capabilities (including those related to voice and speech) must be carefully evaluated.

For example, while it is clear that unique methods of surgical treatment may be employed dependent on characteristics of a specific laryngeal tumor (e.g., size, location, extent of involvement of adjacent structures, etc.), procedures not only differ across surgeons, but more importantly across patients (Gates, Ryan, Cantu, & Hearne, 1982; Gates, Ryan, & Lauder, 1982). This is clearly evident in the area of conservation surgery (i.e., partial laryngectomy) for cancer of the larynx. In this instance, use of a particular type of conservation laryngeal surgery cannot be assumed as identical from patient to patient. Therefore, attempts to collapse data obtained from a truly heterogeneous population are difficult if not impossible. The consequences of this heterogeneity is also directly observed in the area of postsurgical vocal capabilities in these individuals (Weinberg, 1982, 1985). Yet elimination of the malignancy is the first step in the rehabilitation process. Understanding what structures are removed, what remains, and what is reconstructed would appear to have important clinical implications for the speech-language pathologist who must address postsurgical alterations in the patient's voice and speech capabilities.

Laryngeal Carcinoma: A Continuing Problem

Since Billroth's account of surgical removal of the entire larynx due to cancer in 1873, the literature is replete with reports of the resulting profound communication deficit. In 1980, the American Cancer Society (Silverberg, 1980) estimated that approximately 10,500 new cases of laryngeal cancer would be diagnosed each year in the United States. It was also estimated that 3,500 deaths due to laryngeal cancer would occur in 1980. Ten years later, the American Cancer Society (1993) estimated that approximately 13,000 new cases of laryngeal cancer would be diagnosed. Based on these data from the most recent 10-year period, it is not unreasonable to assume that this trend will continue into the 21st century. Despite increases in the overall occurrence of laryngeal cancer (American Cancer Society, 1991), the number of individuals who will survive at least 5 years after diagnosis and treatment will also likely increase over this period. This is in part a function of the increased occurrence of malignant neoplasms, increased life expectancy, as well as overall improvements in the early diagnosis of laryngeal cancer (Byrne et al., 1992; Endicott et al., 1989).

As a diagnostic category, carcinoma of the larynx has been estimated to account for less than 5% of all malignancies which are identified in the human system (Norante & Rubin, 1978; Silverberg & Lubera, 1989). Nevertheless, laryngeal carcinoma appears to be the most frequently occurring cancer within the group of malignancies diagnosed in structures of the head and neck (Bryce, 1985). Bailey (1985a) has stated that laryngeal cancer accounts for approximately 1 in 74 of all malignancies that are diagnosed. Although all forms of cancer carry a significant chance that some degree of altered function will occur, laryngeal cancer also carries the potential for the loss of the primary mechanism of human communication. The loss of one's larynx has pronounced and far-reaching effects that cross boundaries of anatomical, physiological, psychological, and social dimensions (Amster et al., 1972; Johnson, Casper, & Lesswing, 1979; Kitzing & Toremalm, 1970; Sanchez-Salazar &

Stark, 1972). The inability to verbally communicate affects the individual's social and family adjustment (Amster et al., 1972; Gardner, 1966; Watts, 1975), and their ability to maintain economic independence (Ranney, 1975).

Bailey (1985a) has stated that if appropriately managed, "laryngeal cancer is the most frequently cured malignancy of the aerodigestive tract" (p. 257). Appropriate management is often facilitated when the malignancy is identified early in its development (Gates, Ryan, Cooper, Lawlis et al., 1982; Gates, Ryan, & Lauder, 1982). Based on this information, it would appear that laryngeal cancer could be considered an infrequent problem with a high probability of cure (Bailey, 1985a; Bryce, 1985), particularly in the early phases of the disease. If a laryngeal cancer is detected early, the individual has an excellent chance of both survival and maintenance of ability to verbally communicate (Bryce, 1985; Fee & Goffinet, 1985). Should the malignancy be diagnosed at later stages, the consequences are substantial from a variety of perspectives (Lowry, Marks, & Powell, 1973). This includes a high probability that more extensive partial surgical resection (e.g., near-total laryngectomy) will be undertaken or perhaps total laryngectomy. Therefore, the potential for significant postsurgical alteration in voice is also quite high.

The Sequelae of Laryngeal Cancer

As with any other disease process, the diagnosis of cancer has dramatic effects on both the individual who receives such a diagnosis, as well as on his or her friends and family (Gilmore, 1986; Salmon, 1986a, 1986b). These effects go well beyond that of the malignancy itself. Regardless of site of lesion, the social stigmata which frequently occurs following the diagnosis of cancer is now gaining more widespread attention in the clinical domain (Quigley, 1989). This stigmatization extends beyond that of the cancer itself; that is, while the "cancer" may stigmatize the patient, the effects and by-products of treatment may also exacerbate this phenomenon and further isolate the individual.

For example, radical ablative surgery for the treatment of laryngeal malignancy may result in rather dramatic physical consequences which may in turn result in numerous associated stigmata (Goffman, 1963). Physical disfigurement in association with cancer also poses a significant challenge to the patient (Dropkin, 1981) in relation to his or her re-entry into the social milieu (Goffman, 1963). This may influence a given individual's resourcefulness during this time of personal crisis (Caruso-Herman, 1989; Sanchez-Salazar & Stark, 1972). The ability to "cope" encompasses a wide breadth of issues both internal and external to the individual as a person. It has been suggested that the individual's ability to cope successfully with a diagnosis of cancer may indeed influence treatment success (Felton, Revenson, & Hinrichsen, 1984; Weissman & Worden, 1975). Further, in many cases, a diagnosis of laryngeal cancer also carries with it a very real possibility that verbal communication will be affected, at least to some degree (Diedrich & Youngstrom, 1966; Snidecor, 1978). The effects of laryngeal cancer on the individual are extensive and multifaceted and possibly poorly understood by many professionals. It is, therefore, important for those who serve individuals who have been diagnosed with laryngeal carcinoma to carefully acknowledge and consider a variety of dimensions during the process of rehabilitation.

Rehabilitation as a Process

Evolving from changes associated with the diagnosis and medical management of laryngeal cancer and the subsequent changes that occur, the laryngectomized individual is faced with the strengths and weaknesses of several speech rehabilitation options (Reed, 1983a, 1983b). As stated by Greene (1947), the patient who must not only confront possible death from cancer but also the loss of his voice "suffers a shock from which he never completely rallies" (p. 39). Although this is always true for those who undergo total laryngectomy, loss of normal vocal capabilities in those who undergo partial laryngectomy procedures must also be considered.

Since the time of Greene's (1947) statement over 40 years ago, the National Institutes of Health (NIH) report that 5-year survival rates have increased approximately 15%. In 1950, approximately 50% of all patients (all ages) succumbed to the cancer within the first 5-year period. Statistics based on data from 1973–1981 (Public Health Service and NIH, 1984) indicate that as of 1981 approximately 65% of all laryngectomized patients survived the same 5 postsurgical years. This trend has been consistently observed into the 1990s. Considering these data in relation to the total number of new cases of laryngeal cancer that are anticipated to occur, it is assumed that an increasing number of these individuals will also survive at least 5 years postlaryngectomy. Therefore, the need to restore functional communication is of even greater importance to the patient and members of his or her family. However, rehabilitation of functional alaryngeal speech is not always successful.

The Loss of One's Voice

If verbal communication is lost entirely as is the case with total laryngectomy, the rehabilitation process becomes even more challenging to those health care providers who work with the patient. Yet this challenge can be met with greater success if a comprehensive, multidisciplinary approach to the care of an individual with laryngeal cancer is undertaken (Gates, Ryan, & Lauder, 1982; Reed, 1983a). It should be obvious that given the potentially devastating effects of laryngeal cancer, that multiple professionals must be involved in the rehabilitation process (UICC, 1980, 1987).

The long-term benefits of multidisciplinary care will certainly enhance the individual's chance of resuming as near-normal a life as possible following surgery and rehabilitative efforts (Reed, 1983a; Salmon, 1986a, 1986b). Thus, the ultimate goal of a combined, comprehensive rehabilitative effort centers around returning the individual to the most productive and least restrictive life-style following treatment. It is, therefore, not unreasonable to assume that the "cure" of laryngeal cancer entails far more than elimination or removal of the cancer. "Surviving" the disease might then be viewed to comprise more than just the number of months postsurgery. In those who are diagnosed with carcinoma of the larynx, it may be safe to say that medical management of the cancer is only the first step of this rehabilitative process (Gates, Ryan, & Lauder, 1982). Thus, qualitative aspects of survival must be distinguished from discrete quantitative outcome measures.

Voice and Speech Rehabilitation

The literature on speech rehabilitation following total laryngectomy reveals great variation in the amount and degree of success. Whereas it has been reported that as many as 60 to 70% of laryngectomized patients acquire esophageal speech following surgery (Horn, 1962; Putney, 1958;

Snidecor, 1975), less than 50% of these patients who have acquired esophageal speech are reported to be successful in the production of "acceptable" speech (Martin, 1963). Aronson (1980) estimated that approximately one-third of all laryngectomized patients are not capable of learning esophageal speech, whether it be due to physical limitations or psychological reasons (Diedrich & Youngstrom, 1966; Gates, Ryan, Cooper, Lawlis et al., 1982, Gates, Ryan, Cantu, & Hearne, 1982). Aronson (1985) also has been clear to acknowledge that "the reasons for success and failure have not been precisely determined" (p. 393). This concern continues to plague the area of clinical inquiry related to alaryngeal speech in general. Although much has been hypothesized, there is not yet a clear indication of why some individuals succeed and others fail.

In contrast to the relatively high success rates indicated by some authors, a report by Schaefer and Johns (1982) indicated that only slightly better than 24% of laryngectomized patients achieve functional esophageal speech. Gates, Ryan, Cooper, Lawlis et al. (1982) have supported the findings of Schaefer and Johns (1982) in a prospective study of 47 patients. Regardless of information provided in the literature, there do not appear to be any consistent criteria established in respect to what constitutes either success or failure in the acquisition of alaryngeal speech.

Although considerable interest in the success-failure debate has been directed toward esophageal speech, there is limited formal information related to successful acquisition and use of artificial laryngeal devices (i.e., the electrolarynx).[2] This observation is curious given that the introduction and use of the tracheoesophageal (TE) puncture technique (Singer & Blom, 1980) and TE puncture voice prosthesis was met with numerous inquiries about

---

[2]There is, however, a reasonable body of data on issues related to a variety of acoustic parameters of artificial laryngeal speech, as well as on listener judgments of this alaryngeal method of speech production (Goldstein, 1978b; Rothman, 1978, 1982).

the success of this alaryngeal method. Generally, TE puncture and use of a TE puncture voice prosthesis appears to result in relatively high success rates (i.e., > 70%). The dimensions that constitute this success, however, are also relatively undefined beyond that of speech "fluency." Clearly a need exists to more explicitly define what constitutes successful postsurgical voice and speech rehabilitation regardless of mode. This need also extends to individuals who undergo partial laryngectomy procedures.

The Patient as a Person

It is fortunate that in recent years, an ever present attention has been directed at factors best described as "quality of life" issues in those individuals who develop cancer (Bailey, 1985a; Quigley, 1989) and those with communicative disorders (Myers & Baird, 1992). Attention to this important area has added another essential facet to the manner in which one views both the treatment and rehabilitative process. This attention also helps to place the disease in the context of human behavior. Over the past several years, considerable research attention has focused on behavioral aspects of cancer prevention (UICC, 1987). Thus, cancer prevention is now becoming heavily grounded in educational endeavors that attempt to address changes in the life-style of individuals. It is interesting to note, however, that this rather practical perspective is also a rather new one.

Shiffman and his colleagues (Shiffman et al., 1991) have noted that in a working meeting of the American Cancer Society on issues pertaining to behavioral and psychosocial research in cancer, only sparse remarks were made regarding "cancer prevention and control." Shiffman and his colleagues go on to state that it is only since approximately 1986 that the potential importance of research efforts that

address the prevention and early detection and diagnosis of cancer have emerged. It is without question that prevention is the key, but it would be folly to assume that prevention will prevail. Some prevention strategies will, however, culminate in success, and extending this success should be actively pursued.

Interestingly, cancer of the larynx is clearly one form of cancer that is influenced by life-style and personal habits (Schleper, 1989; UICC, 1987; Wynder & Stellman, 1977). When this factor is considered with others such as changes in the provision of health care services and its economic impact, an ever changing medical structure, and advances in technology (Conley, 1984), it appears quite possible that the latter half of the 1990s and the start of the next century will serve as a catalyst for significant changes in how cancer as a disease entity is viewed. This new and broader vision will hopefully culminate in reduced occurrences of cancer in those types of malignancy which appear to be (at least in part) preventable. A more comprehensive vision of the nature and extent of care that is provided to the individual who is diagnosed with cancer may also emerge. Those who have suffered cancer of the larynx may provide the ideal motivational scaffold to realize these goals through educational contributions to the community.

The fact remains, however, that cancer of the larynx is a disease that in large part can be prevented. As stated by the UICC (1987) "the use of tobacco accounts for more deaths than all other known causes combined" (p. 31). The problem is not a simple one; specifically, the UICC (1987) has explicitly acknowledged that one of the most important factors in reducing tobacco related deaths centers on an inability to disrupt the "tremendous political and economic influence of the multi-billion dollar tobacco industry around the world" (p. 31). Through aggressive marketing campaigns "Joe Camel" is now more widely recognized by children than "Mickey Mouse." A need clearly exists to decrease the number of young people who use tobacco products. In 1985, the Surgeon General of the United States stated that to achieve "a smoke-free society" in the United States by the start of the 21st century "a total package of motivation, education, and training efforts" would be required (Koop, 1985, p. 1581). It is without question that continuing efforts are essential if this goal is to be successfully met.

Summary

Significant advances in the treatment of laryngeal cancer have occurred over the past century. The most significant advances have been observed during the past 40 years. The use of conservative surgical approaches for treatment of specific laryngeal tumors is the most significant advance from a postsurgical perspective. These techniques have offered less extensive resections with good long-term survival. Along with the development of new and less radical approaches to the treatment of laryngeal cancer, an increasing awareness of the patient as opposed to the disease has also emerged. As patterns of laryngeal cancer continue to change over the next several decades, a concept of what constitutes comprehensive postsurgical rehabilitation must also change. This need is guided by both the increasing number of women who will be diagnosed with laryngeal cancer, as well as the potential for the speech-language pathologist to encounter both younger and older patients. As a broader vision of patient care arises, issues underlying quality in addition to quantity of life will come to the forefront. These issues will clearly influence the evaluation of what constitutes successful postoperative rehabilitation in those individuals who are diagnosed with laryngeal cancer.

The Nature of the Problem: Circa 1990s

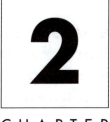

CHAPTER

In recent decades, fundamental understanding of cancer as a disease process has increased dramatically. This naturally has led to improved understanding of the various cancers that occur throughout the body. Concurrent with these fundamental advances is a more sophisticated understanding of the unique nature of cancer of the larynx and the aerodigestive tract (i.e., oral cavity, pharynx, trachea, and esophagus). Factors that potentially underlie or encourage the malignant process across a variety of anatomical sites have been the focus of substantial scientific inquiry.

This is particularly true regarding cancer of the aerodigestive tract, and more specifically, cancer of the larynx. Information obtained empirically ultimately provides clear and often overwhelming information regarding the relationship between smoking and excessive alcohol consumption and the development of pathobiologic alterations of squamous epithelial tissue. The general public is now also better informed about cancer relative to 20 years ago due to rather substantial dissemination of information via the news media.

The purpose of this chapter is to provide information on several areas related to the development of laryngeal cancer. This includes a discussion of the contemporary view on the development of cancer and its biological progression. Additional information is also provided on broad issues pertaining to demographic characteristics associated with laryngeal cancer. Finally, information related to the etiology of malignant change within the larynx is presented with a particular focus on the relationship between smoking and alcohol consumption.

Cancer as a Process: Basic Perspectives on the Progression of Malignant Disease

Dorland's Illustrated Medical Dictionary (1974) clearly and explicitly defines cancer as "a cellular tumor the natural course of which is fatal" and defines malignant (cancer) cells as those which "exhibit the properties of invasion and metastasis" (p. 252). This unambiguous, formal definition is likely to correspond quite well to that of the layperson. That is, if asked the question "What is cancer?" many individuals would offer a rather accurate description of cancer as a disease entity. However, many would generate their definitions with a focus on the end or terminal stages of the disease (i.e., once cancer occurs it is likely to be fatal). Many might also suggest that the diagnosis of a malignancy is the result of a "new" and somewhat "acute" pathological event. Cancer is, nevertheless, believed to be a long-term cellular process.

Based on the plethora of data gathered and information obtained into the broad category of cancer as a pathological process, the contemporary viewpoint of malignant changes within the human body is indeed long-term in nature. Although cancer results from "a multistage process and is multifactorial" (UICC, 1987, p. 50) two specific events are believed to underlie malignant change. Cancer results from specific factors of *initiation* and *promotion* (UICC, 1987). According to the UICC (1987) initiation is the result of:

> a variety of chemical, physical and virological factors which produce a permanent, irreversible (in most instances) alteration in a certain proportion of cells (initiated cells) within the organism and these cellular alterations occur soon after exposure to these factors. (UICC, 1987, p. 50)

In contrast, promotion is a process that:

> occurs subsequently to initiation, usually requiring chronic exposure to promoting agents, and there is substantial evidence that this is a reversible process and that a substantial interval of time could elapse between initiation and promotion without affecting the efficiency of the promoting agents. (UICC, 1987, p. 50)

Cancer is not only thought to be a multistage, long-term mechanism of pathological change but substantial biological variability in malignant change may also exist. Cancer as a disease process has been suggested by the Union Internationale Contra Le Cancer (UICC) to possibly exhibit four distinct biologic phases. It is believed that each of these phases represents a unique and specific stage in the process of malignant change in human systems. It is important to acknowledge that individual cellular types of cancer (e.g., squamous cell, basal cell, etc.) and the anatomical site in which they are first observed clinically exhibit very different natural histories. Thus, the growth or proliferation rate for cancer cells may vary by cell type (Mahadevan & Hart, 1990). Each type of cancer appears to have a rather well-defined pattern and rate of growth which influences changes in the progression of the disease once it is detected clinically. Malignant conditions within the larynx (those that derive from squamous epithelial tissue) also conform to this set of assumptions. Similar to cancers in other anatomical sites, laryngeal cancer is also believed to be a long-term process with a relationship to specific initiating and promoting factors (UICC, 1987).

Oncologists now believe that substantial evidence exists to support the notion that many forms of malignant change are the product of a four-stage pathological process (UICC, 1987). This process may

---

[1]Also known as the International Union Against Cancer

occur over the course of more than 40 years. This view of cancer development is based on numerous conceptual models of the disease. In the *Manual of Clinical Oncology* (UICC, 1987), members of the UICC termed these four stages as the: (1) *induction phase,* (2) *in situ phase,* (3) *invasion phase,* and (4) *dissemination phase.* With exception of genetically based cancers in children and those cancers associated with exposure to radiation (i.e., leukemias) the *induction phase* of malignant change is believed to require anywhere from 15 to 30 years. In cancers that appear related to one's exposure to carcinogenic agents in the environment, many years may elapse before a cancer is detectable (UICC, 1987).

In their discussion of cancerous changes which occur in the larynx, Fee and Goffinett (1985) have stated that changes in epithelial tissue, whether *atypical* or *dysplastic* in nature, are likely a response of the epithelial tissue to "deal with some noxious stimulus" (p. 141). Fee and Goffinet go on to state, however, that atypia and dysplasia may at times be observed in individuals who have no history of exposure to agents believed to be associated with malignant change. Although dysplastic changes within the malignant cell may occur over the course of this induction phase, the extent and degree of dysplasia is viewed as a long-term process which will eventually culminate in an identifiable cancer (UICC, 1987).

The second phase in the malignant process, the *in-situ* phase, is believed to occur in a period of from 5 to 10 years following the completion of the induction phase. This phase represents a point in the malignant process where structural (cellular) changes in tissue may be observed. These cellular changes may be verified through pathological evaluation. Despite the presence of dysplastic changes in epithelial cells, in-situ changes may not always be viewed as cancer. More typically, in-situ changes are often judged to be *microinvasive* according to pathological assessment and may be defined as *precancerous.*

When one considers that this in-situ phase may extend over the period of a decade, the potential for successively increased dysplastic change may involve changes in the severity and/or extent of the dysplasia. Therefore, in-situ changes appear to precede extensive, invasive cancers because of the long-term cellular deviation. In fact, Bailey (1985b) has stated that a "significant percentage" (p. 229) of lesions of the larynx that are confirmed pathologically as carcinoma in-situ will ultimately become invasive in nature. This potential for the evolution of invasive carcinoma of the larynx is believed to increase substantially in the case where increased in-situ microinvasion is observed or where diffuse, multiple lesions are identified (Bailey, 1985b).

The problem encountered with in-situ carcinoma of the larynx is that it is often difficult to diagnose, particularly when associated with changes on the vocal folds (Keane, 1985). Despite a rather unambiguous pathological definition of in-situ carcinoma, some controversy exists about whether such changes should be conservatively monitored (Hintz et al., 1981) or aggressively managed to eliminate all tissue identified (Doyle & Flores, 1977; Doyle, Flores, & Douglas, 1977). Bailey (1985b) believes that carcinoma in-situ of the larynx must be considered as a perilous lesion which threatens the individual's laryngeal function (protective and communicative) and perhaps his or her life. This opinion appears to be shared among the vast majority of laryngologists.

The third phase in the development of cancer is the *invasion phase.* This phase of the process is characterized by the rapid multiplication of malignant cells. With the increased number of such cells, tumors increase in size and extend their destructive margins. It is in this stage of the malignant process that malignant cells penetrate soft tissue and frequently gain access to the lymphatic and vascular systems. At this point in the process, local malignant cells can spread to either *regional* or *distant* sites via the process termed *metastases.* The UICC (1987) has stated that the "elapsed time between the start of invasion and the existence of established metastases may vary from a few weeks to several years" (p. 4). Therefore, the invasive stage of cancer represents a point in the process where cancerous cells exhibit a biologic predilection to proliferate, invade adjacent tissues which are unable to resist the aggressive tendency of the tumor, and to become disseminated within the body.

The final stage of the malignant process is the *dissemination phase.* It is in this stage of the process where substantial opportunity exists for metastatic disease. This stage may occur over a period of from 1 to 5 years. This stage of the cancer process may have been preceded by many years of premalignant change according to the UICC (1987). Concerns regarding metastatic dissemination of malignant cells is of critical importance from both cancer treatment and prognostic perspectives.

Demographics and Laryngeal Cancer: Shifting Patterns

From a demographic perspective, cancer as a broad pathological process transcends age, gender, race, ethnic origin, nationality, religion, or social class boundaries. Within Western cultures in the 20th century, there is evidence that cancer is the second leading cause of death, surpassed only by heart disease (American Cancer Society, 1990; UICC, 1987). Each year in the United States, more than 50,000 individuals are diagnosed with cancer of the head and neck. Of these individuals about 25% (13,000) will ultimately succumb to the disease (Endicott et al., 1989). Specific patterns or trends do at times, however, emerge and may cluster for subgroupings of one or more factors. For example, while the breast is a common site of cancer in adult women, it is not a cancer subsite that is exclusive to females.

Similarly, although historical record indicates that laryngeal cancer is predominately a disease of adult men, it is not exclusive to this group of individuals.

Viewing data on the incidence of squamous cell carcinoma of the head and neck, it has been estimated that the yearly incidence of such malignancies as a diagnostic class is approximately 20 per 100,000 people in the United States (Ernster, 1988; Silverberg & Lubera, 1989). When cancer data are inspected unique relationships between the location of the primary cancer and the individual's age and gender must always be considered (Carniol & Fried, 1982; DeRienzo et al., 1991; UICC, 1987). These data may then be collapsed into a database from which relative increases in the incidence of cancer and, therefore, the related mortality may be inferred. Epidemiological research on cancer has provided a valuable context from which one can view the variability associated with the incidence of the disease. Many researchers also believe that such information provides the basis of "preventative oncology" (UICC, 1987).

The second factor that must be recognized and considered regarding apparent changes in cancer incidence is related to striking improvements in medical technology during the past 20 years. Due to these advances, early detection and identification of tumors has been enhanced considerably. Detection of smaller tumors is now improved, and in cases of early diagnosis a corresponding increase in postdiagnosis survival may also be observed. Thus, a clear distinction must be made when evaluating incidence and mortality data related to cancer. The consequences of this distinction are twofold.

First, early detection of a laryngeal malignancy carries with it an improved chance that it may be treated successfully (Bryce, 1985; DeSanto, 1985; Neel & DeSanto, 1986). Second, early detection suggests that should treatment prove to be unsuccessful, the time period from initial diagnosis to death may be increased commensurately. If a malignant change is diagnosed early in its course, mortality from the disease may differ from past data as a direct result of the early diagnosis. That is, early diagnosis results in time increases at the front end of the problem, and hence, may appear to extend the time from diagnosis to death should the individual succumb to disease. As the UICC has stated, "Advances in treatment of cancer and the resulting increase in the cure rate make mortality statistics an increasingly inadequate reflection of the incidence of the disease" (p. 7).

If one views a broad base of data on the number of new diagnoses of laryngeal cancer (incidence) and death (mortality) associated with the disease, it might appear that cancer is occurring with greater frequency than in previous decades of this century. Two specific factors are believed to have a significant influence on this apparent increase in the frequency of cancer. First, the seeming increase in cancer as a disease is certainly related to a rather dramatic increase in life expectancy since the early 1900s. With the exception of several types of cancer, malignant change is, in general, a disease of aging (Endicott et al., 1989).

Greater than one-half of all individuals in the United States who have a confirmed diagnosis of a malignancy of the head and neck are 60 years of age or older (Endicott et al., 1989). Therefore, as the population increases in age, the proportional incidence of cancer may also increase. It is important to note, however, that the relationship between aging and cancer must also consider the anatomic location of the malignant change (e.g., lung, larynx, etc.), as well as the individual's gender. Norante and Rubin (1978) reported that the peak incidence of laryngeal malignancy was observed in the fifth and sixth decades of life. This has been confirmed in more recent reports (American Cancer Society, 1990). When one evaluates the literature on laryngeal cancer, this age range is not uncommon in a majority of those individuals who are diagnosed with cancer at this site. Although this pattern of incidence appears stable for males

it may be changing for females (Carniol & Fried, 1982; DeRienzo et al., 1991; Morbidity and Mortality Report, 1986; UICC, 1987; United States Department of Health and Human Services, 1984; Wynder, Fujita, Harris, Hirayama, & Hiyama, 1991).

Gender Considerations

The literature has traditionally posited that laryngeal cancer exhibits a strong prevalence in older adult males. In fact, in their summary related to head and neck tumors, Norante and Rubin (1978) state that 95% of laryngeal cancers occur in males. Laryngeal cancer in adult females has been observed infrequently relative to other sites and types of cancer and has therefore, been viewed as a rare occurrence relative to the reported incidence in men. Data on the estimated prevalence of all types and sites of cancer in the United States have recently been reported by Byrne et al. (1992).

The data presented in the Byrne et al. (1992) report were based on personal reports via a questionnaire to a random sample of more than 47,000 households in 1987, with more than 44,000 responses obtained. Briefly, questions posed pertained to whether any type of cancer had been diagnosed in the respondent, what "type" of cancer, "where" in the body it was located, at what age diagnosis occurred, and whether any other type of cancer had been diagnosed. Unfortunately, one of the broad cancer "site and type" categories was a combined grouping of lung and laryngeal malignancies. Thus, the estimated prevalence data are subject to contamination by a distinct group of cancers (i.e., lung cancer). They may, however, be strongly influenced by similar potentially related factors such as cigarette smoking (UICC, 1987). Based on the data reported by Byrne et al. (1992), the estimated prevalence of lung/larynx cancer in male respondents was 199 per 100,000 and for female respondents 90 per 100,000. Therefore, current data suggest that the estimated prevalence is twice as great for males when compared to females. It is again, however, important to point out that two potentially independent cancer anatomical subtypes were combined in this report.

Based on an extensive evaluation of cancer registry data from Birmingham and West Midlands, Great Britain, Robin et al. (1989) reported that the incidence of laryngeal cancer in females has increased over the past 30 years. Whereas a gender ratio of 10.1:1 for the incidence of laryngeal cancer for males was determined for the 5-year period comprising 1957 to 1961, data from the 5-year period from 1977 to 1981 revealed that this ratio had decreased to 5.3:1. Although slight increases in overall incidence were observed for males between 1957 and 1981, rather dramatic increases were noted for females over this same period of time. Similar (regionally based) data are unavailable for North Americans, but there is reason to believe that this trend would also emerge (Silverberg, 1984). For example, in a retrospective analysis of 537 individuals who had been diagnosed with early carcinoma of the larynx that was confined to the glottis, Berger, van Nostrand, Harwood, and Bryce (1985) found an incidence ratio of 9:1 (482 males vs. 55 females). Bailey (1985a) has also stated that between approximately 1965 and 1985 the male-to-female ratio for laryngeal cancer was halved from 12:1 to 6:1. Shifts in societal trends are believed to account for a substantial amount of this ratio change. These data suggest that changes in the smoking and drinking behavior of women has resulted in systematically decreasing male-to-female ratios.

Causes of Malignant Change in the Larynx

The literature has identified several concomitant factors that may influence the development and progression of malignant change in the larynx and other sites of the body. We are confronted daily with reports of numerous potentially carcinogenic agents that we may be exposed to in some manner. According to the UICC (1987) several issues pertaining to one's potential exposure to carcinogenic agents must be considered in relation to the development of cancer.

It is clear that "the nature, amount, and concentration of the carcinogen" (UICC, 1987, p. 3), as well as the temporal duration that one is exposed to such carcinogenic agents can influence the tendency toward malignant change. The UICC (1987) has also identified the anatomical site(s) on which the carcinogen may act and "the presence of other carcinogens or co-carcinogens" (p. 3) as determining factors. This may in turn increase the chance of developing a cancer. The prevailing consensus of information gleaned from the literature in oncology suggests that cancer has often been viewed as a relatively short-term cellular abnormality. However, as noted, it is more likely the result of a multiphase evolution that occurs over many years (UICC, 1987).

When considering laryngeal cancer, there is incontrafutable evidence that links smoking to the development of malignant change in the lungs and larynx (Falk et al., 1989; Guenel, Chastang, Luce, Leclerc & Brugere, 1988; Hinds, Thomas, & O'Reilly, 1979; UICC, 1987; Wynder, Covey, Marbuchi, & Johnson, 1976; and others). This link is also believed to be synergistic and "multiplicative" (UICC, 1987, p. 22) when smoking and alcohol consumption are combined (Cann, Fried, & Rothman, 1985; Moore, 1971; Schottenfeld, Gantt, & Wynder, 1974). Even though the link between smoking and cancer is clearly indicated as a risk factor (particularly in relation to malignancies within the lungs and in the larynx), laryngeal cancer does not always occur in individuals who are smokers. Ward and Hanson (1988) presented data from 19 individuals who had no smoking or drinking history, all of whom developed carcinoma of the larynx. Similar data have been presented by Carniol and Fried (1982) and Morrison (1988). Yet smoking does increase one's chance of developing malignant changes in particular anatomical sites (e.g., laryngeal, oral, pharyngeal, bladder, and pancreas) (UICC, 1987).

Despite clear evidence related to the smoking-cancer link, the mechanism of this causative relationship is not yet well understood (Endicott et al., 1989) and co-contributing factors must be assessed. Factors that potentially influence the development of cancer regardless of the system involved have been broadly termed "environmental factors." According to the definition provided by the UICC (1987) "environment" includes anything that may interact with the individual and which may influence biological structure (i.e., dysplastic cellular changes within a given anatomical site). This includes environmental exposure to dietary contamination of food sources and drink; exposure to smoke, radiation, and drugs; exposures which occur in the work setting; aspects of lifestyle and sexual behavior; and the expansive area of potential carcinogenic agents that are found in association with pollution of air, water, and soil (Endicott et al., 1989; UICC, 1987). These environmental factors are often found in combination. Thus, efforts to clearly identify single sources of carcinogenesis in relation to causation of particular cancers is frequently difficult due to combinatorial interaction.

Smoking, Drinking, and Laryngeal Cancer

In the development of laryngeal cancer, numerous causative agents have been identified (Burch, Howe, Miller, & Semenciw, 1981; Graham et al., 1981; Hinds et al., 1979; Muscat & Wynder, 1992; Norante & Rubin, 1978; Robin et al., 1989; Wynder, Bross, & Day, 1956; Wynder et al., 1976;

UICC, 1987). Two specific factors, smoking and alcohol consumption, appear to have strong links to malignant change in squamous cell epithelium in the larynx. As mentioned previously, these two factors must be viewed together from a causative perspective. Wynder et al. (1976) reported that for those individuals who smoked more than 35 cigarettes per day the "relative risk" of developing a laryngeal malignancy was 7 times greater when compared to nonsmokers. In those individuals who smoked more than 35 cigarettes daily *and* consumed more than 7 ounces of alcohol daily, the relative risk became 22 times greater when compared to those who did not smoke or drink (Wynder et al., 1976). Although smoking and excessive alcohol consumption do appear to be factors in a large number of patients who develop laryngeal tumors, exposure to other agents in the environment may also precede malignant change.

Exposure to co-contaminants such as asbestos or other agents (typically related to occupation) by patients who are diagnosed with laryngeal cancer provide confounding variables that often make definitive cause-and-effect relationships difficult (Muscat & Wynder, 1992). Even if definitive relationships between a given carcinogen, or a specified interactive combination of carcinogens could be identified via prospective or cohort investigations, researchers continue to face limitations regarding what is termed a "dose response" (UICC, 1987). Simply stated, a dose response refers to an empirically derived association between exposure to a particular carcinogenic agent, in a particular amount, and over a particular period of time, and the onset of malignant change.

It can easily be seen that the ability to distinguish consistent dose response relationships is highly problematic. As awareness of environmental exposure issues and the dangers of smoking has increased over the past 25 years, numerous additional factors that suggest a relationship to laryngeal cancer have also been noted. Many factors including the effects of exposure to second-stream or second-hand smoke (Guyatt, & Newhouse, 1985; Somerville, Rona, & Chinn, 1988; Report of the Surgeon General, 1986), environmental contaminants (Wynder et al., 1976), the influence of gastroesophageal reflux (Morrison, 1988; Ward & Hanson, 1988), and occupational exposures (Hinds et al., 1979; Muscat & Wynder, 1992; UICC, 1987; and others) have been identified as potential contributors to dysplastic change in squamous cell epithelium. These changes may then progress to become a carcinoma. As more widespread awareness of these factors increases we are likely to see more comprehensive and detailed analyses of them in future studies. However, the potential for a causal relationship between smoking and laryngeal and lung cancer is more than just a suspicion.[2] Although the tobacco industry continues its attempt to refute extensive scientific data, the evidence that smoking and cancer are related is absolutely overwhelming. The process of education will be enhanced with continued demographic and epidemiologic investigations that will provide more refined overviews into the process of laryngeal malignancy and tobacco use.

Symptoms of Laryngeal Cancer

Over the years, considerable discussion has taken place in relation to symptoms associated with laryngeal cancer. Given the structure(s) that is/are affected by the tumor, one would clearly expect that some change in either the voice or in the individual's breathing would be noted (e.g., stridor or shortness of breath). Although a change in the voice may indeed be associated with laryngeal tumors, this

symptom is also typically associated with a variety of other upper respiratory difficulties. This includes vocal changes associated with cold and flu symptoms, seasonal changes, allergies, the menstrual cycle, as well as many others. Voice change may be more commonly associated with less serious conditions that influence the larynx and the upper respiratory system. However, laryngeal tumors, particularly those that occur on the membranous portion of the glottis, have the distinct potential of disrupting normal vocal fold motion. As a result of this disruption, changes in the smooth, quasiperiodic vibration of the vocal fold may culminate in some degree of what may be best described as "hoarseness" (Graham, 1983). Numerous reports in the literature have shown that disruptions in vocal fold motion due to anatomical factors (i.e., mass changes in the folds) are frequently related to changes in the character of the acoustic signal (Baken, 1987; Boone & McFarlane, 1988). These acoustic changes, which are a result of altered physiology of fold vibration, also are typically associated with concomitant changes in the perceptual characteristics of the voice. While in and of itself the term hoarseness may have numerous interpretations to a group of listeners, it is a feature specific to a change in vocal quality. This quality change typically involves aspects of vocal harshness and/or some degree of breathiness (Fairbanks, 1960). Accordingly, international cancer agencies list *persistent hoarseness* or *a change in voice* that persists longer than 10 to 14 days as one of the cardinal "warning signs" of laryngeal cancer.

It is interesting to note that in the literature there is little consistency to whether a change in the individual's voice was observed as a precursor to the detection of a laryngeal tumor. In assessing this lack of consistency, two factors are worthy

---

[2] It must be noted that compelling evidence for causal relationships to other forms of cancer (e.g., oral, pharyngeal, esophageal, gastric, etc.) as a consequence of tobacco use are also widespread in the empirical literature (Cullen, 1989; Gray et al., 1992; UICC, 1987).

of discussion. First, it is reasonable to assume that some voice change will be associated with the presence of a laryngeal tumor. This is due to direct mechanical influences on vocal fold vibration for voice production. However, the apparent absence of this symptom by patient report may not always be valid. That is, a change in voice may have occurred, but it may have evolved quite slowly and concurrently with the evolution of the malignancy. Changes in voice, therefore, may have been so negligible from a self-perception point of view that they were not noticed. The patient who does report a change in the voice may have only recently observed the change because it had met a critical, and likely quite salient, level for detection. Voice change is frequently first detected by others who then bring it to the attention of the patient.

The second issue that relates directly to a change in voice associated with laryngeal cancer is perhaps best described as a by-product factor. This implies that voice change may be judged by the patient to be secondary to some other condition that has ultimately brought him or her to the physician for medical assessment. For example, a given patient may note a change in voice, but these changes may be initially disregarded as a consequence of other symptoms. This includes frequent coughing, perceived need to clear the throat, ear pain, shortness of breath, a "catch" in the voice, or swallowing difficulties. It is likely, however, that a majority of individuals who are diagnosed with laryngeal malignancies do exhibit some change in vocal

quality. If voice change is noted, it may be differentiated from that of normal speakers using acoustic and perceptual profiles (Murry & Singh, 1982). Yet it is important to note that acoustic and perceptual characteristics of laryngeal cancer do not appear to exhibit a unique profile from that of other nonmalignant mass-type lesions of the vocal fold.

Summary

Information on the development of malignant change now ascribes to the belief that cancer is a long- rather than a short-term process. Though cancer is a multistage process, it appears to conform to a four-phase model. This model involves the progression from induction to the final stage of dissemination to distal anatomical sites, a process that may take many years.

Although historical information suggests that laryngeal cancer predominantly has been a disease of older adult males, this trend appears to be changing. Specifically, increasing numbers of females are being diagnosed with laryngeal cancer. It is believed that this pattern of change is a direct result of behavioral patterns associated with smoking and drinking by women over the past 30 years. The relationship between smoking and drinking and the development of laryngeal cancer is well supported through empirical study. These two factors substantially increase the relative risk of an individual for malignant change in the upper aerodigestive tract.

Diagnosis and Treatment of Laryngeal Cancer: An Overview for the Speech-Language Pathologist

3

CHAPTER

For the individual suspected of having laryngeal cancer, issues pertaining to confirmation of whether the pathological change is benign or malignant is essential. The initial step in such assessment is the clinical examination of the patient which will most often lead to a tissue biopsy (Batsakis, 1979; Hinton & Myers, 1991). In some instances, more sophisticated methods of evaluation may be undertaken. Once a formal diagnosis of cancer is confirmed specific recommendations for treatment can be offered.

The purpose of this chapter is twofold and addresses broad issues related to (1) the diagnosis and (2) medical management of laryngeal cancer. This information will provide the speech-language pathologist with an improved understanding of the diagnostic and management process. An overview of the basic clinical examination by the laryngologist and advanced diagnostic methods are presented. A discussion of tumor invasion and spread, the

lymphatic system, and the classification of disease also will be presented. This information forms the foundation for understanding *conservative* and *radical* approaches to surgical management of laryngeal cancer. Finally, a brief review of information on neck dissection and radiation therapy will be provided.

Regarding surgical management options information presented in this chapter focuses on the most common types of surgical procedures employed for treatment of laryngeal cancer. This information is based on a substantial body of literature from surgical specialists. An attempt has been made to identify the most common surgical procedures used in association with particular types of laryngeal malignancy. It is essential to note, however, that variation does exist regarding specific terminology, as well as unique variations undertaken by each surgeon. Thus, use of a term such as "vertical hemilaryngectomy" may not always represent the identical surgical procedure; rather, this category of partial laryngectomy typically denotes general aspects of a procedure (i.e., which structures are *usually* removed and which are *usually* retained and resected). Procedures described herein are done in "classical" format.

Basic details pertaining to the larynx and related structures involved and resected are noted. By doing so, it is hoped that the speech-language pathologist, as well as those professionals outside of communicative disorders can develop an appreciation for the anatomical changes that occur with a given subtype of surgery for laryngeal cancer. With this information at hand, it is hoped that a clearer, more precise, and more practical understanding of the postsurgical consequences on voice and speech production can be achieved.

Diagnosis of Laryngeal Cancer

The Clinical Examination

Clinical examination of the patient by an otolaryngologist is essential for individuals suspected of laryngeal cancer. Although more advanced diagnostic methods may be utilized for diagnosis, fundamental information will be provided during the physician's clinical examination (McWilliams, 1991). This includes acquiring a detailed history of the patient's present and past health status including the course of the presenting problem. Symptoms such as a change in voice, stridor, or shortness of breath, as well as ear pain or difficulty in swallowing will be noted. Information on smoking and drinking history will also be obtained.

The physician will then conduct a physical examination of the patient. This includes comprehensive assessment of the ears, oral and nasal cavities, the pharynx, hypopharynx, and larynx (McWilliams, 1991). The laryngeal examination typically involves an indirect mirror exam and frequently includes use of flexible and/or rigid endoscopy. Stroboscopy may also be useful in determining abnormal movement of the vocal folds (Hirano & Bless, 1993; Hirano, 1981). Characteristics of the lesion and its location and size are noted. More detailed information on the physical examination of the patient can be obtained in several general otolaryngologic texts (Myers, 1991a, 1991b).

Particular attention is paid to gross movement of the vocal folds as *fixation* of a fold may indicate infiltration of the tumor into the body of the fold or its neural supply. The patient's neck will be carefully examined to identify the presence of palpable lymph nodes which may signal regional spread of disease. Should a malignancy be suspected once the examination is completed, direct laryngoscopy and biopsy will be recommended. Kirchner (1985) strongly supports the use of direct laryngoscopy, particular in those individuals for whom conservation surgical approaches might be considered. In patients who have an extensive lesion that appears to have a significant chance of being malignant, surgery may be scheduled immediately with biopsy performed during surgery.

Advanced Diagnostic Methods

Imaging Techniques

Following clinical examination, more sophisticated methods of evaluation may be performed on patients with suspected or confirmed malignant lesions of the larynx. The most widely used techniques include *computerized tomographic* (CT) scanning and *magnetic resonance imaging* (MRI). CT scanning has been used since the late 1970s for the evaluation and diagnosis of laryngeal cancer (Bergman, Neiman, & Warpeha, 1979; Mancuso, Calcaterra, & Hanafee, 1978; Mancuso, Hanafee, Juillard, Winter, & Calcaterra, 1977). Although use of CT is common, reports on the use of MRI have begun to emerge over the past several years (Hoover, Calcaterra, Walter, & Larrson, 1984). Several studies have assessed the value of various imaging modalities in the detection of head and neck malignancy (Gussack & Hudgins, 1991; Mafee, Schild, Valvassori, & Capek, 1983). The primary advantage of these procedures from those used previously (e.g., lymphangiography) are that they are noninvasive and offer greater interpretive potential (Som, 1987).

Gussack and Hudgins (1991) outlined the relative advantages and disadvantages of CT and MRI procedures for diagnosis of recurrent head and neck tumors. CT appears to have the advantages of (1) providing reliable anatomical architecture, (2) clearly defining lymph nodes, (3) not being contaminated by motion artifacts, (4) providing excellent bony detail, and (5) offering an improved image with use of contrast enhancement. Disadvantages of CT include (1) streak artifacts, (2) inability to distinguish recurrent malignancy from postinflammatory tissue changes, (3) reduced posttreatment specificity, and (4) limitations in acquiring varied imaging planes (e.g., altering patient position).

In comparison, MRI has the advantages of (1) providing excellent imaging of soft-tissue structures, (2) clearly defining lymph nodes, (3) permitting multiplane imaging, (4) not requiring ionizing radiation, (5) permitting contrast enhancement, and (6) detailing patency of the carotid artery. Disadvantages include (1) motion-related artifacts (e.g., patient movement, coughing, swallowing, etc.), (2) lack of imaging specificity, (3) cost, and

(4) decreased levels of patient acceptance (Gussack & Hudgins, 1991).

Application of Imaging Techniques in Head and Neck Cancer

When imaging techniques are recommended, it is done with two specific goals in mind. The first seeks information that identifies discrete areas where malignant disease is suspected. The second seeks information on the entire neck area (Som, 1987). Imaging protocols that seek diagnostic information on the entire neck are of greater value in cases where a known malignancy exists (Som, 1987). More extensive imaging protocols may exhibit benefits in the detection of metastatic disease (Johnson et al., 1981). However, imaging of the greater neck region is more beneficial in that *occult disease* may be identified outside of where the primary lesion (local disease) is located.

Data suggest that CT has some site-specific anatomical sensitivity which is most notable for detection of primary (initial) compared to recurrent tumors. Specifically, identification of recurrent head and neck tumors may be complicated by several factors which often result from treatment of the earlier malignancy. Factors which may confound sensitivity include development of postsurgical scar tissue, radiation fibrosis, tissue edema, and anatomical confounds following use of reconstructive surgical procedures (Gussack & Hudgins, 1991).

CT has been shown to correlate well with whole-mount pathological specimens following surgical removal of the larynx (Mafee et al., 1983). CT scanning has also been investigated in conjunction with other diagnostic methods including cinelaryngoscopy and laryngography (Ward, Hanafee, Mancuso, Shall, & Berci, 1979). Kirchner (1985, p. 199) has suggested that CT might offer the "ideal" method of documenting the extent and *potential invasive characteristics* of a laryngeal tumor through use of "pretreatment" CT protocols. However, Kirchner (1985) acknowledges practical limitations of such imaging that relates directly to "vagaries of ossification" associated with the cartilaginous framework of the larynx (Kirchner, 1985, p. 199). Because of this problem, cartilaginous areas invaded by tumor and those that are incompletely ossified may be difficult to differentiate.

Use of CT scanning for evaluation of cancer spread to cervical lymph nodes has been reported since about 1980 (Mancuso, Maceri, Rice, & Hanafee, 1981). CT appears to have varied rates of sensitivity for successfully identifying tumors and their spread (Som, 1987). MRI scanning, however, may have greater application as a pretreatment diagnostic procedure that improves identification of potential cancer dissemination. This is a result of the MRI ability to more clearly define lymph nodes (Gussack & Hudgins, 1991). Although imaging procedures generally appear to offer advantages from diagnostic and management viewpoints relative to tumor specification, there are currently inconclusive data regarding the potential value of imaging for identifying regional spread of disease via lymphatic dissemination (Som, 1987).

Evolution of Laryngeal Cancer

It has been estimated that approximately three-quarters of all laryngeal malignancies arise from the true vocal fold (Bailey, 1985a). This offers greater opportunity for early diagnosis and treatment. Because of the location for a majority of laryngeal carcinomas, the potential for detection of an early "warning signal" is high; however, this warning is not always respected (UICC, 1987). Changes in the cellular structure of the vocal folds is believed to alter mass characteristics of the fold in addition to the biomechanical vibratory properties associated with phonation. This may create one of the classic warning signs for laryngeal cancer—a change in voice quality. If a glottic carcinoma is identified early, 80 to 90% of patients will respond favorably to conservative treatment approaches (Bailey, 1985a; Biller, 1987; Norante & Rubin, 1978).

In-Situ Carcinoma of the Larynx

In Chapter 2, reference was made to one particular phase of the malignant process, the in-situ stage. This phase may be viewed as an important early stage in the development of laryngeal cancer. Yet in-situ carcinoma of the larynx presents with "no distinctive clinical appearance" (Hintz et al., 1981) (p. 746). Nevertheless, several changes may be noted before in-situ carcinoma is confirmed (Bailey, 1985b; Batsakis, 1979). Changes include hyperplasia and keratosis, and/or keratosis with atypia and dysplasia.[1] These changes may be detected as small, discrete tissue abnormalities or as diffuse changes found on one or both vocal folds. Silver (1981) has stated that in in-situ carcinoma:

> Squamous epithelium is replaced by cells of malignant morphological pattern that do not invade the basement membrane. The entire thickness of epithelium is replaced. There is a fine diagnostic line between severe epithelial dysplasia and carcinoma in situ. (p. 15)

Although these changes may not always precede in-situ carcinoma and more

---

[1]"Keratosis" may exist with or without cellular atypia, and, thus, may exist concomitantly in cases of carcinoma in situ; however, it should be viewed as an independent change in the epithelial cells of the larynx rather than one which is co-dependent with carcinoma in situ.

widespread malignant microinvasion, such changes may precede a more serious disease process (Bailey, 1985b). Silver (1981) has emphatically stated that:

> Carcinoma in situ is considered a malignant, not a premalignant, lesion, containing all the generally accepted cytological criteria of malignancy, except invasion. (p. 25)

If one considers that a majority of laryngeal tumors occur (and are detected) on the glottis, the relationship between in situ cellular change and the potential continuation to microinvasive malignant disease cannot be discounted.

DeSanto (1974) suggested that if untreated, many individuals with in-situ carcinoma of the larynx will eventually present with invasive lesions. Thus, in-situ changes do not transgress basement membrane. Changes to epithelial tissue of the vocal fold have been documented in individuals with smoking histories (Auerbach, Hammond, & Garfinkel, 1970). In-situ carcinoma is, therefore, a serious dysplastic change in laryngeal tissue which if it progresses may become invasive cancer.

Tumor Growth and Invasion

Once malignant microinvasion occurs in the larynx, cells proliferate with an increase in tumor size. Once a tumor is detected questions related to extent of tumor invasion, and/or the spread of malignancy, are paramount. The exact nature of tumor invasion is only clearly identified during pathological assessment of the tumor (Batsakis, 1979). It is accepted that the earlier a diagnosis of laryngeal malignancy occurs, the better the patient's chances are of survival and cure of the disease. Early diagnosis also offers potential

for application of nonsurgical treatment approaches such as use of radiation (Perez & Marks, 1985) or use of limited surgical resections (Bailey, 1985a).

Whole Organ Section Investigations

The invasion of carcinoma into structures surrounding the primary tumor and the pattern of its spread offer many insights into treatment. The foundation for documenting the spread of cancer in the endolarynx or adjacent structures (e.g., hypopharynx) finds its basis in detailed pathological examination of excised larynges. Pathological investigation of this type are termed *whole organ sections*[2] that involve serial sectioning and examination of the entire larynx. This work was pioneered by Tucker (1961) and provides information on the structural relationships between various anatomical components of the larynx and has offered invaluable information on the pathological consequences of laryngeal tumors. As such, particular structures (e.g., cartilage and connective tissue) which serve to "compartmentalize" the larynx can be documented as barriers to the spread of carcinoma (Kirchner, 1989; Silver, 1981). This work has had a dramatic impact on the surgical treatment of laryngeal cancer and has served to guide conservative surgical approaches.

According to Kirchner (1989) whole organ techniques demonstrate "how the lesion invades various components of the larynx, and how one part of the larynx relates to another (p. 661)." The critical importance lies in the fact that a three-dimensional assessment of the tumor can be determined (Kirchner, 1989). Thus, the extent of a tumor below its visually observed surface can be identified, and tumor invasion into adjacent cartilaginous components of the larynx can be specified (Kirchner, 1989). Whole organ investigations

---

[2]Whole organ sections are not done as a routine procedure in most cases of laryngeal cancer.

have contributed significantly to the understanding of the type and extent of treatment that may be best for particular tumors of the larynx.

The majority of reports on whole organ sections of the larynx in relation to cancer have been provided by Kirchner and his colleagues (Kirchner, 1969, 1984, 1989; Kirchner & Carter, 1987; Kirchner, Kirchner, & Sasaki, 1989). Additional work has been undertaken by van Nostrand and his colleagues (van Nostrand & Brodarec, 1982; Olofsson & van Nostrand, 1973). In his article entitled "What Have Whole Organ Sections Contributed to the Treatment of Laryngeal Cancer?" Kirchner (1989) summarized his whole organ section evaluation of 442 laryngeal specimens gathered over 15 years (1964–1979). Kirchner (1989) reported that clinical staging via visualization of the tumor by the examining physician was imprecise in 40% of specimens (Kirchner, 1989; Pillsbury & Kirchner, 1979). Further, when inaccuracies where observed they were "nearly always one of underestimation" (Kirchner, 1989).

Clinical staging was, therefore, inadequate in almost one-half of the specimens examined. When underestimation occurred, it typically involved cartilaginous invasion or extension of the tumor into the pre-epiglottic space. Evaluation of data from the subsequent 10-year period (1980–1989) indicated that inaccuracies in clinical staging of tumors decreased to 22%, and a "sharp decline" in understaging was observed. Kirchner (1989) directly attributed this reduction in underestimation to data from whole organ sections findings.

Kirchner (1989) suggested that data from whole organ sections sensitized the laryngologist to those types of tumors "whose surface appearance reflects a high probability of deep invasion, framework destruction, or extension of cancer into the pre-epiglottic space." For example, clinical features of vocal fold movement such as whether the fold is mobile, restricted in movement, or fixed, may provide valuable information on the invasive nature of the tumor. Tumor extension and invasion may also be restricted due to anatomical constraints (i.e., compartmentalization) indicating site-specific tendencies for patterns of disease spread (Kirchner, 1989; Pressman, 1956; Pressman, Dowdy, & Libby, 1956; Pressman, Simon, & Monell, 1960; Skolnik et al., 1975; Tucker, 1961; van Nostrand & Brodarec, 1982).

Pathological Evaluation of Tumors

Pathological assessment of a tumor provides information on its histologic characteristics and serves to differentiate the type of tumor (e.g., squamous cell, oat cell, etc.) While several varieties of laryngeal malignancies exist, the majority are squamous cell carcinomas (Batsakis, 1979). On histological evaluation of a tumor a grading is provided. This "grading" provides details on how the *tumor cell line* is differentiated from the *host cell line* (site of origin).

Histologic grading of carcinoma was originally posited by Broders (1926) as a method of describing tumors. Using Broders' system a tumor is assessed for a number of features. The essence of Broders' tumor-grading procedure involves identification and quantification of the ratio of malignant cells to those of host tissue. As the ratio of tumor cells increases relative to host cells, it becomes more *differentiated*. Most histopathologic evaluations of a tumor will identify malignant cells as poorly, moderately, or well differentiated. Generally, well differentiated cancer cells tend to be less aggressive relative to those that are poorly differentiated. Poorly differentiated tumors are also more resistant from a treatment perspective.

Dissemination of Laryngeal Cancer

The potential spread of a tumor in the larynx or outside of the laryngeal compartment has significant clinical and prognostic implications. Although a given tumor may be rather large, issues related to its location and involvement of adjacent anatomical structures is of critical importance. Generally, the larger a tumor the greater its potential for spread outside of the laryngeal compartment (Skolnik et al., 1975). If disease spreads into the neck (lymphatic nodes) or to distant sites (i.e., metastasis), survival is often reduced (Johnson et al., 1981). Characteristics of the tumor, therefore, must be carefully evaluated by the surgeon from both treatment and prognostic perspectives. To provide a general framework from which treatment for laryngeal cancer evolves, it is beneficial for the speech-language pathologist to have a basic understanding of neck anatomy and of the lymphatic system.

Questions related to the pattern(s) of tumor growth and spread associated with laryngeal carcinoma have been fruitful areas of anatomical and oncological inquiry over many years. Research has provided the foundation for many surgical treatments used today. If clear patterns of tumor growth and spread can be identified, the utility of conservation (i.e., partial laryngectomy) surgical procedures can be better evaluated (Kirchner, 1975).

Defining and describing patterns of tumor extension may provide information regarding which types of tumors (i.e., location, size, and extension) might be most suitable for partial laryngectomy procedures. However, this decision is ultimately based on the relative success rates associated with both partial and total laryngectomy (or radiation therapy) for a given tumor. For a partial laryngectomy to be realistically considered by the surgeon and patient, reasonable evidence to support the notion that a partial procedure will successfully control continuation or recurrence of the malignancy must exist. As noted by Bailey (1985a), "preservation of the patient's life commands a higher priority than the preservation of laryngeal function" (p. 260). Thus, indications for the consideration, use, and evaluation of partial laryngectomy procedures are a

direct outgrowth of research on tumor growth and spread both within and outside (i.e., the lymphatic system) the larynx.

An Overview of the Lymphatic System

Som (1987) has provided comprehensive information on the lymphatic system of the head and neck and has stated that gathering detailed information about cervical lymphatics is a challenge to the radiologist. According to Som (1987) the lymphatic system of the cervical region is a "closed system" that allows capillary drainage from soft tissues of the neck. The capillary mechanism of the lymphatic system flows directly into larger capillaries which enter individual lymph nodes. A secondary level of lymphatic drainage also exists between adjacent lymph nodes and lymphatic chains (groupings of nodes) in the neck.

Lymphatic chains collectively drain into the venous system of the neck with terminal drainage into the thoracic duct. As a result of this two-tiered closed drainage system, all lymphatics must flow through "at least one, and usually several" lymph nodes prior to outflow via the thoracic duct (Som, 1987). Consequently, the potential exists that lymph which emanates from a region where a tumor is located may be spread via lymphatic drainage (Pressman, 1956; Pressman et al., 1956; Pressman et al., 1960). This possibility is of great concern as a mechanism of metastatic spread of cancer via neck lymphatics.

The most prominent problem that influences one's ability to develop a functional appreciation for the lymphatic system of the head and neck as it relates to cancer is that of nomenclature. Som (1987) has stated that this problem is a function of the use of several classification systems for cervical lymphatics, and a "rather loose intermixing" of nomenclature from one system to the next. A broad grouping of head and neck lymphatics as outlined by

McMinn, Hutchings, and Logan (1981) is presented in Table 3–1.

Lymphatic Groups

Som (1987) has stated that of approximately 800 lymph nodes in the human body, approximately 300 are found in the cervical region with approximately 150 nodes located on either side of the neck. Due to the number of cervical nodes, they are typically divided into four or five distinct nodal groupings or chains. The most superior of these lymph node groups is termed the *pericervical ring* in that these nodes surround the region that grossly separates head and neck structures. Nodes which comprise the pericervical ring include eight groupings: the occipital, mastoid, parotid, facial, retropharyngeal, submaxillary, submental, and sublingual lymphatics. These groups generally receive lymph from those soft tissues that correspond to their names. Som (1987) suggested that of these eight pericervical lymphatic groups, the retropharyngeal, submaxillary, and submental are of clinical importance in considerations of head and neck cancer. A summary of each of these lymphatic groups is provided in Table 3–2.

The next level of lymph nodes below the pericervical grouping are termed the *anterior cervical* and the *lateral cervical* groupings. The anterior cervical lymph nodes are located inferior to the hyoid bone in close proximity to structures of the primary airway (larynx and trachea). The *anterior cervical chain* can be subdivided into two subgroups (Som, 1987); the *anterior or superficial jugular* is contiguous with the jugular vein and associated strap muscles of the neck, and the *juxtavisceral* chain is closely associated with the larynx, thyroid gland, and the tracheoesophageal region.

The *lateral cervical* lymph nodes are distributed throughout perimeter structures that define the boundary of the posterior triangle of the neck and serve as the main lymphatic drainage for the other neck nodes. The lateral cervical nodes are located posterior to the sternocleidomastoid muscle with these nodes subdivided into chains that correspond with their location (see Table 3–2).

Information suggests that early identification of laryngeal cancer carries an increased chance that disease will not spread via the lymphatic system. According to Norante and Rubin (1978), if spread does occur in association with laryngeal cancer a general pattern of metastatic behavior may be observed. If lymphatic dissemination of cancer occurs, the metastases will most often first be observed in the *jugulodigastric* lymphatic chain (Norante & Rubin, 1978). Further, Norante and Rubin (1978) state that metastatic spread of laryngeal cancer is frequently noted to "progress

TABLE 3–1.
Broad Groupings of Cervical Lymphatics.

Lymphatic Chains	Area Served
Occipital, retroauricular, parotid, buccal	Superficial tissues of head
Submandibular, submental, anterior cervical, superficial cervical	Superficial tissues of neck
Retropharyngeal, paratracheal, lingual, infrahyoid, prelaryngeal, pretracheal	Deep tissues of neck

Source: Adapted from McMinn et al., 1981.

TABLE 3–2.

Summary of Lymphatic Subgroups Located in the Pericervical Nodal Chain.

Group	Location	Number	Drainage From	Drainage To
Occipital	At posterior junction of head and neck, base of cranium	3–10	Occipital region	Spinal accessory chain of lateral cervical nodes
Mastoid	Posterior to ear	1–4	Parotid and parietal areas, and skin of the ear	Inferior parotid and superior internal jugular chains of lateral cervical nodes
Nuchal Nodes	Beneath tendon of trapezius	1–3		
Parotid	Superficial to and with the parotid gland	7–19	Skin of forehead and temporal areas, mid- and lateral face, ear, external auditory canal, and eustachian tube, posterior cheek, buccal region, gums and parotid gland	Internal jugular chain of lateral cervical nodes.
Facial Group	In subcutaneous tissues of face, along path of external maxillary artery and anterior facial vein	5–10	Eyelids, cheek, mid-facial region	Submandibular nodal group
Retropharyngeal Medial	Near midline, posterior to upper pharynx (at C_2 level)[a]	1–2	Oro- and nasopharynx, palate, nasal fossae, paranasal sinuses, and middle ear	Superior internal jugular group of lateral cervical nodal chain
Lateral	Near lateral, posterior pharyngeal wall, along path of longus capitus and longus coli muscles	1–3	Oro and nasopharynx, palate, nasal fossae, paranasal sinuses, and middle ear	Superior internal jugular group of lateral cervical nodal chain
Submandibular (submaxillary)	Submandibular triangle lateral to anterior belly of digastric	3–6	Lateral chin region, lips, cheek, and nose, anterior nasal fossae, gums, teeth, palate, anterior tongue, medial eyelids, subman-	Internal jugular group of lateral cervical chain

(continued)

TABLE 3-2. (continued)

Group	Location	Number	Drainage From	Drainage To
			dibular and sublingual glands, and floor of mouth	
Submental	Submental triangle of neck in association with mylohyoid muscle and anterior belly of digastrics	1–8	Chin, lower lip, cheek, anterior gums, floor of mouth and anterior tongue	Submandibular and internal jugular group of the lateral cervical chain
Sublingual	In a lateral grouping associated with anterior and lingual vessels, and as a medial group between the genioglossus muscles	Inconsistent	Tongue and floor of mouth	Submandibular and submental group and internal jugular group of lateral cervical chain
Anterior Cervical (2 divisions)	In infrahyoid region of neck between the carotid sheaths			
Anterior (Superficial) Jugular	Along interior jugular vein in superficial neck fascia	1–4	Skin and muscles of anterior neck	Thoracic duct or anterior mediastinal groups on left side, and into lowest internal jugular chain or highest intrathoracic group on the right
Justavisceral	Near larynx, thyroid gland, and tracheoesophageal grooves	6–16	Supraglottal and infraglottal larynx pyriform sinuses, thyroid gland, trachea, and esophagus	Same as anterior jugular group
Prelaryngeal, prethyroid, pretracheal and lateral tracheal				
Lateral Cervical				
Superficial, deep, internal jugular or deep cervical Superficial	Along external jugular vein, superficial to sternocleidomastoid muscle	1–4		

Deep

Internal jugular (deep cervical), spinal accessory (posterior triangle), and transverse cervical (supraclavicular) groups

Group	Location	Number	Drains	Drainage
Internal Jugular	Close to internal jugular vein, most below level posterior belly of digastric muscle and above course of omohyoid muscle	15–40		
Subdivisions: Superior (upper) or supraomohyoid and infraomohyoid				
Supraomohyoid	Anterior and lateral to internal jugular vein		Parotid, submandibular, submental, and retropharyngeal, and some anterior cervical nodal groups	Lymphatic duct, subclavian or internal jugular vein on right side, in each thoracic duct, or subclavian or internal jugular vein on left
Inframomohyoid	Either anterior, medial, or posterior to internal jugular vein			
Spinal Accessory	Along course of spinal accessory (CN–XI) nerve	4–20	Occipital and mastoid nodes, parietal and occipital scalp, nape of neck, lateral neck, and shoulder	Transverse cervical group, with some drainage to internal jugular chain
Transverse Cervical (supraclavicular)	Along transverse cervical vessels, connecting posterior triangle group with the internal jugular chain	1–10	Posterior triangle group, subclavicular group, skin of anterior-lateral neck, and upper anterior chest	Similar to that of internal jugular group

Source: Adapted from Som, 1987.
aMay be found as low as hyoid bone

stepwise to lower jugular nodes and to remain regional for some time." Thus, the metastatic process in the larynx is to some degree limited by the character of the lymphatic systems which serve these specific structures, as well as those providing drainage for regions that surround the larynx (Batsakis, 1979; Som, 1987).

The relatively independent lymphatics that serve the supraglottis, glottis, and subglottis, as well as the vertical halves of the laryngeal structures also provide a mechanism which influences metastatic behavior (Pressman et al., 1960). Whereas extrinsic laryngeal structures have a rich and comprehensive distribution of lymphatics, intrinsic laryngeal structures have much more restricted and confined lymphatics (this is particularly true of the vocal folds). Consequently, in cases of glottic cancer, spread to the uninvolved contralateral vocal fold is rare.

Classification of Disease

Diagnosis and classification of malignant disease by the physician involves a multifaceted process that begins when a patient's history is obtained. Clinical classification of disease, although an important factor in determining treatment options, cannot be viewed independently from other factors such as the patient's age and general health status (Bailey, 1985a; Hinton & Myers, 1991). As noted, categorization of tumors may be conducted in microscopic fashion using histologic techniques for quantification (e.g., level of differentiation). Information related to biological structure and variation of tumors provides a critical component in the identification and treatment of laryngeal cancer (Bataskis, 1979). Classification of tumors can also be done using more macroscopic criteria related to characteristics of the tumor, its invasion, and spread as viewed clinically through the eyes of the laryngologist (Berger et al., 1985; Hinton & Myers, 1991). This may provide

valuable information regarding the treatment and prognosis of specific classes of laryngeal tumors.

Considerable attention has been directed toward classification of the primary tumor and its possible spread via the lymphatic system. While classification may be beneficial from a strict pathological perspective, greater issues of patient care emerge if a universal classification system is used. Reliable and nonambiguous methods of tumor description at the clinical level may permit clustering of relatively homogenous subject populations. This may then serve to identify which methods of treatment are most effective, which are not, and which may be used in a combined fashion with the best long-term results for the individual (Becker, 1989). Historically, problems with classification systems have centered around the inability to effectively describe a given tumor. This has consequently led to poor communication regarding specific characteristics of tumors, and, hence, decreased the ability to evaluate and compare data on specific types of treatment and resulting survival and morbidity (UICC, 1987).

Clinical Systems of Classifying Laryngeal Tumors

Over the years, several systems for classifying malignant disease have been proposed. Modification of these classification systems has evolved due to difficulties and/or inconsistencies that emerged and were identified with earlier systems. Berger et al. (1985) suggested that clinical staging of tumors may result in an error rate that may range from 10 to 25%. This error may involve either *overstaging* or *understaging* of the tumor (Kirchner, 1989).

Ideally, any tumor classification system seeks to avoid ambiguity not only in the terminology associated with a given system, but in its direct use with a given patient. That is, if clear, nonambiguous specifications for clinically classifying the location and extent of a malignancy can be developed and used universally, treatment and prognosis are likely to be enhanced. Development and use of a well-defined classification system ultimately reduces the potential for error which occurs across observers (Warr, McKinney, & Tannock, 1984). The development of tumor staging systems must be "simple, reproducible, and scientifically valid" (Baker, 1985, p. 87). With this goal in mind, two systems of clinical staging deserve further discussion.

Clinical Staging of Laryngeal Cancer

In the broad spectrum of literature related to laryngeal cancer, two particular classification methods exist as primary *clinical staging* systems. The first was based on recommendations provided by the *American Joint Committee on Cancer*[3] (AJCC) and the second by the *Union Internationale Contra Cancer*[4] (UICC). AJCC guidelines have undergone several revisions over the past 30 years (see AJCC, 1962, 1978, and 1983 for changes during this period) with each revision reflecting greater sensitivity to specific tumor characteristics (e.g., features of VF fixation). The value of these revisions have been reflected in increased overall sensitivity of successive staging systems. Specifically, Tucker, Alonso, and Speiden (1971) assessed the correlation between clinical and pathological staging of laryngeal tumors by comparing stage levels obtained using the 1962 and 1972 AJCC systems. Based on results from 100 laryngeal cancers, Tucker et al. reported a higher correlation between clinical and pathological stages when employing the revised system; this was interpreted to reflect improved overall sensitivity of the revised classification system (Kirchner, 1989).

Despite similarities between guidelines provided by the AJCC and UICC, several differences exist. To facilitate international communication about clinical staging, these two committees sought to resolve differences and ambiguities between their independent systems with hope of developing a joint recommendation by 1986. However, reference to both systems (i.e., AJCC and UICC) are found in the literature dependent on the author(s) and the date of investigation. Regardless of which clinical classification system is used, the goals are quite consistent. Keane (1985) summarized these objectives as (1) providing better methods of communicating information about the state of specific cancers, (2) aiding the decision-making process related to treatment, (3) assisting in determining a patient's prognosis, and finally, (4) providing a method for comparing treatment effectiveness.

Generally, both the AJCC and UICC systems use the "TNM" system that provides information on the tumor, associated lymph nodes, and the presence of metastatic malignant disease. Identification and classification of the tumor (T) category provides details on lesion size and extent, the node (N) category provides information on the extent of regional malignant spread in the cervical lymphatic compartment, and the metastasis (M) category identifies distant spread of the disease.

Clinical staging is an extremely valuable tool, but it is not without limitations (Kirchner, 1989; UICC, 1987). Issues related to how well it classifies the "spectrum of lesions" that constitute laryngeal carcinomas as a clinical entity are always of concern. The TNM systems have been cited as an "inadequate method of quantifying tumors that range from quite early in their development to those that are clearly advanced carcinomas" (DeSanto, Pearson, & Olsen, 1989). The primary cause of this inadequacy, according to DeSanto et al. (1989) is a result of a "merging of stages" and a system which cannot, for example, differentiate between "late stage T2 or early stage T3" tumors.

---

[3]Formerly identified as the American Joint Committee for Cancer Staging and End Results Reporting.
[4]Also referred to as the International Union Against Cancer.

Tables 3–3, 3–4, and 3–5 outline specific definitions provided by the AJCC (American Joint Committee on Cancer Staging and End Results Reporting, 1978) for the T category, as related to squamous cell carcinomas in the supraglottal, glottal, and subglottal regions, respectively (Norante & Rubin, 1978).[5] By using the terms supraglottal, glottal, and subglottal, the laryngeal compartment can be segmented anatomically (Biller, 1987; Silver, 1981); this segmentation is then frequently carried over in relation to surgical options (i.e., consideration of specific types of partial laryngectomy procedures). For referential purposes, *glottal* represents the true vocal folds and the anterior and posterior commissures.

For comparative purposes, the recommended staging system for glottic and supra- and subglottic lesions proposed by the UICC (1987) are provided in Tables 3–6 and 3–7, respectively.

Information on the clinical staging of lymph node (N) involvement as outlined by the AJCC and UICC are provided in Tables 3–8 and 3–9, respectively. Though less detailed, the UICC system may offer

advantages from a clinical perspective. Finally, Table 13–10 presents staging categories for distant metastasis. This category is similar across the AJCC and UICC systems. Regardless of staging system, the N and M categories provided are applicable to all malignancies within the upper aerodigestive system (AJCC, 1978; UICC, 1987). Using the TNM staging system, information from all three categories leads to disease "stage" groupings related to the overall state of the cancer. A stage grouping can then be used in determining patient prognosis. A summary of these groupings according to the AJCC is presented in Table 3–11.

Factors Influencing Treatment

The confirmation of laryngeal malignancy and the amount of tumor extension exhibited will in many cases require some surgical intervention. Nonsurgical treatment, particularly the use of radiation as a

TABLE 3–3.
Anatomical Staging for Primary Tumors (T) of the Supraglottis.

Primary Tumor Categories
TX   Tumor cannot be assessed by rules
T0   No evidence of primary tumor

Classification of Supraglottal Malignancies
T1S   Carcinoma in situ
T1   Tumor confined to region of origin with normal mobility
T2   Tumor involves adjacent supraglottal site(s) or glottis without fixation
T3   Tumor limited to larynx with fixation and/or extension to involve postcricoid area, medial wall of pyriform sinus, or pre-epiglottic space
T4   Massive tumor extending beyond the larynx to involve oropharynx, soft tissues of neck, or destruction of thyroid cartilage

Source: From AJCC, 1978, O. H. Bearhs & M. H. Myers (Eds.), *Manual for staging cancer*, Philadelphia, PA, J. B. Lippincott, reprinted with permission.

---

[5]The term "specific definitions" has been used in reference to the TMN classification system, but it is necessary to note that clear separation between categories is at times ambiguous. Thus, as noted by DeSanto et al. (1989) some tumors may fall somewhere in between two definitions, and clinical classification may then result in some degree of *understaging* or *overstaging*.

primary treatment modality, is typically recommended only for a small percentage of cancerous lesions, usually those that are quite early in origin (Bailey, 1985a).

Therefore, for a majority of patients with laryngeal cancer some surgical resection will be necessitated. Surgical resection may range from limited, well-localized

TABLE 3–4.
Anatomical Staging for Primary Tumors (T) of the Glottis.

Primary Tumor Categories

TX   Tumor that cannot be assessed by rules
T0   No evidence of primary tumor

Classification of Glottic Malignancies

T1S   Carcinoma in situ
T1   Tumor confined to vocal cord(s) with normal mobility (including involvement of anterior and posterior commissures)
T2   Supraglottic and/or subglottic extension of tumor with normal or impaired cord mobility
T3   Tumor confined to the larynx with cord fixation
T4   Massive tumor with thyroid cartilage destruction and/or extension beyond the confines of the larynx

Source: From AJCC, 1978, O. H. Beahrs & M. N. Myers (Eds.), *Manual for staging cancer,* Philadelphia, PA, J. B. Lippincott, reprinted with permission.

TABLE 3–5.
Anatomical Staging for Primary Tumors (T) of the Subglottis.

Primary Tumor Categories

TX   Tumor that cannot be assessed by rules
T0   No evidence of primary tumor

Classification of Subglottic Malignancies

T1S   Carcinoma in situ
T1   Tumor confined to the subglottic region
T2   Tumor extension to vocal cord(s) with normal or impaired cord mobility
T3   Tumor confined to larynx with cord fixation
T4   Massive tumor with cartilage destruction extension beyond the confines of the larynx, or both

Source: From AJCC, 1978, O. H. Beahrs & M. N. Myers (Eds.), *Manual for staging cancer,* Philadelphia, PA, J. B. Lippincott, reprinted with permission.

TABLE 3–6.
Clinical Staging Guidelines for Primary Tumors of the Glottic Larynx.

T1   Tumor limited to vocal cord(s) with normal fold mobility; may involve anterior or posterior commissures.
T1a   Tumor confined to one vocal cord fold.
T1b   Tumor involves both vocal folds.
T2   Tumor extends to supraglottic and/or subglottic regions; vocal fold mobility remains.
T3   Tumor limited to larynx but vocal fold demonstrates fixation.
T4   Tumor invades thyroid cartilage and/or encroaches on other tissues of the larynx.

Source: From UICC, 1987, *Manual of clinical oncology,* 4th, New York, NY, Springer-Verlag, reprinted with permission.

TABLE 3–7.
Staging of Tumors of the Supra- and Subglottal Regions.

T1	Limited and mobile
T2	Extension of tumor to glottis with retained mobility
T3	Fixation of one or both vocal folds
T4	Extension of tumor beyond larynx

Source: From UICC, 1988, *Manual of clinical oncology*, 4th, New York, NY, Springer-Verlag, reprinted with permission.

TABLE 3–8.
Staging Categories for Regional (Cervical) Lymph Node Involvement Associated with Laryngeal Cancer.

N0	No clinically positive nodes
N1	A single clinically positive homolateral node less than 3 cm in diameter
N2	Single clinically positive homolateral node more than 3 cm, but not more than 6 cm in diameter, or multiple clinically positive homolateral nodes, none more than 6 cm in diameter.
N2a	Single clinically positive node more than 3 cm but not more than 6 cm in diameter.
N2b	Multiple clinically positive homolateral nodes, none over 6 cm in diameter.
N3	Massive homolateral node(s), bilateral node(s), or contralateral node(s).
N3a	Clinically positive homolateral node(s), one of which is more than 6 cm in diameter
N3b	Bilateral clinically positive nodes.[a]
N3c	Contralateral clinically positive node(s) only.

Source: From AJCC, 1978, O. H. Beahrs & M. N. Myers (Eds.), *Manual for staging cancer*, Philadelphia, PA, J. B. Lippincott, reprinted with permission.
[a]It is recommended that in this situation, each side of the neck should be staged separately.

TABLE 3–9.
Staging Categories for Regional (Cervical) Lymph Node Involvement Associated with Laryngeal Cancer.

N1	Involvement of movable homolateral regional lymph nodes.
N2	Involvement of movable contralateral *or* bilateral regional lymph nodes.
N3	Presence of fixed regional lymph nodes.

Source: From UICC, 1987, *Manual of clinical oncology*, 4th, New York, NY, Springer-Verlag, reprinted with permission.

TABLE 3–10.
Staging Categories for Distant Metastases of Laryngeal Cancer.[a]

M0	No (known) distant metastases.
M1	Distant metastasis present—specify site(s).

Source: From AJCC, 1978, O. H. Beahrs & M. N. Myers (Eds.), *Manual for staging cancer*, Philadelphia, PA, J. B. Lippincott, reprinted with permission.
[a]The specific site(s) of any distant metastasis will also be identified (e.g., pulmonary, lymph nodes, other).

procedures that may be performed via laser excision (Weisberger, 1991) to those that require the removal of the entire larynx (total laryngectomy) (Silver, 1981). Neck dissection may also be performed dependent on the type of lesion and the philosophy of the surgeon and may vary from limited unilateral to radical bilateral procedures (Silver, 1981).

A general surgical approach is usually identified a priori by the surgeon based on a collection of clinical information and

TABLE 3–11.
Classical Staging Associated with Progression of Cancer and Related Stage Groupings for Cancer (Squamous Cell Carcinoma) of the Larynx Based on Clinical Staging of Disease Using T, M, and N System.

Classical Cancer Stages[a]

Stage 0	In situ cancers, no invasion
Stage I	Early local invasion, no metastases
Stage II	Limited local extension and/or minimal regional lymphatic involvement
Stage III	Extensive tumor and/or regional lymphatic involvement
Stage IV	Locally advance disease, or *any* situation with distant metastases

Cancer of the Larynx and Cancer Stage[b]

Stage I	T1 N0 M0
Stage II	T2 N0 M0
Stage III	T3 N0 M0
	T1, T2, or T3 N1 M0
Stage IV	T4 N0 or N1 M0
	Any T N2 or N3 M0
	Any T Any N M1

Source: From [a]UICC, 1987, *Manual of clinical oncology*, 4th, New York, NY, Springer-Verlag, and [b]AJCC, 1978, O. H. Beahrs & M. N. Myers (Eds.), *Manual for staging cancer*, Philadelphia, PA, J. B. Lippincott, reprinted with permission.

additional diagnostic evidence related to characteristics of the tumor. The procedure ultimately performed, however, may vary considerably based on direct observation of the endolarynx during surgery and detailed pathological assessment. Terminology used herein should be viewed as a template of what occurs during surgery, *not as an absolute and invariant metric.*

Determining the amount of surgical resection required is based on many factors. The most critical relates to the size and location of the tumor, along with careful consideration of its extension into surrounding structures of the larynx. The distribution of lymphatics in each of the three laryngeal regions (supraglottic, glottic, and subglottic), also demonstrate unique profiles regarding the potential for metastatic spread. Thus, the location and extension of a tumor and its relationship to lymphatics contribute significantly to treatment options. As a tumor becomes larger, the chance that total laryngectomy will be required to eliminate the malignancy

with adequate safety margins also increases. Total laryngectomy also carries with it the likelihood that some form of neck dissection will also be required (Bryce, 1985; Hinton & Myers, 1991; Robbins et al., 1991).

Size and Site of Laryngeal Tumors

The location of a laryngeal tumor is specified by (1) where the lesion is observed visually (e.g., posterior region of the left vocal fold) and (2) its location relative to general regions of the larynx (i.e., supraglottis, glottis, and subglottis). In North America approximately 70–80% of all malignancies are glottic (Bailey, 1985a; Bryce, 1985).

Anatomic structure of the larynx and the upper airway provides a straightforward view of lesion location. Attention centers on whether the lesion is confined to the glottis or whether it extends superiorly (supraglottal) or inferiorly (subglottal) (Biller, 1987). Extension of the tumor in the anterior-posterior or lateral plane is also considered (Kirchner, 1989; van Nostrand & Brodarec, 1982). Determination of these features guide method of treatment. It may also impact decisions concerning the patient's prognosis. Dependent upon the location and extent of the tumor, surgical options may involve removal of an early, discrete, and apparently well-localized lesion via use of the laser (Ossoff, Sisson, & Shapshay, 1985; Strong, 1975; Weisberger, 1991) to those requiring partial resection (Silver, 1981), to those which require total laryngectomy and associated radical neck dissection and reconstructive surgery (Silver, 1981).

Glottic Carcinoma

Bailey (1985a) has provided an excellent review of management options for individuals diagnosed with carcinoma confined to the glottis. Bailey emphasized that the patient's life demands a "higher priority" over a desire to maintain laryngeal structure and function, but one must always consider the posttreatment period. That is, Bailey (1985a) notes that management of glottic tumors must strive to achieve the "highest quality of life obtainable after treatment" (p. 260). Although *quality of life* is not defined, such a reference appears to supersede simple quantitative aspects of treatment.

In those with no evidence of metastatic spread, Bailey (1985a) states that an 80 to 90% treatment success rate can be achieved. This high degree of success exists using either limited surgery or radiation therapy as the primary (and sole) modality of treatment (Harwood et al., 1980; Pellitteri et al., 1991; Perez, Holtz,

Ogura, Dedo, & Powers, 1968; Silver, 1981; Stewart, Brown, Palmer, & Cooper, 1975; Vermund, 1970). Thus, *conservative surgical approaches* to management of glottic carcinoma yield excellent success provided the lesion is detected early, and metastasis has not occurred. Kirchner (1985, p. 199) states that early glottic carcinomas (i.e., T1 lesions) are frequently superficial and do not typically exhibit invasion into the vocal ligament or the conus elasticus. For T1 tumors, the incidence of regional spread (neck) is about 2%, increasing to about 17%, 25%, and 65% as T-stage is upgraded (Skolnik et al., 1975). Such lesions respond favorably to either radiation therapy or localized limited surgical resection (Silver, 1981).

Subgroups of Glottic Cancers

According to Bailey (1985a) a subgroup of about 20 to 25% of all individuals diagnosed with carcinoma of glottic origin will exhibit tumors that are not confined to the membraneous glottis. In this subgroup the tumor will involve regions of the anterior commissure. This type of tumor may be better managed through use of treatment modalities that differ from those for "true" glottic tumors[6] (i.e., no anterior or posterior extension on the vocal fold). A second subgroup of about 20% will exhibit tumor extension into supraglottal structures. Bailey (1985a) states this type of tumor extends to involve one-half of the ipsilateral ventricular (false) vocal fold. A third subgroup of approximately 20% demonstrates extension into subglottal regions; extension usually exceeds 5 millimeters (mm) from the true vocal fold. The fourth and final subgroup accounting for about 15 to 20% of those with glottic lesions exhibits encroachment of the tumor into

---

[6]This is due to laryngeal lymphatics; specifically, if the anterior commissure is threatened or in fact violated the potential for malignant spread in the larynx is increased. Therefore, management will often involve at least partial resection of the contralateral hemilarynx.

cartilaginous structures (i.e., either the vocal process and/or body of the arytenoid cartilage ipsilaterally). Based on information provided by Bailey (1985a) glottic carcinoma may be segmented into five distinct diagnostic (tumor based) subgroups. A summary of subgroupings is provided in Table 3–12.

Determining Diagnostic Subgroups

Categorical subgrouping of individuals with glottic carcinoma is strongly influenced by anatomical reference points. From a management viewpoint, extension of a tumor almost always dictates how much of the larynx will be excised, and, consequently, how much tissue remains (Silver, 1981). Reasonable excisional margins must be maintained to avoid violating the tumor itself or leaving occult tumor cells behind. It is, however, an understanding of how cancer spreads within the larynx that mandates what surgical approaches are pursued (Kirchner, 1970, 1975, 1985, 1989; Kirchner & Carter, 1987; Ogura, 1955).

Clinical data suggest that when glottic carcinoma extends to and involves the cartilaginous framework of the larynx (e.g., portions of the arytenoid cartilage),

cancer recurrence may be more prevalent in this group following treatment by radiation alone (Chung & Sagerman, 1989; Strong, 1976). In contrast, lesions which are diagnosed relatively early in their development may be treated successfully through use of either limited surgical resection or radiation therapy (Kirchner, 1985; Silver, 1981; Weisberger, 1991). Application of radiation therapy as a primary treatment modality may also be less limiting from a voice production perspective relative to even limited surgical resections. Finally, information has suggested that early T1 N0 glottic tumors may be treatable through use of the laser (Elner & Fex, 1988; Koufman, 1986; McGuirt & Kaufman, 1987; Ossoff et al., 1985; Strong, 1975).

Restriction of Vocal Fold Mobility

Regarding tumor extension and invasion of adjacent cartilaginous structures in the larynx, one diagnostic issue is of extreme importance. Evaluation of suspected laryngeal malignancies always seeks to determine whether movement is intact in the involved vocal fold. Abnormal or sluggish movement of the vocal fold, or more critically, nonmovement of the vocal fold has significant clinical

TABLE 3–12.
Diagnostic Subgroups of Individuals Identified with Glottic Carcinoma.

Subgroup	Description
1	Approximately 15 to 20% have tumor confined to unilateral membranous glottis (true vocal fold).
2	Approximately 20 to 25% have tumor which extends to the anterior commissure of the glottis.
3	Approximately 20% have supraglottic extension involving the inferior one-half of the ventricular fold.
4	Approximately 20% have subglottal extension into the conus elasticus.
5	Approximately 15% to 20% have posterior extension of tumor to ipsilateral arytenoid cartilage.

Source: Adapted from Glottic Carcinoma by B.J. Bailey (pp. 257–278) in *Surgery of the larynx,* B.J. Bailey and H.F. Biller (Eds.), 1985, Philadelphia: W.B. Saunders, reprinted with permission.

implications. Nonmovement or *fixation* of a vocal fold frequently indicates that invasion involves deep penetration into the muscular structure of the fold (the vocalis muscle and paraglottic space) or deep cartilaginous invasion (cricoarytenoid joint). Prognosis may then be less favorable (UICC, 1987). This may be determined using stroboscopic evaluation as part of the clinical assessment protocol (Hirano, 1981; Hirano & Bless, 1993). If true fold fixation is confirmed, total laryngectomy is frequently recommended (Silver, 1981; Bailey, 1985a).

Prognosis

Large lesions of the larynx (squamous cell carcinomas) typically have a poorer prognosis relative to smaller lesions (Johnson et al., 1981; UICC, 1987). If carcinoma extends into or through the cartilaginous framework of the larynx, or should it infiltrate submucosal tissue below the primary tumor, the chance of metastatic spread to the lymphatic system is increased substantially (Kirchner, 1975, 1985; Ogura, 1955; Sessions, 1976). Thus, more extensive lesions exhibit an increased potential for more extensive resection of the endolarynx.

Bailey (1985a) has identified three considerations that must be evaluated by the surgeon in determining the appropriate treatment modality. These three preoperative considerations impact directly on the patient's potential survival following diagnosis. Specific considerations include: (1) tumors confined to a single true vocal fold are believed to have less than 5% chance of metastatic spread to cervical lymph nodes (Kirchner, 1985; Skolnik et al., 1975); (2) in those who exhibit fixation of a vocal fold, invasion of tumor into cartilage, or tumor invasion outside the "interior" compartment of the larynx, a 30 to 40% chance of metastatic spread to the lymphatic system exists, and this is typically associated with a 5-year survival rate of less than 50%; and (3) of those with glottic carcinoma (unspecified by subgroup), approximately 20% will develop a second primary tumor (approximately 6% will occur in the larynx or laryngopharynx with the remaining secondary tumors being identified in the head and neck, lung, gastrointestinal, or urinary systems) (Batsakis, 1979; Myers, 1991a, 1991b; UICC, 1987).

A Review of Surgical Treatment Options: Factors Underlying Choice of Treatment Modality

In their discussion of the embryologic development of the larynx, Lawson and Biller (1985) succinctly stated the importance of subdividing the mechanism into three distinct anatomical regions: the supraglottis, glottis, and subglottis. This segmentation has significant implications for the identification, diagnosis, management, and long-term survival of the individual who presents with a laryngeal tumor. Specifically, Lawson and Biller state:

> The three areas serve as barriers to the vertical spread of tumors and, in addition, the biological behavior of neoplasms and their pattern of spread at each anatomical site are different. This compartmentalization of the larynx also provides an anatomical basis for partial laryngectomy surgery. (p. 234)

Conservation Procedures

One of the earliest questions following diagnosis of laryngeal cancer relates to lesion extension. This question is asked in relation to the patient's prognosis and as it pertains to the potential for conservative rather than radical ablative surgery (Bailey,

1985a). Biller (1987) defined conservation laryngeal surgery as "that type of laryngeal surgery which adequately removes the tumor yet preserves the phonatory, respiratory, and protective functions of the larynx" (p. 38). Conservative approaches for treatment of laryngeal cancer may involve direct consideration of factors that impact quality of life (Bailey, 1985a).

Once specific details of the tumor (size and extension) are known the surgeon can carefully assess the patient's candidacy for conservative surgery. Bryce (1985) has noted that larger tumors (e.g., T3) that result in impaired vocal fold mobility or clear fixation pose a substantial area for disagreement among head and neck surgeons as to which treatment method is most appropriate. Despite limitations, conservative surgery may be suitable for certain tumors that are "specialized and extended" (Bryce, 1985, p. 194). However, the limits of such conservative applications for laryngeal carcinoma have been expanded considerably in the past decade (e.g., near-total laryngectomy). Johnson et al. (1981) have suggested that if malignant cells are detected in a regional cervical lymph node, the number of patients who will survive 5 years postdiagnosis will be reduced by 50%. This figure is reduced further if more than a single node is invaded through metastatic spread (Chung & Sagerman, 1989; Reed, Mueller, & Snow, 1959).

Ultimately, the physiologic goal of conservative surgery is to maximize the patient's opportunity to maintain some degree of phonatory function, to retain adequate sphincteric function of the upper airway for protective purposes (i.e., prevention of aspiration), and to maintain swallowing so that nutrition is maintained without supplemental measures (Biller, 1987; Pearson, 1981; Pearson, Woods, & Hartman, 1980; Ward, 1988). This decision is in large part a function of a comprehensive, and well-defined evaluation of the laryngeal malignancy (Hinton & Myers, 1991). It has been estimated that somewhere between 50% and 70% of all laryngeal malignancies may be surgically treated using conservation procedures (Schechter, 1986; Schechter & El-Mahdi, 1984). The surgeon must, however, carefully and comprehensively assess conservation surgery for cancer of the larynx along two dimensions: (1) the curability or survival associated with the procedure, and (2) the ability to retain functional integrity of the resected laryngeal mechanism (Bailey, 1985a; Biller, 1987; Ward, 1988).

In cases where reconstruction of the glottis is necessitated due to partial surgical excision, several goals may be targeted either individually or in combined fashion. Bailey (1985c) identified four primary goals including enhancement of voice, improvement of glottic competence to prevent aspiration, restoration of the airway in cases where respiration has been impaired due to primary surgery, and finally, for the prevention of infection or tissue change at the site of the resection.

Goals of Conservation Laryngeal Surgery

As noted, conservation surgical procedures seek to remove all aspects of the tumor and maintain safe surgical margins while concurrently maintaining sphincteric and phonatory functions of the larynx postsurgically. According to Friedman, Katsantonis, Siddoway, and Cooper (1981) three distinct anatomical-physiological requirements must be achieved to meet these goals postsurgically. The first demands that at least one arytenoid cartilage remains mobile on its cricoid articulation. The second requires reconstruction of the endolarynx to be completed so that an adequate amount of tissue "bulk" is provided in the posterior glottal region, thus, decreasing potential complications related to aspiration. The third seeks an adequate glottal aperture so that respiration is not impeded. In other words, the glottis cannot be reduced to the point where inspiratory capabilities are reduced. From a functional voice production perspective, these three goals are indeed additive. These requirements would also appear to influence factors associated with myoelastic-aerodynamic events (Titze, 1980) that may occur in the reconstructed mechanism (see Moon & Weinberg, 1987). If any of these goals are not met, the speaker's overall speech and voice proficiency may be reduced commensurately.

Indications for Conservation Laryngeal Surgery

For specific tumors of the larynx, treatment success using conservation surgery is comparable to that observed with total laryngectomy (Goepfert, Lindberg, & Jesse, 1981). It can be universally stated that more extensive surgical resections associated with conservative approaches are likely to result in an increased potential for postsurgical complications (Ward, 1988). Even the most conservative surgical approaches such as the laryngofissure and cordectomy technique is subject to complications.

With accumulation of additional data in the future the relative success of conservation surgery as an independent treatment entity can be compared to combined methods of treatment such as surgery and radiation (Campbell & Goepfert, 1989; Goepfert, 1984; Goepfert et al., 1981). Success of conservation procedures must address aspects of whether a greater chance of "cure" exists in addition to reductions in patient morbidity as a result of surgery. Hence, consideration of less radical procedures may provide the individual with fewer functional consequences. This ultimately impacts the individual's quality of life, provided that cancer control is not sacrificed. These concerns are considerable given the extensive impact that total laryngectomy has on one's life.

The decision to pursue more conservative treatment options, however, does require that the most accurate information

on the extent of the tumor into adjacent soft tissue or the cartilaginous framework of the larynx is available to the surgeon (Hinton & Myers, 1991). Clinical staging of the tumor offers important information in this regard (Becker, 1989; Kirchner & Som, 1971a; Myers, 1991a, 1991c; UICC, 1987). This concern always supersedes the desire to retain some postsurgical phonatory capacity and the preservation of a good airway. The desire to retain vocal capabilities is essential to the overall success of the patient's long-term rehabilitation; however, adequate surgical margins must be achieved to eliminate future spread or recurrence of cancer.

Development of Conservation Surgical Procedures for Laryngeal Cancer

Attempts to develop conservative surgical approaches for management of laryngeal carcinoma have existed since Billroth's first report of total laryngectomy (Biller, 1987). The development of conservative approaches transpired in a period that preceded information about intrinsic pathogenesis of tumor growth and spread. That is, information on the presence of deep invasion of tumor into underlying muscular and/or cartilaginous structures in the larynx was frequently unknown. Early approaches in many instances, however, had merit in relation to contemporary understanding of tumor biology and potential for invasion of adjacent structures (Pressman, 1956; Pressman et al., 1956, 1960). Careful observation of tumors often dictated what structures would be excised and which would be retained to maintain functional integrity of the postsurgical laryngeal system. Although many procedures used today have been modified to some extent, conservation laryngeal surgery evolved along two anatomical (surgical) planes dividing the larynx (Biller, 1987).

Approaches to Anatomically Segmenting the Larynx

The "planes" alluded to by Biller (1987) distinguish two basic types of conservative surgical treatment. The term *vertical partial laryngectomy* refers to procedures that involve glottic lesions; the term *horizontal partial laryngectomy* refers to procedures employed when a supraglottal tumor exists (Kirchner & Som, 1971b; Silver, 1981). The terms vertical and horizontal denote the *general plane of resection*. These planes of reference subdivide the larynx into left and right, or upper and lower sections. This system of categorization is apparent in many conservative methods reported in the literature; however, features of the tumor mandate the "true" margins of resection. The two planes (Biller, 1987) do not account for partial resections in the anterior-posterior or superior-inferior planes for either the vertical or horizontal procedures (Silver, 1981). These terms should, therefore, not be assumed as all inclusive.

Complications Associated with Conservation Laryngectomy

The introduction of conservation surgical procedures brought with it a new vision from both treatment and rehabilitative perspectives. It must be noted, however, that conservation procedures do have considerable limitations (Hinton & Myers, 1991) and carry the risk of significant complications (Ward, 1988). Further, revision or completion (total) laryngectomy at a later time may be necessary should the procedure prove unsuccessful in eliminating the malignancy (Biller & Som, 1977; Myers & Ogura, 1979; Ward, 1988).

Biller (1987) suggested that the commonly noted complication of postsurgical stenosis of the reconstructed larynx, as well as other problems, may have become more evident as extent of surgical resection has increased. Extended surgical resections have a greater chance that a functional laryngeal mechanism (both sphincteric and phonatory) cannot be created. Thus, a fine line may exist with conservation surgical procedures; finding the balance between the requirements of conservation laryngeal surgery is contingent on each patient's clinical and pathological presentation (Hinton & Myers, 1991). This is particularly true in cases of vertical partial laryngectomy. Extensive vertical partial resections must ensure safe surgical margins, but attempts to preserve phonatory, respiratory, and sphincteric (protective) functions of the larynx may not be realistic (Bailey, 1985a, 1985c; Hinton & Myers, 1991; Ward, Berci, & Calcaterra, 1977). It is critical for the speech-language pathologist to acknowledge the importance between postsurgical glottal competence and the overall sphincteric capacity of the larynx following conservation procedures. This relationship must always be considered in the course of postsurgical speech and voice rehabilitation. Due to increased levels of resection, Biller (1987) has stated that a "plateau" may have been reached in conservation surgery; thus, the chance of encountering a variety of postsurgical complications may be increased.

Ward (1988) has identified complications that may occur with conservation laryngectomy procedures, as well as the potential causative factors associated with them. The complications identified (Ward, 1988) may be subdivided into three primary categories: those which occur at the time of the surgery or in the immediate postsurgical period, those which occur in the intermediate postsurgical period, and those which occur or persist well after the patient has been discharged. The speech-language pathologist who works with patients who undergo partial or total laryngectomy procedures must be keenly aware of changes that may suggest postsurgical infection (pain, edema, etc.) and immediately refer the patient to his or her surgeon for timely evaluation. A summary of these complications can be found in Table 3–13.

Although several complications noted by Ward (1988) (e.g., tissue sloughing, development of granulation tissue) may occur with inadequate surgical reconstruction, newer reconstructive procedures (i.e., those that retain an adequate vascular supply and postsurgical lymphatic drainage to reconstructed tissues) with conservation laryngectomy may reduce these complications. Complications in the postoperative period such as development of laryngeal stricture or stenosis may be reduced by inserting a laryngeal keel (removed once re-epithelialization has occurred) in procedures like the antero-frontal partial laryngectomy (Kirchner, 1975; Som & Silver, 1968).

Partial Laryngectomy Procedures

Surgical techniques for glottic cancers have been identified using nomenclature that includes *cordectomy (laryngofissure)*, *hemi-laryngectomy*, *vertical partial laryngectomy*, and *extended frontolateral laryngectomy*. These procedures may be recommended for those who exhibit discrete, superficial glottic carcinoma (up to T2) or for those who have more extensive T1 lesions involving the arytenoid or extending to the anterior commissure (Bailey, 1985a; Biller, Ogura, & Pratt, 1971; Neel, Devine, & DeSanto, 1980; Silver, 1981; Som & Silver, 1968). Another procedure termed *supraglottic subtotal or horizontal partial laryngectomy* is appropriate for lesions of the supraglottis that do not encroach on the glottis. Each of these procedures will be presented and discussed in the subsequent section.

Cordectomy

Tumors that appear well-localized to a single vocal fold which maintains it's mobility may be considered for conservative

---

TABLE 3–13.
Complications Associated with Conservation Surgical Procedures for Laryngeal Cancer.

Complications Occurring at the Time of Surgery or in the Immediate Postoperative Period
Paralysis of neural innervation to larynx
Stenosis of larynx and/or airway
Edema
Infection
Tissue Sloughing

Complications Occurring in the Intermediate Postoperative Period
Development of granulation tissue
Improper healing of surgical site

Complications Occurring or Persisting Into the Postoperative Period Following Discharge
Scarring
Swallowing difficulties (dysphagia)
Aspiration
Recurrence of malignancy

Source: Adapted from Ward, P.H. (1988), Complications of laryngeal surgery: Etiology and prevention, *Laryngoscope, 98,* 54–57, The Laryngoscope, St. Louis, MO, with permission.

surgical management using a partial laryngectomy procedure termed a *cordectomy* and *laryngofissure* (Kirchner, 1975; Sessions, Maness, & McSwain, 1965; Silver, 1981). In cases where *cordectomy* is considered, careful preselection of patients is necessary. Bailey (1985a) has suggested that the following factors always be considered when this type of procedure is considered: (1) the tumor cannot be larger than 5 mm, (2) it must be confined to the middle third of the true vocal fold and must be located on the free margin of the fold, (3) the vocal fold must be mobile, and (4) tumor margins must be confirmed. Although these tumors can be managed successfully via surgery they also respond quite favorably to other forms of treatment, most notably radiation treatment (Bailey, 1985a; Goepfert et al., 1981; Hinton & Myers, 1991; Wang, 1983). Further, cordectomy may be undertaken on an infrequent basis today (Silver, 1981).

Cordectomy involves entrance into the endolarynx via a vertical incision, termed a *laryngofissure*, at the midline of the thyroid cartilage following tracheostomy. This is shown in Figures 3–1 and 3–2.

The tumor is then resected from the inner perichondrium of the thyroid lamina, superiorly to the region of the laryngeal ventricle, inferior to the free margin of the involved vocal fold, and then posteriorly (Kirchner, 1975; Silver, 1981). The area of resection during tracheotomy and laryngofissure is shown in Figure 3–3; further details are provided in Silver (1981). Therefore, the laryngofissure involves re-sectioning of a tissue wedge that includes the entire tumor and sufficient tissue margins. Resection usually does not involve the anterior region of the ipsilateral vocal fold to reduce the chance of a laryngeal web (Kirchner, 1975). The general surgical sequence of this procedure as reported by Silver (1981) is shown in Figures 3–4 a–f.

Hemilaryngectomy

The term *hemilaryngectomy* has traditionally implied that one-half of the larynx is removed surgically. This terminology defines partial laryngectomy procedures that are applied in the superior-inferior or vertical plane. Hemilaryngectomy is

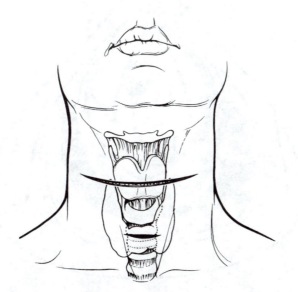

Figure 3–1. Transverse incision and tracheotomy site associated with laryngofissure and cordectomy. (From *Surgery for cancer of the larynx and related structures* by C. E. Silver, 1981, New York: Churchill Livingstone. Reprinted with permission.)

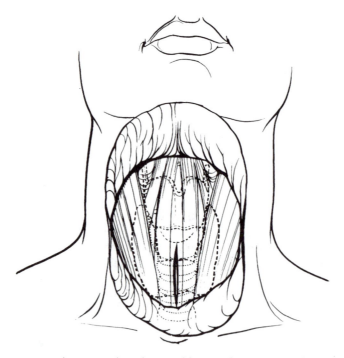

Figure 3–2. Entrance to larynx and trachea and laryngofissure (vertical incision). (From *Surgery for cancer of the larynx and related structures* by C. E. Silver, 1981, New York: Churchill Livingstone. Reprinted with permission.)

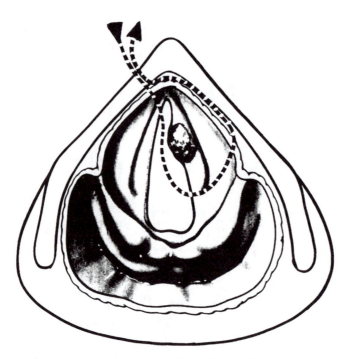

Figure 3–3. Area of glottic resection associated with laryngofissure and cordectomy. (From *Surgery for cancer of the larynx and related structures* by C. E. Silver, 1981, New York: Churchill Livingstone. Reprinted with permission.)

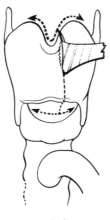
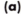

(a)

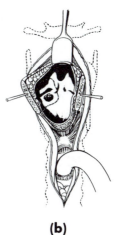

(b)

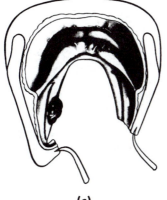

(c)

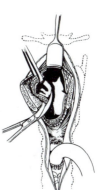

(d)

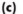

(e)

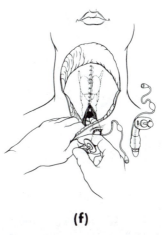

(f)

Figure 3–4. **(a)** Thyroid cartilage is separated just off midline contralateral to involved side. **(b)** Larynx is entered to expose tumor. **(c)** Superior view representing separation of thyroid cartilage relative to location of tumor. **(d)** Excision of tumor and adjacent tissue. **(e)** Superior view of larynx following resection via cordectomy. **(f)** Closure is undertaken and tracheostomy tube is positioned following resection. (From *Surgery for cancer of the larynx and related structures* by C. E. Silver, 1981, New York: Churchill Livingstone. Reprinted with permission.)

used for both T2 and T3 lesions (Silver, 1981). Kirchner (1985) has stated that hemilaryngectomy may be appropriate in a small number of cases of glottic carcinoma where vocal fold fixation is apparent. However, Kirchner (1985) states that tumor extension *cannot* exceed more than 1 centimeter (cm) inferiorly in both the anterior and middle regions of the larynx. An example of the region of excision for hemilaryngectomy is shown in Figure 3–5. From an anatomical perspective, hemilaryngectomy has been interpreted to imply resection via sagittal section of the larynx. True and complete hemilaryngectomy resections in the vertical plane are

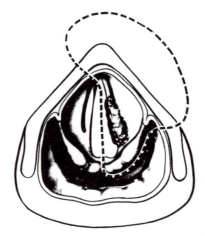

Figure 3–5. Area of excision associated with hemilaryngectomy. (From *Surgery for cancer of the larynx and related structures* by C. E. Silver, 1981, New York: Churchill Livingstone. Reprinted with permission.)

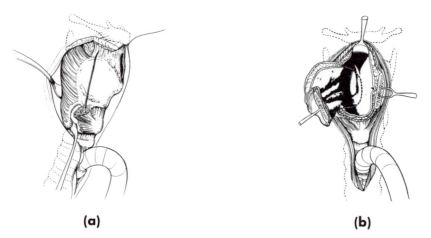

(a)   **(b)**

Figure 3–6. **(a)** Following entrance to laryngeal region, the thyroid cartilage is incised (thyrotomy) on lateral-posterior region. **(b)** Larynx is entered through thyrotomy and area to be incised is identified. **(c)** Tumor and adjacent tissue is resected with separation of cricoarytenoid joint. **(d)** Midsection of remaining lateral-posterior thyroid cartilage is prepared as a cartilage flap. **(e)** Cartilage flap is positioned on posterior aspect of cricoid cartilage and sutured in place. **(f)** Mucosa from pyriform sinus covers cartilage flap with associated reconstruction and closure. **(g)** Closure of strap muscles and anterior neck region. (From *Surgery for cancer of the larynx and related structures* by C. E. Silver, 1981, New York: Churchill Livingstone. Reprinted with permission.)

uncommon (Bailey, 1985a). However, numerous modifications of hemilaryngectomy have been reported (Rothfield, Johnson, Myers, & Wagner, 1989). Thus, modified hemilaryngectomy procedures such as the vertical or fronto-lateral laryngectomy are more common and have greater flexibility in their application (Silver, 1981). The procedural surgical sequence for hemilaryngectomy is shown in Figures 3–6 a–g; additional details can be found in Silver (1981).

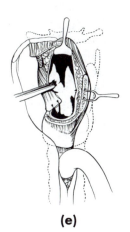

(c)

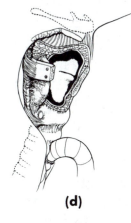

(d)

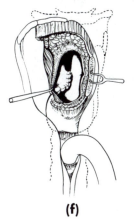

(e)

(f)

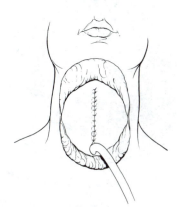

(g)

Figure 3–6 continued

Vertical Partial Laryngectomy

Sasaki (1983) has addressed the indications and applications of *vertical partial hemilaryngectomy* for tumors involving one-half of the larynx; however, involvement cannot restrict vocal fold mobility. Sasaki also suggests that vertical hemilaryngectomy may be appropriate in cases where the tumor has been staged from T1 to those of early T3 tumors where radiotherapy is not indicated. An example of the excised region associated with vertical partial laryngectomy is shown in Figure 3–7.

Expanding the Definition of Vertical Partial Laryngectomy

Bailey (1985a) has expanded the definition of *vertical partial laryngectomy* into three distinct surgical subtypes. Bailey believes that one of these three modifications will be appropriate for a variety of glottic tumors. Determining which modification is most appropriate is primarily contingent on tumor extension on the membranous vocal fold. Remember that in cases where laryngofissure and cordectomy is appropriate, a strict criterion for its application is related to restriction of the lesion to the middle third of a single vocal fold, with clear tumor margins and full vocal fold mobility. Extension of the tumor (most notably into the subglottal region and the potential invasion of portions of the arytenoid cartilage) influences which surgical subtype may be most applicable. These surgical subtypes have been termed Basic Types 1, 2, and 3 (Bailey, 1985a).

Basic Type 1 (Ipsilateral Tumor)

From a superior view, the Basic Type 1 vertical partial laryngectomy procedure involves removal of cartilage and soft tissue from the midpoint of the thyroid cartilage (thyroid prominence) posteriorly to a point which is approximately 3 mm anterior to the superior cornua of the ipsilateral thyroid cartilage. When anterior

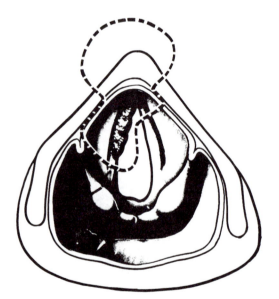

Figure 3–7. Area of resection associated with vertical partial (frontolateral) laryngectomy. (From *Surgery for cancer of the larynx and related structures* by C.E. Silver, 1981, New York: Churchill Livingstone. Reprinted with permission.)

encroachment of the tumor is suspected (i.e., toward the anterior commissure), Sasaki (1983) suggests that the anterior resection occur just off midline contralateral to the tumor. This resection includes removal of the ipsilateral vocal process. This procedure is used when the tumor *is restricted to the middle third of the vocal fold*. In instances where the tumor extends posteriorly along the membranous fold, the entire arytenoid cartilage on the involved side must be resected (Bailey, 1985a). From a frontal view, resection occurs from the top of the ipsilateral thyroid alae down to and including subglottal tissue to the superior aspect of the cricoid. Using the *Basic Type 1* surgical procedure the entire vocal fold is removed along with sufficient tissue margins in the anterior-posterior, as well as inferior-superior planes (Bailey, 1985a).

Basic Type 2 (Ipsilateral Tumor with Extension to Anterior Commissure of Larynx)

This vertical partial laryngectomy procedure has application when a glottic tumor extends anteriorly to the anterior commissure. It is similar to the Basic Type 1 resection; however, anterior extension of the resection moves beyond the midline of the thyroid cartilage to include an area that comprises approximately one-third of the contralateral thyroid lamina (Bailey, 1985a). The resection takes place approximately 2–3 mm contralaterally on the vertical plane. This extended resection relates to the anterior extension of the tumor on the membranous fold. The use of a partial contralateral resection requires removal of contralateral portions of soft tissue structures, namely the anterior sections of the ventricular and true vocal folds and the anterior subglottal region.

Basic Type 3 (Extension of Tumor to Contralateral True Vocal Fold)

This procedure is simply an extension of Basic Types 2 and 3. Use of this method is

appropriate when extension of the tumor is confirmed to cross the anterior commissure (Bailey, 1985a). Extension may also involve up to one-third of the contralateral true vocal fold (anterior). Tumor extension across the commissure requires resection on the contralateral aspect of the hemilarynx to be extended approximately 4–5 mm. This is termed an *anterior commissure technique* (Kirchner & Som, 1975; Som & Silver, 1968). The area of resection is shown in Figure 3–8. All remaining surgical resections are similar to those used in the Basic Type 1 and 2 techniques. Accordingly, more extensive resection of contralateral soft tissue structures (i.e., ventricular and true vocal folds and subglottal tissue) is undertaken.

Modifications of Basic Types 1, 2, and 3

Evaluating the three vertical partial laryngectomy procedures outlined by Bailey (1985a) it is apparent that application of these types of procedures requires that the tumor is confined to the vocal fold. Although the tumor may indeed extend to, or in fact cross, the anterior commissure of the larynx, carcinoma is confined to the membranous portion of the vocal fold. When the tumor extends beyond the confines of the membranous glottis to include either a cartilaginous structure of the larynx or involve some portion of the subglottis, several modifications of the basic subtypes of vertical partial laryngectomy procedures are recommended (Bailey, 1985a).

The first modification is indicated for those who have subglottal extension of the carcinoma; subglottal involvement may extend up to 2–3 mm. As such, the inferior-superior resection must be adjusted to accommodate subglottal extension (Kirchner, 1985). However, the anterior-posterior resection may be identical to that employed with either of the three subtypes of vertical partial laryngectomy (Bailey,

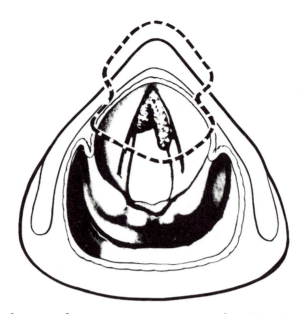

Figure 3–8. Area of resection for anterior commissure procedure. (From *Surgery for cancer of the larynx and related structures* by C. E. Silver, 1981, New York: Churchill Livingstone. Reprinted with permission.)

1985a). In cases of subglottal tumor extension, therefore, considerably more tissue must be resected in the inferior plane. Consequently, resection includes approximately one-half of the superior cricoid cartilage.

The second modification outlined by Bailey (1985a) applies to tumors that extend posteriorly on the true vocal fold and invade the arytenoid cartilage. This invasion is typically confined to the vocal process of the ipsilateral cartilage. Because the tumor extends posteriorly, the Basic Type 1 vertical partial laryngectomy is applicable, but the entire ipsilateral arytenoid cartilage is also resected.

Use of vertical partial laryngectomy procedures is contingent on numerous considerations. Gathering information on the true degree of tumor extension (Batsakis, 1979; Hinton & Myers, 1991; Silver, 1981) has important implications to the individual and his or her potential postsurgical voice and speech capabilities. Although various subtypes and/or modifications of this type of surgery exist, they are not employed where tumor extension exceeds 2–3 mm into the subglottis or

where posterior invasion results in vocal fold fixation (Bailey, 1985a).

If this guideline is violated more aggressive surgical treatment is necessitated (Kirchner, 1985). More aggressive methods frequently result in more limited postsurgical vocal capabilities and a real possibility for some degree of physical disfigurement and associated stigmatization (Dropkin, 1981, 1989; Goffman, 1963). The importance of these issues in association with conservation laryngeal surgery has not been addressed in the literature. Yet this issue may have dramatic implications for the total rehabilitation of some individuals who select such treatment options.

Limitations of Partial Vertical Laryngectomy

Although aspects of tumor resection relative to subglottal tumor extension must meet specific criteria for successful application (Kirchner, 1985), limited information is available regarding tumor extension above the glottis. Specifically, are vertical partial laryngectomy procedures applicable in cases where the carcinoma extends into the laryngeal ventricle? This type of extension may be a limiting factor for vertical partial laryngectomy, but it may not be entirely exclusionary as individuals with small primary tumors in the ventricle may be candidates for conservative surgery (Bailey, 1985a). Nevertheless, comprehensive evaluation of the tumor and its spread (Batsakis, 1979) must be carefully evaluated prior to considering conservation procedures as potential treatment options (Kirchner, 1969, 1975, 1989).

Extended Partial Laryngectomy

Modifications of classic partial laryngectomy procedures are likely to be common in patients with laryngeal cancer. The primary determining factor in these cases relates to the location and extent of the tumor, as well as related pathological characteristics (Batsakis, 1979). The extent of resection is, similar to all other procedures outlined, guided by the need to maintain adequate tumor-free margins (Sessions, 1980). More extended partial laryngectomy procedures, therefore, may fall into a category best described as extended hemilaryngectomy. This type of procedure is then variable depending on the characteristics of the tumor, its margins, and overall extension.

Antero-Frontal Partial Laryngectomy

Another extension of the conservation surgical procedures outlined previously has been termed the *antero-frontal partial laryngectomy*. This procedure is performed using an approach termed the anterior commissure technique (Kirchner, 1975; Som & Silver, 1968) and is recommended for tumors that involve the glottis bilaterally (see

Figure 3–9). That is, the carcinoma crosses the anterior commissure to involve the membranous segment of both true vocal folds. When a tumor crosses the anterior commissure, the vocal folds must retain normal movement or exhibit only limited reductions in mobility for the antero-frontal procedure to be considered. Inferior tumor extension at the anterior commissure cannot exceed 1 cm. If it does, the potential for tumor invasion into the cricothyroid membrane is substantial (Kirchner, 1975), and the procedure is not applicable. Clinically staged T2 lesions may be considered for the antero-frontal partial laryngectomy. The surgical sequence for the anterior commissure technique as outlined by Silver (1981) is shown in Figure 3–9 a–d.

Although this technique has been reported by several authors with modification, Kirchner (1975) reported the following standard procedural protocol. Entrance to the endolarynx is achieved by performing a bilateral thyrotomy (vertical incisions are made approximately 1 cm off the thyroid midline). The thyrohyoid membrane which lies beneath the bilateral thyrotomy incisions is subsequently incised. The endolarynx is then entered through the cricothyroid membrane which lies at the anterior midline of the cricoid cartilage. Tissue is then excised from the perichondrium of the thyroid. The degree of resection in the posterior plane is contingent on tumor extension (Kirchner, 1975). Obviously, this procedure is most appropriate when carcinoma is confined to anterior aspects of the glottic larynx; posterior extension in the presence of a transglottic tumor would necessitate more aggressive surgical resections (e.g., near-total laryngectomy or total laryngectomy).

Extended-Fronto-Lateral Laryngectomy

The *extended fronto-lateral laryngectomy* is recommended when carcinoma involves

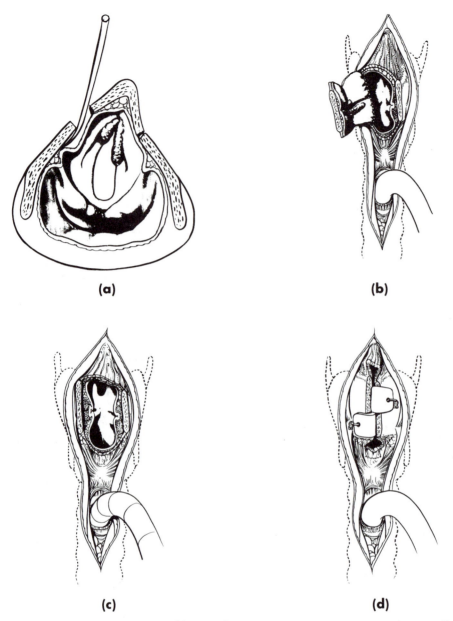

(a)

(b)

(c)

(d)

Figure 3–9. (a) Superior view of larynx depicting anterior commissure technique. **(b)** Anterior commissure and associated mucosa is incised. **(c)** View of larynx following removal of anterior commissure. **(d)** Closure of larynx following anterior commissure resection. Note laryngeal keels which are affixed to thyroid cartilage for closure; keels are removed 6–8 weeks following initial resection. (From *Surgery for cancer of the larynx and related structures* by C. E. Silver, 1981, New York: Churchill Livingstone. Reprinted with permission.)

the entire anterior-posterior length of the vocal fold (T2 and T3 lesions) including the vocal process (Kirchner, 1975; Silver, 1981). Reduction in vocal fold movement does not limit its application; however, fixation requires additional consideration. If fixation is observed the extended fronto-lateral procedure can only be used if the tumor does not extend more than 1 cm inferiorly on the fold. If the tumor extends beyond this distance, concerns related to safe surgical margins have been raised (Kirchner, 1975; Kirchner & Som, 1971a). This is particularly important in the posterior portion of the fold because of the potential to invade the cricoid cartilage (Kirchner, 1975; Ogura & Biller, 1969). The extended fronto-lateral laryngectomy *is not* suitable for glottic carcinomas with an excessive degree of inferior extension (i.e., > 1 cm), particularly in association with the cartilaginous glottis. The region of resection for extended fronto-lateral laryngectomy is shown in Figure 3–10.

The method for the extended fronto-lateral laryngectomy is as follows. Initially, the external perichondrium is excised from the thyroid lamina on the side of the tumor. This is followed by creation of a vertical thyrotomy lateral to the midline of the thyroid contralateral to the tumor. Thus, although the attachment for both vocal folds at the anterior commissure is resected a section of contralateral thyroid lamina and vocal fold remains. In the superior-inferior plane, the larynx is sectioned above at the margin of the ventricular vocal fold and below at the margin of the superior cricoid cartilage.

When the surgical resection involves excision on one arytenoid cartilage, Bailey (1985a) has stated that reconstructive procedures to increase "bulk" in the area of such extended resections are essential to reduce potential aspiration complications. Thus, extended fronto-lateral partial laryngectomy may require sufficient glottic reconstruction to maintain the patency of the endolarynx for respiratory purposes, as well as for achieving adequate postsurgical voice production.

Additional Considerations

Individuals who exhibit moderate to severe chronic obstructive pulmonary disease (COPD) may not be suitable candidates for vertical partial laryngectomy (Becker, 1989). This issue has considerable clinical implications from a rehabilitative perspective. If one recalls that one of the basic goals of conservation laryngectomy is to maintain an adequate airway, resections similar to those reported may be contraindicated (Ward, 1988). When potential complications of postsurgical stenosis are considered jointly with these factors (i.e., poor

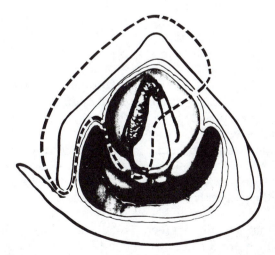

Figure 3–10. Area of resection for extended frontolateral laryngectomy. (From *Surgery for cancer of the larynx and related structures* by C. E. Silver, 1981, New York: Churchill Livingstone. Reprinted with permission.)

pulmonary capacity and reduction in aperture of postsurgical airway), careful and serious consideration is required. Additionally, should the individual pursue a total laryngectomy as a treatment option, pulmonary status may limit the choice of postsurgical rehabilitation options. That is, COPD has been suggested to be a contraindication for use of the tracheoesophageal puncture voice prosthesis (Andrews, Mickel, Monahan, Hanson, & Ward, 1987). Thus, a broader vision of the rehabilitation process must always come to the forefront of all individuals who are diagnosed with laryngeal carcinoma, no matter how limited or extensive.

Despite which vertical partial laryngectomy procedure (and related modifications) is anticipated by the surgeon several factors with rehabilitative implications must be considered. First, regardless of preoperative assessment the potential always exists that tumor invasion will be more extensive than originally believed. In this instance an anticipated partial laryngectomy may become a total laryngectomy. Thus, the surgeon will frequently request permission to undertake this more radical procedure. When this possibility is likely more specific preoperative information on both procedures (partial and total laryngectomy) and the postsurgical sequelae would be in order. However, this type of situation requires careful coordination of efforts between the surgeon and the speech-language pathologist. It is particularly important that the patient understands the postsurgical communication consequences for each procedure. This information should be provided by the speech-language pathologist once the surgeon discusses the proposed surgery with the patient. The speech-language pathologist must ensure that the patient has been clearly advised regarding the status of his or her condition and the potential degree of surgical resection. Therefore, direct communication between the surgeon and the speech-language pathologist is essential.

Near-Total Laryngectomy

The desire to use partial laryngectomy procedures is frequently applied in cases where lesions are early in their evolution, or where tumor extension is not widespread. Partial laryngectomy procedures must be guided by the need to provide an adequate surgical resection with clear and safe margins. The primary goals of surgical management are frequently at odds in cases of larger and more extensive malignant lesions of the larynx. However, Pearson and his colleagues (Pearson, 1981; Pearson et al., 1980) sought to extend the boundaries of the surgical resection while at the same time creating a surgical speaking shunt for postoperative communicative purposes. The procedure that was offered was termed the *near-total* laryngectomy.

The near-total procedure may be employed as primary treatment for a variety of laryngeal tumors including glottic lesions with cord fixation, subglottal lesions, and supraglottal tumors that exceed the prerequisites for classic supraglottic laryngectomy (Pearson, 1981). Additionally, near-total laryngectomy may also be applicable in those who present with tumors of the pyriform sinus provided that the postcricoid and cricopharyngeal regions are spared from tumor extension (Pearson, 1981). Thus, the procedure typically involves extensive resectioning to provide disease-free surgical margins.

Briefly, near-total laryngectomy involves maintaining a mucosal tissue strip on the side contralateral to the tumor once it has been resected. The typical resection involves the tracheal wall, approximately two-fifths of the subglottis, a segment of an innervated true vocal fold with its arytenoid and the ventricular and aryepiglottic folds. Once the resection is complete the remaining tissue is reconstructed into a "shunt" which connects the trachea and the pharynx, and a permanent tracheostoma is created. Thus, near-total laryngectomy provides a reconstructed tissue conduit that permits pulmonary air to be diverted from the trachea to the upper airway for speech purposes when the tracheostoma is closed. Successful development of functional voice following the near-total laryngectomy procedure has been reported to be as high as 95% (Keith, Pearson, Thomas, & Lipton, 1988; Keith, Thomas, & Pearson, 1987). The advantages of near-total laryngectomy lie in its potential application to larger and more extensive laryngeal tumors without sacrificing oncologic safety, as well as the potential for the maintenance of an intrinsic mechanism for postsurgical voice and speech production.

Rationale for Near-Total Laryngectomy

The development and use of near-total (subtotal) laryngectomy (Pearson, 1981) found its major rationale in that some large tumors of the larynx may be amenable to less than total laryngectomy. The near-total procedure which was initially introduced by Pearson and colleagues (Pearson, 1981; Pearson et al., 1980) has been employed for glottic tumors staged as T3 or T4 lesions and for carcinoma of the pyriform sinus staged at either T1, T2, or T3. According to DeSanto et al. (1989) near-total laryngectomy may bridge the gap between the potential for undertreatment of such lesions through application of "classic partial" laryngectomy procedures and the potential for overtreatment exhibited by total laryngectomy.

Despite this bridging between conservative and total laryngectomy, the decision to use near-total laryngectomy is still guided by principles of oncologic safety. DeSanto et al. (1989) have conceptualized the use of near-total laryngectomy "as an alternative to laryngectomy for patients who are candidates for conventional conservation surgery but are physiologically compromised by age or general health"

(p. 4) or when safe surgical margins cannot be guaranteed using conservation laryngectomy. In their opinion, total laryngectomy is required on oncological grounds only for lesions of the glottis, supraglottis, or laryngopharynx that result in the fixation of a vocal fold. DeSanto et al. (1989) also suggest that total laryngectomy may be appropriate in a subgroup of individuals who exhibit less advanced (T1 and T2) supraglottic or laryngopharyngeal tumors and whose age or general physiologic condition would limit the use of partial laryngectomy procedures and associated risks of postsurgical aspiration.

Horizontal Supraglottic (Subtotal) Laryngectomy

The *horizontal supraglottic laryngectomy* (Kirchner, 1975) is indicated for those who exhibit carcinoma of the epiglottis or the ventricular vocal fold, provided it does not extend across or enter the ventricle or encroach on the anterior commissure. If these criteria are met, a barrier to inferior extension of the carcinoma into the thyroid cartilage is believed to exist (Kirchner, 1975; Kirchner & Som, 1971b). However, carcinoma involving the epiglottis and/or the ventricular vocal fold that extends inferiorly to involve the laryngeal ventricle or the anterior commissure will not meet these anatomical criteria. Carcinoma that spreads in such a fashion must be considered as *transglottic* (McGavran et al., 1961). Kirchner, Cornog, and Holmes (1974) demonstrated that once the carcinoma becomes transglottic its potential for invasion into the thyroid cartilage is high. Primary supraglottic tumors that become transglottic have been shown to be very aggressive with considerable potential for cartilaginous infiltration and invasion (Kirchner, 1969, 1985; Kirchner & Som, 1971b; McGavran et al., 1961). Consequently, a safe resection margin may be obtained through the ventricle and anterior commissure approach. An example of the general area of resection for supraglottic subtotal laryngectomy (Silver, 1981) is shown in Figure 3–11.

The horizontal supraglottic laryngectomy involves creation of a horizontal (apron) incision in the thyroid cartilage at or about the level of the ventricle once the external perichondrium is stripped in a downward fashion. Thus, with removal of the upper section of the thyroid alae excision of the pre-epiglottic space can be achieved. Most of the hyoid bone is also resected with only the greater cornu of this structure on the side which is least involved left intact postsurgically. The general procedure of supraglottic subtotal laryngectomy is shown in Figures 3–12 a–c (Silver, 1981).

Total Laryngectomy

Laryngeal tumors judged unsuitable for conservative surgical approaches will require a total laryngectomy (Hinton & Myers, 1991; Silver, 1981). With a majority

of advanced tumors, (i.e., T3 lesions or greater) conservative approaches do not permit safe surgical margins; advanced lesions require a wide-field approach for purposes of oncologic safety (Kirchner, 1985; Silver, 1981). An example of such a tumor is shown in Figure 3–13.

Total laryngectomy involves removal of the entire laryngeal framework (thyroid, cricoid, arytenoid cartilages, and the epiglottis), as well as all intrinsic membranes and muscles including the vestigial cartilages (Silver, 1981). This generally includes removal of the hyoid bone, associated strap muscles of the neck, and one or more superior tracheal rings (DeWeese & Saunders, 1977; Silver, 1981). Thus, total laryngectomy involves surgical removal of the laryngeal valve from the superior aspect of the airway. The trachea is then brought anterior in the midline of the neck and sutured into place. This results in complete and total (functional) separation of the primary airway and the oral, pharyngeal, and upper digestive pathways. The area of resection is shown in Figure 3–14. The general surgical sequence for total laryngectomy is shown in

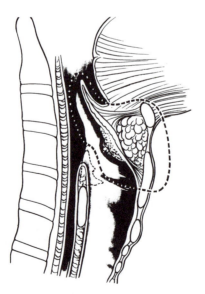

Figure 3–11. Area of resection for supraglottic subtotal laryngectomy. (From *Surgery for cancer of the larynx and related structures* by C. E. Silver, 1981, New York: Churchill Livingstone. Reprinted with permission.)

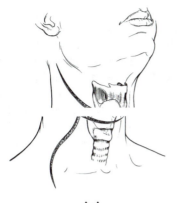

(a)

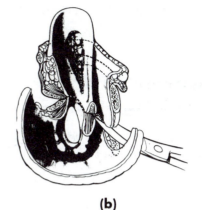

(b)

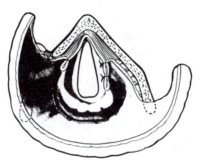

(c)

Figure 3-12. **(a)** Neck incisions typically used with supraglottic subtotal laryngectomy. **(b)** Resectioning of supraglottal mucosa. **(c)** Supraglottic region following resection. (From *Surgery for cancer of the larynx and related structures* by C. E. Silver, 1981, New York: Churchill Livingstone. Reprinted with permission.)

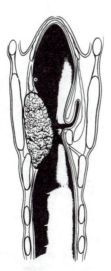

Figure 3-13. Tumor requiring total laryngectomy. (From *Surgery for cancer of the larynx and related structures* by C.E. Silver, 1981, New York: Churchill Livingstone. Reprinted with permission.)

Figure 3–15 a–g (for further details, see Silver, 1981).

Multimodality Approaches to Treatment

Once a diagnosis of advanced disease is confirmed and additional clinical information obtained management options can be evaluated. With large lesions this will usually indicate total laryngectomy. Yet use of surgery as the sole treatment approach for more extensive tumors is rare. As a tumor increases in size, multimodality approaches to treatment are often considered. Consideration of multimodality treatment protocols are also influenced by histological information obtained from biopsy.

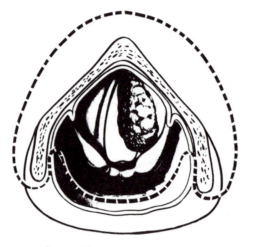

Figure 3–14. Area of resection for total laryngectomy. (From *Surgery for cancer of the larynx and related structures* by C.E. Silver, 1981, New York: Churchill Livingstone. Reprinted with permission.)

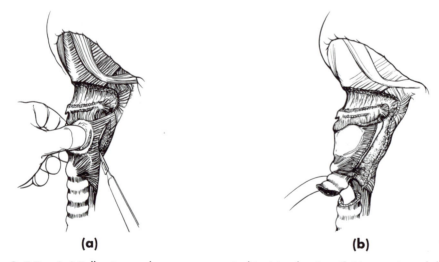

(a)   **(b)**

Figure 3–15. **(a)** Following neck entrance, surgical incision begins. **(b)** Larynx is mobilized and separated from trachea. **(c)** Resection of larynx from hypopharynx. **(d)** Incisions are completed and larynx is removed in its entirety. **(e)** Hypopharyngeal defect following removal of larynx. **(f)** Closure of hypopharynx. **(g)** Construction of tracheostoma and postoperative closure. (From *Surgery for cancer of the larynx and related structures* by C. E. Silver, 1981, New York: Churchill Livingstone. Reprinted with permission.)

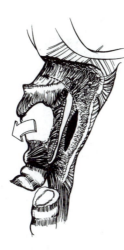
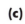

(c)

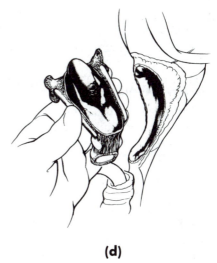

(d)

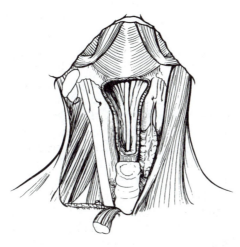
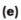

(e)

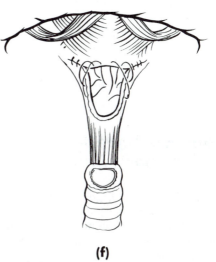

(f)

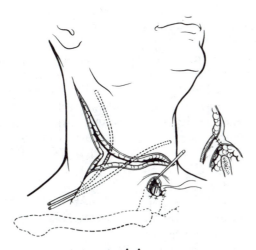

(g)

Figure 3–15 continued

Large tumors or those that are poorly differentiated histologically exhibit a greater propensity for dissemination of disease (Weisler, Weigel, Rosenman, & Silver, 1989). Consequently, it has been suggested that the probability of observing metastatic spread within the neck is increased, and, therefore, combined therapy is often recommended (Becker, 1989; Chung & Sagerman, 1989).

Combined therapy routinely involves either neck dissection and/or radiation therapy (Chung & Sagerman, 1989). Clinical staging of lymph node involvement (N category) which suggests a negative neck (i.e., N0) may exhibit an error rate of 20 to 30% (DeSanto, Holt, Bearhrs, & O'Fallon, 1982; Weisler et al., 1989). This suggests that combined treatment, particularly in larger tumors with apparently negative nodal involvement may be justified (Chung & Sagerman, 1989; Myers, 1991a).

Rationale Underlying Multimodality Treatment

Surgical removal of lymphatics has generally been undertaken to eliminate or prevent the spread of cancer when a tumor has been identified in any region of the human body. In laryngeal cancer neck dissection has been employed. It is more common to see a patient who has had a total laryngectomy and some form of concomitant neck dissection than it is to see an individual who has undergone total laryngectomy alone (Myers, 1991c). Due to cervical lymphatics, the use of radical or *en bloc* neck dissection has frequently been used in treatment for laryngeal cancer (Robbins et al., 1991).

Although total laryngectomy removes all structures that are potentially in the field of malignancy for the larynx proper, neck dissection is believed to provide an extended zone of treatment in an attempt to eliminate potential cervical metastases (DeSanto et al, 1982; Rabuzzi, Chung, &

Sagerman, 1980). However, data indicate that radical neck dissection does not always prove successful in eliminating occult disease (DeSanto et al., 1982; Myers, 1991a, 1991c).

Neck Dissection

Due to lymphatic compartmentalization within and around the larynx considerable attention has been directed toward removal of cervical lymphatics in the neck region (Myers, 1991b, 1991c; Robbins et al., 1991). This surgical procedure has been broadly termed and discussed as *neck dissection*. Neck dissection has historically involved the removal of all cervical lymphatic chains, hence, the term *radical neck dissection* has emerged. The primary goal of radical neck dissection is to eliminate all cervical (regional) metastases that may be present. Evidence suggests that as tumor size increases the potential for nodal involvement also increases (UICC, 1987), which may increase the chance for recurrent disease (Chu & Strawitz, 1978).

Since its introduction in the early 1900s (Crile, 1906), radical neck dissection was almost always performed with total (wide-field) laryngectomy. As surgeons began using more conservative surgical approaches to management, modifications in the neck dissection also emerged (Kirchner, 1985). Although radical neck dissection continues to exist in classic form, less ablative and more selective neck dissections have emerged with the desire of many surgeons to employ conservation surgery whenever possible (Wenig & Applebaum, 1991).

Guidelines for Neck Dissection

Once the choice of a radical neck dissection is abandoned, description of what structures are removed in a given neck dissection vary. Problems with inconsistent descriptions of neck dissection are primarily twofold. First, two patients who undergo surgery that falls under the same classification terminology may be left with different residual structures. Second, and perhaps most importantly, poor definition and specification of the extent and degree of neck dissection provides a substantial confound in monitoring oncologic treatment of that patient (UICC, 1987). Therefore, in 1988 the Committee for Head and Neck Surgery and Oncology of the American Academy of Otolaryngology-Head and Neck Surgery formed a subcommittee to address issues pertaining to neck dissection terminology (Robbins et al., 1991).

Six specific goals were presented by the Committee: (1) to develop standardized terminology for surgical neck dissection while maintaining traditional terms such as radical and modified neck dissection; (2) to specifically define lymphatic and nonlymphatic structures removed with a given dissection procedure; (3) to standardize terms used to describe cervical lymphatics, with particular emphasis on lymphatic groups most susceptible to metastatic disease; (4) to define both clinical and surgical boundaries of cervical lymphatics dissected; (5) to limit the number of terms used to classify dissection procedures while maintaining a comprehensive system for classification; and (6) to develop a classification system that correlates with cervical metastatic spread of the disease and satisfies acceptable standards of cancer control (Robbins et al., 1991; UICC, 1987). To meet their objectives, a six-level, anatomically based definition for the boundaries of lymph node groupings that are removed in a traditional radical neck dissection was developed. The anatomical breakdown of lymphatic groups are provided in Table 3–14 which provides a nonredundant and well-defined regional compartmentalization of the cervical lymphatics including the submental and submandibular groups, the upper, middle, and lower jugular groups, the posterior triangle group, and the anterior compartment group.

Emerging Concepts in Terminology

The Academy's recommendations on neck dissection (Robbins et al., 1991) were influenced directly by four underlying principles. First, radical neck dissection was judged to be "the standard basic procedure for lymphadenectomy" (Robbins et al., 1991, p. 602); they believed traditional radical neck dissection provided the basis for classification of all other procedures. Consequently, it was recommended that the term "modified radical neck dissection" be employed when "one or more nonlymphatic structures" (p. 602) that is/are traditionally excised in a radical neck dissection is preserved. From a conceptual standpoint, recommended nomenclature differentiates radical and modified procedures based on the preservation or removal of nonlymphatic components. However, two additional classifications for dissections were proposed. The first, termed "selective neck dissection," pertains to a dissection where one or more lymph node groups typically removed during a radical procedure is/are preserved. It is important to note that the selectivity of this type of procedure can be further divided in specific dissection subtypes. The fourth and final classification was termed "extended radical neck dissection." This involves the surgical removal of additional lymphatic and/or nonlymphatic structures along with a traditional radical procedure. The specifics of the radical, modified radical, selective and extended radical neck dissection procedures as developed and outlined by Robbins et al. (1991) are provided in Appendixes A, B, and C, respectively.

TABLE 3–14.
Anatomical Boundaries for Cervical Lymph Node Regions
Associated with Radical Neck Dissection.

Level I: The Submental and Submandibular Groups

Submental Group
Lymph nodes within the triangular boundary of the anterior belly of the digastric muscles and the hyoid bone.

Submandibular Group
Lymph nodes within the boundaries of the anterior and posterior bellies of the digastric muscle and the body of the mandible. The submandibular gland is included in the specimen when the lymph nodes within this triangle are removed.

Level II: Upper Jugular Group

Lymph nodes located around the upper third of the internal jugular vein and adjacent spinal accessory nerve extending from the level of the carotid bifurcation (surgical landmark) or hyoid bone (clinical landmark) to the skull base. The posterior boundary is the posterior border of the sternocleidomastoid muscle and the anterior boundary is the lateral border of the sternohyoid muscle.

Level III: Middle Jugular Group

Lymph nodes located around the middle third of the internal jugular vein extending from the carotid bifurcation superiorly to the omohyoid muscle (surgical landmark), or cricothyroid notch (clinical landmark) inferiorly. The posterior boundary is the posterior border of the sternocleidomastoid muscle, and the anterior boundary is the lateral border of the sternohyoid muscle.

Level IV: Lower Jugular Group

Lymph nodes located around the lower third of the internal jugular vein extending from the omohyoid muscle superiorly to the clavicle inferiorly. The posterior boundary is the posterior border of the sternocleidomastoid muscle, and the anterior boundary is the lateral border of the sternohyoid muscle.

Level V: Posterior Triangle Group

This group comprises predominantly the lymph nodes located along the lower half of the spinal accessory nerve and the transverse cervical artery. The supraclavicular nodes are also included in this group. The posterior boundary is the anterior border of the trapezius muscle, the anterior boundary is the posterior border of the sternocleidomastoid muscle, and the inferior boundary is the clavicle.

Level VI: Anterior Compartment Group

This group comprises lymph nodes surrounding the midline visceral structures of the neck extending from the level of the hyoid bone superiorly to the suprasternal notch inferiorly. On each side, the lateral boundary is the medial boarder of the carotid sheath. Located within this compartment are the perithyroidal lymph nodes, paratracheal lymph nodes, lymph nodes along the recurrent laryngeal nerves, and precricoid lymph nodes.

Source: From Robbins, et al., (1991), Standardizing neck dissection terminology, *Archives of Otolaryngology Head and Neck Surgery, 117,* 601–605; copyright 1991, American Medical Association, reprinted with permission.

Radiation Therapy

The use of radiation therapy for laryngeal cancer is well documented (Keane & Cummings, 1986). Radiation therapy is the treatment of choice with specific types of laryngeal malignancies, particularly early glottic cancer (Silver, 1981). If a glottic tumor meets specific criteria, radiation therapy may be equally as successful as surgery via a cordectomy (Chung & Sagerman, 1989; Hinton & Myers, 1991; Kirchner, 1975; Silver, 1981; Wang, 1983). Neel et al. (1980) have presented outcome data on 182 patients with well-defined cancers confined to the vocal fold and suggest that a 95% success rate may be observed. As a tumor increases in gross size, radiation may become less effective (Chung & Sagerman, 1989). When success rates between radiation therapy and surgery (hemilaryngectomy) were compared for T2 lesions, Kirchner and Owen (1977) reported that surgery resulted in a cure rate (71%) that was doubled from that of radiation therapy. The application of radiation treatment for early carcinomas of the larynx also offers the opportunity for the patient to retain phonatory function with minimal alteration. Although voice changes following radiation treatment may occur due to shrinkage of the tumor and/or radiation-induced tissue edema (Miller, Harrison, Solomon, & Sessions, 1990), it is agreed that overall changes in voice quality following radiotherapy are not typically substantial (Beckett, 1969; Karim et al., 1983; Murry, Bone, & Von Essen, 1974; Stoicheff, 1975; Stoicheff, Ciampi, Passi, & Fredrickson, 1983).

Use or radiation in recent years has been increasingly apparent, particularly in cases where a conservation procedure was employed. Nevertheless, considerable discussion exists in the literature on the use of radiation treatment for carcinoma of the larynx (Chung & Sagerman, 1989). The overall response of a tumor to direct radiation treatment may be determined by characteristics of the tumor proper (cell type, differentiation, etc.) and/or "immunosuppressive" characteristics of the host (Batsakis, 1979; Nordman, Joensuu, Kellokumpu-Lehtinen, Minn, & Mantyla, 1990). Although such issues are beyond the scope of this discussion, it is important to acknowledge that the success of radiation therapy cannot be viewed in a discrete, direct response context. Rather, numerous factors, many of which likely remain unidentified, may influence the response of a given tumor to radiation and determination of whether local malignancy has been successfully eradicated from the host.

In cases of squamous cell carcinoma confined to a single true vocal fold (i.e., no extension beyond the membranous portion of the fold), radiation therapy as a primary modality has been suggested to have comparable results to that of surgery alone (Bailey, 1985a; Hinton & Myers, 1991; Silver, 1981). Though controversial, tumors in the region of the anterior commissure, sometimes referred to as "horseshoe" tumors, also may be treatable using radiation (Kirchner, 1970; Som & Silver, 1968). Lesions that potentially extend to the cartilaginous part of the glottis, cross the anterior commissure, or threaten the subglottal region, will typically require combined treatment approaches (surgery and radiation) (Chung & Sagerman, 1989).

Bailey (1985a) has suggested that the occurrence of second primary tumors are observed twice as frequently in individuals who receive radiation treatment for glottic carcinoma. These secondary primary tumors may occur earlier in this group of patients. Where a recurrence of glottic carcinoma is observed in individuals who have received primary radiation therapy, use of vertical partial laryngectomy may be highly successful in selected populations of patients (Wagenfield & Bryce, 1979). *Salvage* surgery (total laryngectomy) in attempts to control the recurrent cancer may also be pursued (Hinton & Myers, 1991; Myers & Ogura, 1979).

The recurrent (secondary) tumor has to display six specific clinical criteria for the surgeon to consider vertical partial laryngectomy. These tumor-based criteria are (1) the recurrent tumor must be confined to a single vocal fold, though it may involve the anterior commissure; (2) the arytenoid cartilage must be tumor free; (3) if subglottal extension is noted, it cannot exceed 5 mm; (4) tumor invasion cannot involve cartilage of larynx; (5) no vocal cord fixation (i.e., fold must remain mobile); and (6) the location of the recurrent tumor must "correlate closely" with the primary tumor (Biller et al., 1971; Campbell & Goepfert, 1989). Berger et al. (1985) have used "moderate" doses of radiation treatment in the management of T1 glottic lesions and have outlined several advantages. These advantages are summarized in Table 3–15.

Role of Radiotherapy

Radiation has also been employed postoperatively to control occult disease and may be used in combination with surgery including neck dissection. The use of postoperative radiation may be recommended with several goals in mind. As a comprehensive treatment program for management of head and neck cancer in general, radiation has been shown to offer excellent results (Hinton & Myers, 1991). The use of radiotherapy in the comprehensive management of laryngeal cancer may take many forms (Myers, 1991b; Silver, 1981). For example, radiation may be used as a primary treatment modality or it may be used before or following surgery for removal of the tumor. Radiation may also be used in cases where information suggests that the neck is clinically negative (i.e., free of disease) (Batsakis, 1979). Although the literature related to laryngeal cancer in general has shown the efficacy of radiotherapy for early glottic tumors,

the use of radiation therapy as a primary method of treatment for more advanced tumors is less specific (Nordman et al., 1990). That is, concerns about the usefulness of radiation therapy as a primary treatment modality have been raised. As the duration and dosage levels of radiation increase, the chance that complications may arise in secondary interventions should the malignancy recur are increased substantially (Berger et al., 1985; Mintz, Gullane, Thomson, & Ruby, 1981).

Prophylactic Versus Adjunctive Radiotherapy

DeSanto et al. (1982) have identified two classes of radiation treatment, *prophylactic* and as an *adjunct to neck dissection*. The rationale underlying radiotherapy as a prophylactic treatment emanates from a belief that microscopic metastatic cells that exist in the lymphatics of the neck may not always be detected via clinical evaluation (Batsakis, 1979). Thus, lymph nodes within the neck may "harbor metastatic foci" (DeSanto et al., 1982, p. 502) that may not be detected clinically (e.g., palpation of cervical chains). In fact, DeSanto et al. noted that about one-third of "clinically negative" necks were found, on later examination using histopathological methods, to have signs of metastatic spread. It is believed that if the primary tumor is radiosensitive and responds favorably to radiation therapy, any occult cells

TABLE 3–15.
Advantages of Moderate Doses of Radiation Therapy as Primary Management Modality in Early Glottic Carcinoma in Comparison to Traditional Dosage Levels.

1. Malignancy is controlled in majority of patients.
2. Larynx is retained with concomitant "natural" voice.
3. Complications of radiotherapy (tissue necrosis) is reduced.
4. Identification of recurrent tumors may be enhanced because of reduced tissue edema.
5. Increased success of secondary "salvage" surgery in those individuals who exhibit recurrent disease.
6. Frequency of severe postsurgical complications is not increased.

Source: Adapted from Berger et al., 1985, Failure analysis of T1 glottic carcinoma treated with radical radiotherapy for cure with surgery in reserve (pp. 195–199), in P.B. Chretien, M.E. Johns, D.P. Shedd, E.W. Strong, & P.H. Ward (Eds), *Head and neck cancer*, Philadelphia: B.C. Decker.

disseminated into the lymphatic channels will also be eliminated.

Rabuzzi, Chung, and Sagerman (1980) provided data on the use of prophylactic neck irradiation in patients with a variety of head and neck cancers (oral, oropharyngeal, hypopharyngeal, and laryngeal) and reported use of radiation in prophylactic form for subclinical (i.e., N0) necks resulted in low rates of lymph node metastases. While they identified 18 (13%) of all patients ($n = 139$) studied as "failed" radiation cases, Rabuzzi et al. stated that about 85% (13 of 18) demonstrated recurrent and persistent disease. They believed that these patients demonstrated metastatic spread as a result of incomplete control of the primary cancer. Thus, only 5 of 126 patients were classified as "pure failures" following prophylactic neck irradiation.

The second type of radiation treatment may be utilized as a primary therapy modality or in combination with neck dissection. This type of radiation use is appropriate in cases where involvement of the cervical lymphatics is confirmed. In an adjunctive role, radiation therapy is used to eliminate metastatic cells so that the chance of their release during neck dissection is reduced (DeSanto et al., 1982). In cases where radiation precedes surgical resection there exists a higher incidence of delayed wound healing, sloughing, and the potential for carotid artery erosion and the development of pharyngeal fistulae. In contrast, use of radiotherapy in a postoperative capacity seeks to eliminate any disease existing in areas peripheral to surgical resection (DeSanto et al., 1982). Thus, postoperative radiation attempts to destroy remnants of the primary malignancy and those cells that may be dispersed into lymphatic channels.

The use of radiation for the prophylactic management of suspected neck disease associated with laryngeal cancer has also been a controversial area of inquiry. This controversy centers around whether occult disease is present. Although there has been some suggestion that the physical examination of the neck may be inefficient (< 40% correct detection) in the detection of cervical nodal disease (DeSanto et al., 1982; Rabuzzi et al., 1980), data have also shown that a physical examination performed by an experienced clinician may exhibit similar levels of sensitivity to that obtained with CT scanning (Feinmesser, Freeman, Noyek, & Birt, 1987; McWilliams, 1991). Despite these differences, considerable interest exists regarding what is the best method of addressing potential neck disease. However, whether prophylactic radiotherapy and/or neck dissection provides the most attractive method of treatment is still unresolved.

Given that application of radiation may take several forms in relation to when it is provided to the individual (preoperatively, postoperatively), specific advantages and disadvantages may be found with each. Perez and Marks (1985) have provided an excellent review of the literature related to radiotherapy in the treatment of laryngeal cancer and have outlined the relative advantages and disadvantages, a summary of which is provided in Table 3–16.

Complications of Radiation Therapy

The potential for complications during or subsequent to radiotherapy may be observed for treatments used on either a prophylactic basis or in association with radiation as primary treatment modality for specific types of laryngeal carcinoma. Complications associated with radiation as an independent therapy modality are limited, but complications may become more prevalent in cases where combined treatments are employed. That is, complications are more likely to be observed in patients who undergo surgery and receive radiotherapy regardless of whether the radiation is provided pre- or postoperatively (DeSanto et al., 1982; Perez & Marks, 1985). Complications following surgical

TABLE 3–16.
Advantages and Disadvantages of Pre- and Postoperative Radiotherapy.

Preoperative Advantages
1. "Inactivation" of tumor cells disseminated as a result of surgical resection.
2. Improved vascularization and oxygenization.

Preoperative Disadvantages
1. Tumor shrinkage may result in inadequate margins associated with the surgical resection.
2. Potential complications related to tissue healing.

Postoperative Advantages
1. No "distortion" of surgical field.
2. Size and extent of tumor can be accurately assessed at time of surgery.
3. No complications in tissue healing.

Postoperative Disadvantages
1. Oxygenization of cells may compromised because of fibrosis or disrupted vascularization as a consequence of surgery.

Source: From Perez, C.A., & Marks, J.E. (1985), Radiation therapy for carcinoma of the larynx (pp. 417–433), in B.J. Bailey and H.F. Biller (Eds.), *Surgery of the larynx,* Philadelphia: W.B. Saunders, reprinted with permission.

salvage include infection, tissue necrosis (particularly in relation to reconstructed flaps), fistula, and pulmonary problems (Bailey, 1985a; DeSanto et al., 1982). Other problems include abscess, granulation tissue, and cartilage necrosis (Kirchner, 1970).

When radiation is used for prophylactic purposes to "sterilize" the neck, thus reducing the chance of occult metastatic spread, several common complications or side effects may be noted. Specifically, generalized irritation of the skin may be reported by the patient. Tissue fibrosis may also be observed in various degrees of severity. Skin irritation may be a temporary problem, but tissue fibrosis is likely to be permanent with greater degrees of fibrosis observed with larger doses of radiation. Tissue fibrosis may be a complicating factor in speech rehabilitation, particularly in patients who undergo total laryngectomy and wish to use a transcervical artificial larynx.

Chemotherapy

The use of chemotherapeutic agents for management of head and neck cancers is found most frequently in patients who demonstrate advanced malignancies (UICC, 1987; White, 1991). However, application of chemotherapy for laryngeal cancer is noted less often than that associated with other sites. This is due to the general effectiveness of surgical and radiotherapy either alone or in a combined treatment protocol. Additionally, coexisting illnesses or problems must be carefully assessed by the physician as toxicity associated with chemotherapy may pose significant contraindications (Goodman, 1989). Thus, application of chemotherapy may serve a palliative role in cancer management (Myers, 1991b; White, 1991).

In patients with advanced disease who receive chemotherapy, the speech-language pathologist should strive to provide the most functional method of communication possible. Should verbal communication not be an option, augmentative or alternative approaches should be considered. In such cases, an organized and timely approach to treatment should be emphasized so that the patient is provided with functional communication. This is particularly important in patients who are in the terminal stages of the disease process.

Summary

This chapter has addressed a variety of topics related to the diagnosis and treatment of laryngeal cancer. Information reviewed has focused on aspects of both conservative and radical approaches to treatment. A particular emphasis has been placed on the presentation of specific methods of surgical intervention. Factors associated with biological characteristics of a tumor, its size, and level of extension influence not only options for treatment but long-term prognosis. The specific advantages and disadvantages of distinct types of conservative partial laryngectomy procedures as dictated by features of tumor growth and spread have been presented. This includes laryngofissure and cordectomy, antero-frontal partial (anterior commissure technique), extended fronto-lateral, and horizontal supraglottic laryngectomy. The application of total laryngectomy has also been reviewed. This information provides the speech-language pathologist with an enhanced appreciation of residual anatomical structure and postsurgical functional vocal capacity. Consequently, speech-voice intervention can be structured in accordance with these limitations.

APPENDIX A.
Neck Dissection Classification.

Radical Neck Dissection

Includes:
1. Removal of all ipsilateral cervical lymph node groups extending from the mandible to the clavicle, and from the lateral border of the sternohyoid muscle, hyoid bone, and contralateral anterior belly of the digastric muscle, to the anterior border of the trapezius muscle posteriorly.
2. All lymphatic nodes outlined in levels I through V (see Table 3–14).
3. The spinal accessory nerve (cranial nerve XI), the internal jugular vein, and the sternocleidomastoid muscle.

Excludes:
1. Suboccipital nodes
2. Periparotid nodes except for infraparotic nodes in the posterior region of the submandibular triangle
3. Buccal, retropharyngeal, and paratracheal nodes

Source: From Robbins et al., (1991), Standardizing neck dissection terminology, *Archives of Otolaryngology Head and Neck Surgery, 117,* 601–605; copyright 1991, American Medical Association, reprinted with permission.

APPENDIX B.
Definition of Modified Radical Neck Dissection.

Definition
The modified radical neck dissection involves surgical excision of all lymph nodes routinely removed during radical neck dissection with the preservation of one or more nonlymphatic structures such as the spinal accessory nerve, internal jugular vein, and sternocleidomastoid muscle. Recommended that structures preserved should be identified, for example "modified radical neck dissection with preservation of the spinal accessory nerve."

Source: From Robbins et al., (1991), Standardizing neck dissection terminology, *Archives of Otolaryngology Head and Neck Surgery, 117,* 601–605; copyright American Medical Association, reprinted with permission.

APPENDIX C.
Definition of Selective Neck Dissection and Classification Subgroupings of Neck Dissection.

Definition: Selective Neck Dissection

Selective neck dissection defines any type of cervical lymphadenectomy where there is surgical preservation of one or more lymphatic node groups typically removed in a radical neck dissection. Four distinct subtypes of selective neck dissections are outlined: supraomohyoid neck dissection, posterolateral neck dissection, lateral neck dissection, and anterior neck dissection.

Definition: Supraomohyoid Neck Dissection

Involves removal of lymph nodes within the submental and submandibular triangles (Level I), the upper jugular lymph nodes (level II), and the midjugular lymph nodes (level III). The posterior boundary of the dissection is marked by the cutaneous branches of the cervical plexus, and the posterior border of the sternocleidomastoid muscle. The inferior limit is the superior belly of the omohyoid muscle where it crosses the internal jugular vein.

Definition: Posterolateral Neck Dissection

Involves removal of the suboccipital lymph nodes, retroauricular lymph nodes, upper jugular lymph nodes (level II), middle jugular lymph nodes (level III), lower jugular lymph nodes (level IV), and the nodes within the posterior triangle of the neck (level V). It should be noted that this procedure is typically used in association with cutaneous melanoma of the posterior scalp and neck.

Definition: Lateral Neck Dissection

Involves removal of the upper jugular lymph nodes (level II), middle jugular lymph nodes (level III), and lower jugular lymph nodes (level IV). These lymphatics lie in the lateral aspect of the neck in relation to the posterior triangle and submandibular triangle, and the median (anterior) compartment.

Definition: Anterior Compartment Neck Dissection

Removal of lymph nodes surrounding the visceral structures of the anterior neck. Lymphatics include pretracheal, paratracheal, perithyroidal, and precricoid (level VI) nodes. The superior border of dissection is the hyoid bone, the inferior border is the suprasternal notch, the lateral borders being the common carotid arteries. Note: lymphadenopathy and dissection within the anterior compartment is typically associated with thyroid cancer.

Source: From Robbins et al., (1991), Standardizing neck dissection terminology, *Archives of Otolaryngology Head and Neck Surgery, 117,* 601–605; copyright 1991, American Medical Association, reprinted with permission.

Management of the Patient with Laryngeal Cancer: The Role of the Speech-Language Pathologist

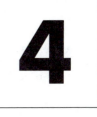

CHAPTER

> They do indeed have cancer, with no choice but to face up to it and have done whatever can be done. They, and their families and friends, are frightened by this disease as by no other, and they come to their rooms fearing pain and death, in need of all the reassurance they can find. (Thomas, 1983, p. 198)

Based on information presented in the previous chapters of this text, it should be clear that the diagnosis and subsequent surgical treatment of laryngeal cancer results in significant alterations in laryngeal anatomy. This change in "form" also results in changes in the functional integrity of the laryngeal mechanism. The purpose of this chapter is to place postoperative consequences of treatment for laryngeal cancer in the context of the relationship between the patient and the speech-language pathologist. This requires that the speech-language pathologist serves the patient in a number of ways. Thus, the focus herein is directed toward several essential services that the speech-language pathologist must offer to the patient.

The roles presented herein are believed to be generic to the clinical process rather than those specific details related to pre- and postoperative counseling; such details will be addressed more comprehensively in later chapters. If the responsibili-

ties outlined in this chapter can be met successfully, the potential for successful rehabilitation is believed to be enhanced. Additionally, the speech-language pathologist must be aware of numerous fallacies that have existed for many years regarding laryngectomy and those who undergo this procedure. Through such understanding a more comprehensive vision of the disease, its treatment, and the rehabilitative journey that the patient will embark on may be appreciated.

The Diagnosis of Cancer and Its Impact on the Patient

Although these changes differ substantially depending on the extent of surgical resection (Hinton & Myers, 1991; Silver, 1981), the effects must be evaluated on an individual patient basis. All individuals who receive a particular type of treatment (e.g., hemilaryngectomy) are not necessarily left with the same residual anatomy or postoperative function. The patient's psychological "being" (Diedrich & Youngstrom, 1966; Shanks, 1986a) must also be considered as an important variable relative to how he or she will adapt to these changes (Dropkin, 1989; Dropkin & Scott, 1983; Gilmore, 1986). Postsurgical changes also have direct implications to the patient and members of his or her family regardless of whether partial or total laryngectomy was performed. However, these concerns are often more significant when total laryngectomy is performed.

In the case of malignant disease the typical interval that has elapsed from the time of diagnosis to that of treatment is quite short. Therefore, the patient frequently must attempt to cope with varied issues over a very brief period. This includes the acknowledgment of cancer, as well as the often dramatic physical consequences of treatment (Dropkin, 1989). In those instances where surgery is undertaken, these consequences must be confronted by the patient in an overnight fashion. The extent of adaptability is certainly influenced by the extent of treatment. For example, total laryngectomy is generally accompanied by greater "shock" than is hemilaryngectomy because of the more obvious disfigurement associated with the former. These changes, however, can be quite debilitating to all patients regardless of how extensive or radical the surgical treatment.

Confronting the Diagnosis

As with any diagnosis of cancer, the patient may enter what has been best described by patients' themselves as a "shutoff" mode. This is true at least to some degree in all patients who are diagnosed with laryngeal cancer. Many patients frequently have reported that once

they heard the physician utter the word "cancer," their ability to comprehend additional information that was provided to them at this time was greatly reduced if not limited entirely (Reed, 1983a). This inability to comprehend such information may be most pronounced if it is provided in close temporal proximity to that of the medical diagnosis (Reed, 1983a). This inability may also be shared by a spouse or loved one who is present at the time the diagnosis; he or she too may miss important details that are presented.

Denial is not uncommon at the time of diagnosis, and it may persist for many months postoperatively (Gates, Ryan, & Lauder, 1982). Care must be taken by all professionals who serve this population to ensure that essential information is presented to and understood by the patient. In doing so, the clinician must acknowledge that the processing and understanding of new information by the individual who has received a diagnosis of cancer will at best be reduced. The speech-language pathologist must also realize that most of the information to be presented is likely to be "complex" for the patient. Few patients have even the most basic knowledge of how voice is produced, the relationship between the airway and the larynx, its relationship to the oral and pharyngeal cavities, and so forth. Thus, *clarity and redundancy* are essential components for the speech-language pathologist to be successful in providing basic information to the patient diagnosed with laryngeal cancer.

Anticipating the Worst and Adjusting to Change

When a health problem exists all individuals will exhibit various degrees of fear in the period leading up to the medical diagnosis. Those who wait for confirmation of a suspected malignancy must also prepare for the worst, knowing that treatment is likely to be aggressive. Once a malignancy is confirmed, the long-term impact of treatment for cancer of the larynx may place additional demands on the patient's ability to acknowledge, cope, and adjust to the problem. That is, any diagnosis of laryngeal cancer has the real potential of disrupting the individual's verbal communication at least to some degree. In those who require total laryngectomy, verbal communication will often be lost entirely at least during the first several weeks postoperatively. Effective verbal communication may be lost over an even longer period for others. In a majority of patients diagnosed with a malignancy in anatomical sites other than the vocal tract, their ability to verbally communicate will likely remain intact in the immediate postoperative period, as well as over the course of their disease should treatment fail. Having the ability to verbalize feelings of disbelief, sadness, frustration, anger, and so forth plays a critical role in confronting and addressing the problem and moving through the recovery and rehabilitation process. Unfortunately, those with laryngeal cancer may not be able to rely on this most basic capability. Therefore, the speech-language pathologist has the potential to offer an invaluable service to the patient, with responsibilities manifest in several specific forms.

The Primary Responsibilities of the Speech-Language Pathologist

The Provision, Interpretation, and Facilitation of Information to the Patient

The speech-language pathologist's role in serving patients with laryngeal cancer is in an idealized form quite multifaceted. Many of these facets may not be realized by the clinician as they frequently cross pre- and postoperative boundaries. The essence of this responsibility addresses three primary, although not necessarily mutually exclusive, areas of patient care. These areas might best be described as the *provision*, *interpretation*, and *facilitation* of information. Specifically, the speech-language pathologist should always play a primary role in the provision of information on what can be expected postoperatively from a voice, speech, and communicative perspective. This includes the provision of information on basic anatomical and physiological changes that may or will occur postoperatively. This function as a provider of information pertains to all patients with laryngeal cancer regardless of the treatment method(s) they undergo (e.g., radiotherapy, conservation surgery, total laryngectomy, or a combination of treatment modalities).

Unfortunately, at times the provision of basic information frequently may be glossed over or covered insufficiently (Blanchard, 1982). In fact, several reports in the literature have suggested that the provision of information in the pre- and postoperative period is insufficient in many cases (Hoops, Clarke, & Martin, 1975; Salmon, 1986a). It is essential, however, for the patient to understand the changes that will be encountered postoperatively, as well as *the reason* for these changes. Patients need not be presented with fine details at this time, yet they must have at least a cursory understanding of why changes will occur.

Although some speech-language pathologists might view this responsibility as a professional duty, it should also be viewed as a common courtesy which addresses the patient as a person. The provision of information in the preoperative period should lay the foundation for the presentation of more detailed information at a later time (i.e., postoperatively). This is particularly true in those who will undergo total laryngectomy. Providing the patient with essential information on the primary anatomical and physiological changes may well form the basis of his or her ability to cope with the increasing demands encountered postsurgically.

The second role that the speech-language pathologist offers to the patient is one of interpretation. That is, it is not uncommon for the patient to miss essential or "key" points that have been presented by others (e.g., the physician, etc.). The speech-language pathologist can, therefore, help to ensure that the patient has been presented with clear and concise information from a variety of sources. The speech-language pathologist must also ensure that misconceptions by the patient and/or members of the family do not exist (Duguay, 1966). In many cases information presented by other professionals is laced with complex notions and terminology. This will require that the speech-language pathologist serves in an *interpretive* capacity to "translate" for the patient. However, it *is not* the duty of the speech-language pathologist to provide information on issues related to medical diagnosis, prognosis, surgical options, and so forth (Reed, 1983a). The primary responsibilities that the speech-language pathologist accepts pertain to communication proper and those areas that relate directly to postsurgical alterations in anatomy and physiology (e.g., neck breathing, loss of smell and taste, etc.) (Diedrich & Youngstrom, 1966; Gardner, 1971; Murrills, 1983; Reed, 1983a; Salmon, 1986a, 1986c). Although others may indeed offer valuable information to the patient, issues related to communication are almost exclusively within the domain of the speech-language pathologist's area of expertise. It should, therefore, be clear that the best patient care evolves from the combined efforts of several disciplines and specialties and the ability of these professionals to successfully communicate with one another.

As noted, the act of interpreting information for the patient must be done in a conscientious manner. Although redundancy in the presentation of information is helpful to most patients, this redundancy should never overstep one's area of expertise. In instances where the patient requests further information on an area that lies outside of the speech-language pathologist's expertise (e.g., "What are the risks associated with my surgery?") or professional mandate, the clinician should simply explain that he or she is unable to answer because it is not within their domain. However, the speech-language pathologist *should assure the patient* that this concern will be brought to the physician's (or other appropriate professional) attention and, hopefully, this information will be provided. Reed (1983a) has very succinctly addressed this common clinical dilemma by stating:

> Very basic information outside the team member's formal area of training may be offered, but questions from the patient or spouse requiring a more technical answer should be referred to the appropriate team member. This policy will help prevent the patient from receiving contradictory information. (p. 112)

In this capacity, the speech-language pathologist is able to establish a presence as a facilitator for the patient. Good follow-up by the clinician involves checking with both parties involved (i.e., patient and health care professional) to confirm that the concern or question raised has been addressed clearly for the patient and/or members of the family.

Because of the potential for contact with the patient in the preoperative period, the speech-language pathologist may also serve in an "interpretive" capacity. That is, patients may ask questions which require some degree of interpretation or explanation. For example, the patient or family member may have heard the term "tracheostoma" used several times in relation to the surgery, yet may not understand what this term refers to or means. The patient might ask the speech-language pathologist for clarification. The speech-language pathologist's ability to interpret, however, should always be governed by good judgment. In this case the clinician would certainly be able to respond to the patient's inquiry. Good judgment should also be accompanied by the clinician's ability to be comfortable saying "I can't answer that" or "I don't know!"; good clinical care in these instances should always be followed by "But, I'll find out!" or an indication that the speech-language pathologist will arrange for the appropriate person to provide information requested.

Regardless of how many patients diagnosed with laryngeal cancer the speech-language pathologist works with, new concerns and questions will always come forth based on individual needs of that patient. Consequently, good judgment, clinical experience and acumen, and an interest in providing the highest quality care that is possible to the patient and his or her family, are never dictated by a single set of rules. Although many issues are of importance to all patients (e.g., airway alteration, etc.), many others will be quite individualized and must be dealt with in a straightforward and commonsense manner (e.g., continuation of a specific avocation such as woodworking). Again, the interpretive role provided by the speech-language pathologist also entails the requirement of seeking out and providing specific information when requested, or arranging for consultation between the patient and other professionals.

The final role that the speech-language pathologist serves is that of a facilitator. The speech-language pathologist must do what the patient cannot do in the early period following surgery. This does not imply that the clinician should establish a situation where dependency is encouraged, but rather one in which the speech-language pathologist and the patient and members of his or her family work together. The speech-language pathologist may in many cases be the patient's only active "advocate" during the early postoperative period when a truly viable method of communication is still limited. In some instances this may require the clinician to use sound intuition in determining if particular information, professional or personal contacts, as well as external support mechanisms are required. The importance of directly contacting the patient at the earliest time postoperatively is essential. Although other professionals will be actively involved with the patient during this period, it is very much medically oriented. Thus, contacting the patient offers the opportunity for personal contact that frequently is not attended to at this time.

In conclusion, the speech-language pathologist serves multiple roles in working with patients who will undergo surgery for laryngeal cancer. Because of the nature of the problem, multidisciplinary approaches are necessary to ensure the most comprehensive care possible. It is the responsibility of the speech-language pathologist to address those areas that impact communication. However, the speech-language pathologist also offers valuable service to the patient via his or her ability to provide, interpret, and facilitate the flow of information. If the patient can be adequately informed in both the pre- and postoperative periods, the patient's ability to cope may be significantly improved during rehabilitation.

Attitudes About Laryngectomy Revisited: A Need for Change

In 1982, Gates and colleagues (Gates, Ryan, Cantu, & Hearne, 1982; Gates, Ryan, Cooper, Lawlis, et al., 1982; Gates, Ryan, & Lauder, 1982; Ryan, Gates, Cantu, & Hearne, 1982) reported results from a comprehensive investigation that addressed a wide range of issues related to the "Current Status of Laryngectomee Rehabilitation." This investigation culminated in a series of four articles that focused on the results of therapy (Gates, Ryan, Cooper, Lawlis, et al., 1982), causes of failure (Gates, Ryan, Cantu, & Hearne, 1982), issues underlying intelligibility of esophageal speech (Ryan, Gates, Cantu, & Hearne, 1982), and finally, on attitudes about the rehabilitation of the individual who undergoes laryngectomy for laryngeal cancer (Gates, Ryan, & Lauder, 1982). Although considerable information was presented in this multiphase project, the information provided regarding attitudinal perspectives should become mandatory reading for all who are involved in the rehabilitation of individuals who undergo laryngectomy. According to Gates, Ryan, and Lauder (1982) attitudes in several areas may prove to have significant impact on the patient's overall rehabilitation following laryngectomy. Regarding attitudinal perspectives, Gates, Ryan, and Lauder (1982) indicated that the primary emphasis of their study sought to:

> discuss our perceptions of the problem by enumerating and discussing twelve postures or attitudes that, we believe, could have an adverse effect on rehabilitation (p. 97).

The influence of 12 specific attitudes that were presented and discussed by Gates, Ryan, and Lauder (1982) continue to have direct implications from which some of the information and philosophy presented in this text evolved. Although aspects of these 12 attitudes or beliefs have been noted in part by others over the years, Gates, Ryan, and Lauder (1982) articulated many issues that, depending on one's philosophy, may in reality underlie what transpires in the clinical domain. Should more open and perhaps more enlightened attitudes be developed by professionals who serve patients who undergo laryngectomy, it would seem that provision of better care would be a natural occurrence.

The attitudes summarized by Gates, Ryan, and Lauder (1982) are of importance

to clinicians because they specify many beliefs that are based on erroneous assumptions. No matter how well-meaning the original intention of such attitudes was, many of these attitudes can only exist as a negative influence on the individual's recovery and rehabilitation following laryngectomy. Although Gates, Ryan, and Lauder (1982) sought to carefully articulate these attitudes so that a change could be fostered, a decade has now passed, and many of these attitudes still prevail explicitly and implicitly in some circles. That is not to say that many who serve patients with laryngeal cancer have not considered the suggestions of Gates, Ryan, and Lauder (1982); they have. However, a continuation of such attitudes at times may be evidenced to occur in a rather unconscious manner. Consequently, the 12 attitudes presented by Gates, Ryan, and Lauder (1982) are worthy of brief presentation and discussion once again. Therefore, each of these "attitudes" as entitled and outlined by Gates et al. (1982d) will be summarized in the subsequent section of this chapter. By doing so, clinicians may be permitted an opportunity to assess their own clinical attitudes and philosophies toward the management of patients who have been laryngectomized.

Attitude One

The first attitude addressed by Gates, Ryan, and Lauder (1982) "Laryngectomy Homogenizes People" outlined difficulties encountered when those who undergo laryngectomy are classified as a group. Although these individuals do share one feature in common, that being that they were diagnosed with cancer of the larynx and underwent surgical treatment to remove the malignancy, they cannot be considered as a homogenous clinical population. As noted by Duguay (1979, p. 424) "each laryngectomized individual is just that—an individual." It was Gates and colleagues' belief that such an attitude "although rarely discussed" (Gates, Ryan, &

Lauder, 1982, p. 97) frequently enters into the clinical pursuit of rehabilitation. Gates, Ryan, and Lauder (1982) state:

> to deal with laryngectomees in a singular rather than in a flexible and individualized manner deprives the patient of the opportunity of having his needs addressed realistically (p. 97).

As such, each patient must be viewed as an individual, and clinical impressions should not be influenced by past experiences with other laryngectomized patients.

The frailty of this attitude is easily seen when the literature on those who undergo laryngectomy is reviewed. Data obtained in a variety of areas show that considerable variability exists across individuals who have been laryngectomized. This is true in those broad areas that encompass both physiological and psychological performance. Thus, clinicians must strive to separate the unique characteristics of each individual patient (Diedrich & Youngstrom, 1966; Duguay, 1979; Gardner, 1971; Shanks, 1979; Snidecor, 1978). Attempts to identify a common set of attributes to characterize patients is difficult if not entirely impossible. It is apparent from the literature that heterogeneity is a cardinal feature of laryngectomy. Therefore, a priori assumptions about laryngectomized individuals should be avoided in all cases. Clinicians should maintain their ability to observe and assess each patient as an individual. This will permit structuring of a rehabilitation program that conforms to the patient.

Attitude Two

This attitude incorrectly assumes that "The 1980s Laryngectomee is the Same as the 1960s Laryngectomee." Unfortunately, Gates, Ryan, and Lauder (1982) point out that while the basic surgical procedure for laryngectomy is essentially unchanged over the past several decades, the progno-

sis for these patients may have changed. Gates, Ryan, and Lauder (1982) note that given earlier diagnosis and the potential detection of smaller malignant lesions, many patients may now be considered for conservation laryngectomy procedures. This is indeed true in the 1990s. Yet they also point out that total laryngectomy may not be the treatment method of choice for larger and more advanced disease. In these cases, multimodality treatment protocols that involve radical surgery (total laryngectomy and neck dissection) and adjuvant therapy (radiation and perhaps chemotherapy) may be pursued (Batsakis, 1979; Becker, 1989; Silver, 1981; Taylor, 1979). Therefore, the laryngectomized individual of today may:

> have a poorer prognosis for cancer control, more treatment morbidity, and a less favorable outlook for recovery than was his 1960 counterpart (p. 98).

The application of such comprehensive multimodality treatment approaches also has implications on postlaryngectomy speech rehabilitation. In fact, Gates, Ryan, and Lauder (1982) state that today's (i.e., 1980s) laryngectomized patient may be less likely to acquire successful esophageal speech when compared to those who were laryngectomized several decades earlier. Unfortunately, insufficient data are currently available to either support or refute this suggestion. Thus, the speech-language pathologist must view and present postlaryngectomy rehabilitation options in a fair an unbiased manner; however, every patient may demonstrate unique characteristics that must be dealt with at the clinical management level. That is, clinical expectations based on data from the past may be wholly inappropriate. Similar to Attitude One, the ability of the clinician to avoid anticipating homogeneity is quite valuable.

The speech-language pathologist should also realize that since the time of the reports by Gates and colleagues (Gates, Ryan, Cantu, & Hearne, 1982; Gates, Ryan,

Cooper, Lawlis, et al., 1982; Gates, Ryan, & Lauder, 1982; Ryan, Gates, Cantu, & Hearne, 1982), a considerably increased interest has emerged in the area of conservation surgical procedures for laryngeal cancer (Biller, 1987; Ward, 1988). As a result, the possibility exists that speech-language pathologist will encounter a larger number of patients who have undergone "salvage" total laryngectomy. That is, those patients in whom a partial laryngectomy procedure has been unsuccessful are frequently treated through use of the more extensive laryngectomy procedure. These patients cannot, therefore, be considered the same as patients who received total laryngectomy as the initial form of surgical treatment. This is also true for patients who experience recurrent disease following radiotherapy (Viani, Stell, & Dalby, 1991). This suggests that treatment "subgroups" of total laryngectomized patients may be seen clinically. Although this may be "era-dependent" in may respects, it is also a function of philosophical approaches to treatment (Harrison, 1990), the surgeon, and the technique employed.

Attitude Three

The third attitude that "Passive-dependency is Characteristic of Laryngectomees" is an outgrowth of common stereotyping of those who are laryngectomized. The incorrect assumption of "homogeneity" expressed in Attitude One may correspond with this belief. The notion that all patients who undergo laryngectomy are helpless and highly depended is indeed ill-founded. Gates, Ryan, and Lauder (1982) acknowledge that some patients do exhibit a "passive-dependent personality", however, they also point out that all patients require time to comprehend and adjust to the crisis with which they are forced to address. All clinicians have worked with highly dependent patients at times, but the majority of patients cope with their shock, disbelief, and grief

in a relatively predictable fashion. The majority of patients are likely to be independent, motivated, and quite resourceful. Therefore, preconceived notions about levels of dependency which again attempt to homogenize the laryngectomized population may be unwarranted and will likely influence the clinical interaction.

This attitude may also be seen to affect the clinician-patient relationship. In fact, if an assumption is made that all patients are dependent, only two possible avenues of clinical interaction are likely to occur. If the clinician accepts the notion of dependency, he or she may respond by modifying the clinical "approach" to one that either plays directly into the patient's perceived (or anticipated) dependency, or one which effectively disengages the clinician from the patient in an attempt to foster independence. In the first instance, the clinician may accept greater levels of responsibility not only in the early period of treatment, but possibly into even the later stages of rehabilitation. This scenario has great potential to limit the patient's ultimate re-entry to the social milieu because he or she may not have been provided with the chance to problem-solve on-line in a more independent manner.

In the second situation, one which is perhaps most critical, a perception of dependency may be met with a response by the clinician of letting patients "fend for themselves." Although patients must be encouraged to assume larger levels of responsibility throughout the progression of the rehabilitation program, the timing of when this occurs is critical. It must be remembered that the patient and members of his or her family are now facing the reality of both the cancer as a disease and the consequences of its treatment. In many cases treatment may continue postoperatively in the form of radiation therapy. Thus, progression of therapy in general, and the patient's ability to *accept and cope* with the increasing demands associated with treatment and rehabilitation, must be viewed with an understanding that other demands coexist. Clinicians must, therefore, carefully consider the issue of independence in relation to both the level of responsibility desired and the timing of its introduction to the patients. The speech-language pathologist must be aware that dependency levels may wax and wane for many patients as they move through the recovery and rehabilitation process. This suggests that a logical and systematic framework for the introduction of a variety of tasks in which the clinician desires independence by the patient be followed; this framework, however, cannot be inflexible in that each patient will require a unique structure for facilitating independence.

Attitude Four

The attitude that "Rehabilitation Begins After Cancer Treatment is Completed" is one based on historical record. Although "rehabilitation" in a formal sense may not in many cases begin until after surgery, radiation, and so forth, it cannot be said that this is the *ideal time* for the process of rehabilitation to begin (Gates, Ryan, & Lauder, 1982). There would appear to be great value in beginning rehabilitation at some point immediately after diagnosis, *but prior to medical treatment.* Rehabilitation takes many forms; in the case of laryngeal cancer, information from a variety of sources (physicians, speech-language pathologist, nurses, etc.) prior to the initiation of medical therapy is the first step in the process of recovery and rehabilitation. In this early time of crisis (Shanks, 1979), information itself, provided that it is offered in a clear and accurate manner (Salmon, 1986c) may be viewed as a primary resource to the patient and members of his or her family.

Attitude Five

This attitude centers around the belief that "Preoperative Counseling by a Laryngec-

tomized Person is Essential for Effective Rehabilitation." Gates, Ryan, and Lauder (1982) state that, in general, a preoperative visitation by a laryngectomized individual may provide the patient with an opportunity to understand what is to take place and might then assist the long-term rehabilitation process. However, these authors also point out three reasons where a preoperative visitation may prove to be "counter-productive" to the rehabilitation process.

First, Gates, Ryan, and Lauder (1982) note that the fear and anxiety often experienced by patients in the preoperative period will often render them incapable of remembering "factual information" presented to them. Second, for some patients exposure to a laryngectomized individual may increase the level of distress and fear they exhibit. Thus, preoperative anxiety may be heightened in some patients. Third, Gates, Ryan, and Lauder stress that perceived differences between the patient and the laryngectomized visitor may be judged by the patient to be a result of surgery rather than one which has its foundation in differences between two individuals. Thus, Gates, Ryan, and Lauder suggest that the preoperative visit by a laryngectomized individual "should not be encouraged routinely" (p. 99). Similar to others (Murrills, 1983; Reed, 1983a; Salmon, 1986a, 1986c) they recommend that such visitations be arranged at the request of the patient. Based on potential shortcomings associated with a preoperative visitation by a laryngectomized individual, clinicians should be keenly aware of the potential consequences of such a visit, and therefore, be prepared to address problems should they arise.

Attitude Six

This attitude rests with the belief that "Rehabilitation is Only for the Patient." Thus, individuals who may provide a valuable resource to the patient (e.g., spouses and partners) may be excluded from all segments of the rehabilitation process (Blanchard, 1982; Duguay, 1966; Gardner, 1961, 1966; Gibbs & Achterberg-Lawlis, 1979). Such an attitude reflects a complete disregard for the comprehensive rehabilitation of the patient and a successful return to family and social roles. Gates, Ryan, and Lauder (1982) state that:

> While patient-oriented programs are a necessity, failure to work also with individuals important to the patient can adversely affect the success of the program (p. 99).

This statement is very true. It should be easy to see that successful rehabilitation following laryngectomy must at a minimum involve members of the patient's immediate family and quite possibly close friends (Square, 1986a). This attitude when coupled with Attitude Four as outlined by Gates, Ryan, and Lauder (1982) will have sufficiently detrimental effects on the patient's long-term outcome in rehabilitation. Without the support of loved ones, clinical management will likely become a more arduous process and the likelihood of addressing patient-specific needs in the rehabilitation program will be decreased. Exclusion of a patient's spouse or partner or family members may neglect their need to understand and adjust to the changes they will observe in the patient. To accept this attitude places the patient who will undergo laryngectomy "at-risk" for both a successful recovery and rehabilitation.

Attitude Seven

Historical bias plays an important role in this attitude which decries "Esophageal Speech is the Primary Goal of Postlaryngectomy Rehabilitation." One need only to assess the literature on esophageal speech success to find merit in disavowing such an attitude. Gates, Ryan, and Lauder along with many others across disciplines believe that esophageal speech provides an excellent form of alaryngeal communication (DiCarlo, Amster, & Herer, 1955; Diedrich & Youngstrom, 1966; Edelman, 1984; Snidecor, 1978). However, they acknowledge that overall success in acquiring esophageal speech may be less than ideal (Aronson, 1980; Schaefer & Johns, 1985). As a result, this myopic view of postlaryngectomy speech rehabilitation must be discarded.

Gates, Ryan, and Lauder's (1982) primary concern rests with the perception that if the patient is unable to successfully acquire esophageal speech, then the "rehabilitation effort" has failed. Such a belief is unfounded. When considered with other information outlined by these authors (see Attitude Two), it can be seen that data obtained in the past may not necessarily provide the most appropriate basis for comparison. If today's patients are indeed different from those of the past, the ability for patients to successfully acquire esophageal speech may be reduced commensurately.

Regarding the consequence of an attitude that posits esophageal speech as the sole measure of success in rehabilitation, one needs to look further into the effects of this attitude upon the patient. Gates, Ryan, and Lauder (1982) have acknowledge the potential impact of this attitude on the patient who is moving through the rehabilitation process by stating:

> those patients who are unable to acquire an esophageal voice or those whose esophageal speech is poor may be looked upon as "failures"—a potentially devastating psychologic circumstance (p. 100).

Therefore, Gates, Ryan, and Lauder (1982) recommend that the surgeon and the speech teacher (whether lay or professional) try to:

> disengage their personal anxieties from the patient's situation and focus their

efforts on the patient's needs rather than on their own desires for success (p. 100).

If esophageal speech is the only metric of success in laryngectomy rehabilitation, then the literature would suggest that speech-language pathologists have been unsuccessful in their clinical endeavors with this population over many years. Surely effectiveness of postsurgical speech rehabilitation should supersede considerations of mode (Diedrich & Youngstrom, 1966; Gates, Ryan, Cooper, Lawlis, et al., 1982; Gates, Ryan, & Lauder, 1982).

Attitude Eight

This attitude maintains that "The Artificial Larynx is a Crutch That Keeps Patients From Learning Esophageal Speech" and it has a long and continuing history in postlaryngectomy speech rehabilitation. It is perhaps the greatest fallacy among the 12 attitudes presented by Gates, Ryan, and Lauder (1982). There is no evidence to support the notion that esophageal speech cannot be obtained if artificial laryngeal speech is acquired (Duguay, 1978; Rothman, 1982). Although the concept of an artificial larynx as a "crutch" may persist in some venues, one should cast aside this simple semantic argument and focus on the goal of rehabilitation—namely, to provide the patient with a useful and serviceable method of postsurgical communication (Berry, 1978a, 1978b; Diedrich & Youngstrom, 1966; Reed, 1983a). Unfortunately, the belief that the artificial larynx is a "last resort" (Luboinski, Eschwege, & Stafford, 1989, p. 165) method of communication continues to be found in the contemporary literature. Gates, Ryan, and Lauder have summarized the danger in adopting such a negative attitude toward the artificial larynx by stating:

To deliberately keep a person voiceless (even if the voice is an electromechanical voice) has psychological consequences

for both patient and family that are potentially devastating (p. 100).

Thus, preventing a patient from using an artificial larynx is contrary to the goals of a successful rehabilitation program following total laryngectomy (Lauder, 1968, 1970; Salmon, 1978a, 1978b. In the case of a speech-language pathologist, it would also appear to be a clear breech of recommendations that guide ethical clinical practice. Adoption of such an attitude is unwarranted and not in keeping with responsibilities of the speech-language pathologist or others who provide care to patients with laryngeal cancer.

Attitude Nine

Gates, Ryan, and Lauder (1982) have identified Attitude Nine as "The Artificial Larynx is an Electromechanical Vibrator Developed by the Western Electric Company." This belief is based solely on inadequate information and is easily rectified. Gates, Ryan, and Lauder note that while not untrue, this view is incomplete. Several types of externally applied artificial laryngeal devices are commercially available for postlaryngectomy speech rehabilitation. However, other devices such as the intraoral artificial larynx also exist (see Chapter 11). As suggested by others (Duguay, 1978; Gates, Ryan, Cooper, Lawlis, et al., 1982; Keith & Shanks, 1986; Salmon & Goldstein, 1978) Gates, Ryan, and Lauder recommend that those who will work with patients on speech rehabilitation following laryngectomy should become acquainted with all commonly available artificial laryngeal devices. The relationship to acoustic and perceptual characteristics must also be understood by the clinician (Goldstein, 1978a, 1978b; Rothman, 1978; Weiss & Basili, 1985; Weiss, Yemi-Komshian, & Heinz, 1979). This will then permit application of the most appropriate device for any given patient. Finally, clinicians should also be aware of clinical modifications that may be used with artificial laryngeal devices (Blom, 1978; Lowry, 1981; Zwitman & Disinger, 1975).

Attitude Ten

The attitude that "Any Esophageal Speaker or Speech Pathologist Can Teach Esophageal Speech" is quite erroneous. Although both lay and professional teachers may excel at esophageal speech training, not everyone can teach esophageal speech (Duguay, 1980). Gates, Ryan, and Lauder (1982) state that the successful teacher of esophageal speech "requires a special skill that must be developed under intensive tutelage and polished by extensive experience" (p. 100). Thus, many speech-language pathologists may have little or no experience in this area of clinical practice. However, speech-language pathologists have the prerequisite knowledge in communication disorders and sciences that can facilitate the development of this additional clinical skill. Nevertheless, special skills must be developed and continually refined for those who teach alaryngeal communication.

Attitude Eleven

This attitude suggests that "Esophageal Speech Teachers are Good Psychologists"; unfortunately, this is not always the case (Rollin, 1987). Gates, Ryan, and Lauder (1982) indicate that while the "speech teacher" may demonstrate an ability to motivate and be supportive of the patient, and may also serve in the capacity of "alleviating the patient's postoperative depression," that psychological counseling efforts must fall to others who are specially trained. In many instances, the interpersonal interaction between the patient and clinician during the therapeutic process serves as valuable indirect method of providing guidance. However, many complex problems throughout the course of recovery and rehabilitation will be encountered by most patients. The speech-language pathologist, therefore, must ensure that appropriate resources who can provide necessary psychological services are made available to the patient. Yet Gates, Ryan, and Lauder (1982) were careful to note that "few psychologists have experience in the problems of laryngectomees" (p. 101). Consequently, they suggest that members of the laryngectomy rehabilitation team educate psychologists about laryngeal cancer and its postsurgical sequelae in an attempt to facilitate and provide appropriate counseling for these patients.

Attitude Twelve

The final attitude outlined by Gates, Ryan, and Lauder (1982) focused on the belief that "Surgeons Should Not Become Involved in Rehabilitation." This believe runs contrary to the needs of an effective program of rehabilitation (Bailey, 1985a; Diedrich & Youngstrom, 1966; Hoops, Clarke, & Martin, 1975; Johnson et al., 1979). It is also essential that the surgeon provide details regarding both the diagnosis and treatment of the disease as this is in his or her purview. This information cannot be presented by others on the rehabilitation team (Reed, 1983a). Involvement of the surgeon also must go beyond that of diagnosis and surgery according to Gates, Ryan, and Lauder (1982). They suggest that the surgeon may also play an "important supportive role" (p. 101) to the patient beyond the early postoperative period (Pearson, 1986). The essence of their role comes into play as a critical member of the *rehabilitation team*, and as such they are encouraged to actively participate with other professionals in the process. Again, combined, multidisciplinary efforts will increase the potential for successful long-term rehabilitation and re-entry into the patient's social milieu.

Summary

The purpose of this chapter has been to outline the role and responsibilities that the speech-language pathologist undertakes in the management of individuals with laryngeal cancer. Although unique responsibilities may exist for patients who undergo partial laryngectomy, and those who undergo total laryngectomy, a broad-based role and set of responsibilities is addressed. Namely, the speech-language pathologist may be seen as a source of mediation for the patient. That is, the speech-language pathologist may best serve the patient through the provision, interpretation, and facilitation of information and its clear communication to the patient. The speech-language pathologist, therefore, is seen to play a critical role in the patient's rehabilitation throughout both preoperative and postoperative periods. This role transcends numerous other capacities in which the speech-language pathologist may serve a primary role. It is apparent that the speech-language pathologist can play a significant role in ensuring that the patient has adequate information on what is to occur. If this goal is successfully accomplished, long-term rehabilitation is likely to be enhanced considerably.

Voice and Speech Treatment Following Partial Laryngectomy

CHAPTER

As presented in Chapter 3, surgical treatment for laryngeal cancer will always result in some degree of structural ablation. The degree of ablation and reconstruction may be considered to exist along of an anatomical continuum. Partial laryngectomy procedures such as the cordectomy may be viewed as quite limited relative to the more extensive "partial" procedures such as the near-total laryngectomy. Further, some surgical procedures may be "extended" based on the surgeon's judgment. In these instances, elimination of the tumor and maintenance of safe oncologic margins may involve removal of more tissue than that of the classic procedure described previously.

Although all surgical procedures for laryngeal cancer require the speech-language pathologist to have a good understanding of the general extent of resection and subsequent reconstruction, the post-surgical system always must be addressed on an individualized basis. The amount of tissue that is surgically removed does not always correlate well with the postsurgical speech and voice outcome. That is, what would appear to be rather minimal resections may result in substantial reductions in vocal capabilities and overall quality. In contrast, rather extensive resections may result in remarkably good postsurgical voice quality. However, it may be safe to say that the more extensive the surgical resection undertaken, the *greater the potential* for postsurgical alteration in the individual's voice (Berke, Gerratt, & Hanson, 1983; Rizer, Schechter, & Coleman, 1984).

It is believed that if limitations and reductions in postsurgical vocal capabilities are identified early in those who receive conservation laryngeal surgery, two specific avenues of clinical emphasis may be pursued. Specifically, the speech-language pathologist should seek to establish treatment goals that are directed toward (1) enhancing residual vocal capabilities and (2) striving to reduce and/or eliminate potential compensatory changes that may develop postoperatively. These goals are of particular importance for patients who undergo conservation laryngeal surgery. This is a result of the need for these individuals to adjust to postsurgical changes that exist in the upper airway. Additionally, in more extensive partial resections (i.e., near-total laryngectomy) the patient must also learn to coordinate voice production with new behaviors such as digitally closing the airway. Regardless of the extent of resection performed, therapeutic goals for those receiving conservation laryngectomy may evolve from procedures used with normal laryngeal speakers. That is, clinical methods that are used in patients who demonstrate voice disorders due to laryngeal pathophysiology may also have utility with those who have undergone surgical treatment for laryngeal cancer.

The purpose of this chapter is to provide an overview of general concerns that the speech-language pathologist must focus on during formal assessment, as well as those that may be addressed in subsequent treatment sessions. To provide a specific focus relative to the broad types of surgical procedures used, issues pertaining to each method will conform to several combined classes of procedures described earlier in Chapter 3. Consequently, (1) *cordectomy,* (2) *vertical partial laryngectomy procedures* (i.e., hemilaryngectomy), (3) *antero-frontal partial laryngectomy and extended fronto-lateral laryngectomy,* and (4) the more extensive *near-total laryngectomy* will be dealt with as a separate categories. Thus, these four clusterings of particular surgical procedures may enhance the general understanding of the types of voice limitations that result from the degree of resection and reconstruction and that may be anticipated in the postsurgical period.

Rehabilitation Following Conservation Laryngectomy

Cordectomy

The traditional application of surgical thyrotomy or laryngofissure with cordectomy (Bailey, 1985; Pressman, 1954; Silver, 1981) is currently encountered on a less frequent basis clinically. The contemporary treatment of choice for small, discrete tumors confined to the glottal margin is radiation therapy (Hinton & Myers, 1991; Myers, 1991b; Silver, 1981; UICC, 1987). The use of laser excision is also gaining popularity for treatment of early glottic cancers (Weisberger, 1991).

At the outset it is important to acknowledge that in a majority of patients voice changes related to cordectomy are often quite minimal. Despite resectioning of the membranous portion of a vocal fold many patients retain excellent vocal skills and voice quality. Occasionally, however, the speech-language clinician will be called on to work with an individual who has undergone a traditional cordectomy. This patient is most likely to be seen well past the time of surgery, perhaps well beyond the immediate postoperative period.

Although these patients are often informed that they will experience some degree of vocal change in the postoperative period, this issue often is not the most important concern they must confront. Further, they are typically informed that their voice will be altered due to the surgery they undergo, and obviously such a change is not unexpected. Hence, voice change is frequently a secondary complaint that may be brought to the physician's attention well beyond the early recovery period.

Referral to the speech-language pathologist for voice evaluation and possible treatment, however, may be based on the individual's complaint of voice change, physical discomfort during voice production, or both in the postoperative period. Given that a period of recovery from surgery is anticipated, early changes seldom draw the patient's or family member's attention. Yet a continuation in voice change that exists several months postoperatively may be perceived as more noticeable than during the early recovery period. It should be remembered that many patients who have early tumors identified are often quite sensitive to voice change; in fact, that may have been the primary complaint that initially prompted them to seek medical evaluation. If patients become "aware" of voice difficulties postsurgically they will likely bring it to the attention of their surgeon. Once the laryngologist rules out any potential recurrent disease, the referral to the speech-language pathologist may take place.

In individuals who undergo cordectomy and are referred many months postsurgery, the generic complaint centers around issues pertaining to changes in voice quality and effort. These issues must be assessed as independent parameters in such a situation. That is, voice quality is a multidimensional feature of voice that comprises global aspects of fundamental frequency (pitch) and intensity (loudness). Clear data on postoperative vocal performance are indeed quite sparse in the literature; therefore, there is not an adequate comparative database to assess the quantitative acoustic changes in voice. Effort, on the other hand, usually relates to the patient's perception that he or she is required to put substantial energy into attempts at voice and speech production. When increased effort is reported, it may be the result of the patient's attempt to overcome a rather closed postsurgical laryngeal valve or as a direct compensation to augment reductions in pitch, loudness, and overall vocal quality.

Treatment: Cordectomy

In patients who undergo cordectomy the speech-language pathologist can assume that at least some degree of change in all parameters of voice is likely. These changes may not be particularly conspicuous in the majority of patients, and hence, do not appear to interfere with verbal communication. In patients who experience more substantial alteration in voice, a comprehensive evaluation is required.

As with any other type of voice disorder, the clinician must sort out whether the patient's primary complaints are anatomically or physiologically based, or a combination of factors. Similar to the speaker with a more common hyperfunctional voice disorder, the "vicious circle" (Boone & McFarland, 1988) of voice disorders following conservation laryngectomy is just as likely to occur. Minor changes in the acoustic signal, such as decreased vocal intensity or a slightly aperiodic (noisy) voice, are not unusual to observe in those who undergo cordectomy. Changes of this nature may be judged to be a direct consequence of surgical ablation and may not be amenable to change via formal therapy. However, patients who, for example, are observed to have increased fundamental frequency, excessively aperiodic voices, or intermittent voice stoppage, and so forth may be experiencing problems that result from physiologic adjustment in the postoperative period. This will require that at least a brief period of therapy be initiated in an attempt to reduce these inappropriate behaviors. Hypofunctional behaviors are less often noted in those who undergo cordectomy; hence, tasks that focus on reducing specific behaviors are more commonly the focus of therapy with this population.

Following assessment which mirrors that of a typical laryngeal voice evaluation (Boone & McFarland, 1988) the speech-language pathologist should seek to identify which vocal behaviors have the greatest impact on voice production. That is, those changes that negatively affect voice quality should be targeted for immediate reduction. A "best voice" approach (Boone & McFarland, 1988) is an ideal approach to reducing negative behaviors. Tasks that are directed toward producing "easy" phonation are generally beneficial. Phonatory tasks that stress easy voice production may be merged with those that are best described as *extended length of utterance* (ELU) tasks.

The primary issue in merging these types of tasks is based on increased length of utterance being frequently incompatible with forced phonation. Controlling rate of speech through tasks that emphasize normal interphrase and sentence pausing also serves to break the patient's desire to push through the utterance. Thus, the essence of treatment for vocal alterations in patients who undergo cordectomy should focus on tasks that facilitate (1) smooth, easy phonation; (2) increasing length of utterance in conjunction with easy phonation; and (3) control of speech rate via phrasing tasks. Use of a variety of facilitation approaches used with other types of voice disorders may also be quite appropriate for particular behaviors. This includes the use of feedback, ear training, and respiration training (Boone & McFarland, 1988). Although not often employed with patients who undergo partial laryngectomy, explaining the problem to the patient may be quite beneficial in facilitating an understanding of the mechanical problem with which he or she must cope during verbal communication.

In patients who experience weak or insufficient voice production following cordectomy the clinician should seek to improve several behaviors. These patients will frequently complain of soft voices. Hypofunction associated with cordectomy is often characterized by a whispered voice. This may be a compensation for somatic discomfort experienced in the early postoperative period that has been maintained over time. Thus, therapy should be directed at increasing approximation of the laryngeal valve (i.e., vocal fold and/or related structures).

Although use of the pushing approach (Boone & McFarland, 1988) has been recommended, care should be exercised to ensure the patient does not overcompensate for a weak voice by forcing air through the postoperative larynx. Feedback via use of a Visi-Pitch[1] may prove particularly valuable in this situation. Specifically, use of a *percent voicing* measure obtained while in the frequency and intensity function of Visi-Pitch analysis routing can provide an index of nonturbulent (voiced) sound production. It is important to note that the goal in such a task *is not* 100% voicing, but rather a balance between voiced and unvoiced sound production. This will require that normative values be obtained on materials used by the clinician prior to initiation of this type of task. However, an extremely tight postsurgical laryngeal conduit may result in a higher percentage of voicing for some patients due to loss of abductory control. Noise from anatomical constriction and/or airway turbulence may also be present.

It should be acknowledged that the previously discussed goals and tasks may be equally applicable to cordectomy via laser surgery (Weisberger, 1991). Despite the method of tumor excision, the speech-language pathologist's goal is to identify problem behaviors whether they be of a hypo- or hyperfunctional nature. Once identified, tasks structured to either increase (hypofunctional) or decrease (hyperfunctional) behaviors can be implemented. Careful data collection is essential for determining treatment effectiveness. However, changes associated with nonsurgical approaches to treatment of early glottic lesions (i.e., radiotherapy) cannot be addressed in similar fashion due to the likelihood that radiation induced changes are likely to be permanent.

---

[1]Kay Elemetrics, Pine Brook, NJ.

Vertical Partial Laryngectomy

Information related to vocal function in individuals who have undergone vertical partial laryngectomy is characterized by substantial interspeaker variability (Blaugrund et al., 1984; Hirano, 1976; Hirano, Kurita, & Matsuoka, 1987; Mihashi, 1977). This category of conservation laryngeal surgery may vary from the true vertical procedure to more extensive vertical procedures that cross the anterior commissure (Silver, 1981). Thus, considerable variation is to be expected from this subgroup of patients.

Information on hemilaryngectomy has been presented by several research teams. Leeper, Heeneman, and Reynolds (1990) presented comprehensive data from seven adult males who received classical vertical hemilaryngectomy for early glottic cancer. Six were treated surgically following recurrence of the malignancy after an unsuccessful course of radiation therapy. All patients were at least 2 years post-

surgery at the time of evaluation which included videostroboscopy, aerodynamic, and acoustic assessment. Additionally, perceptual ratings of voice quality and severity were obtained. Overall, perceptual judgments indicated that voice quality was characterized by "rough, low-pitch, breathy, and constricted" voice quality. Stroboscopic evaluation revealed that five patients exhibited incomplete closure of the glottal area and concurrently demonstrated excessive supraglottal activity. Two patients exhibited either "irregular or narrow" constriction of the glottis and appeared to exhibit increased movement of the remaining vocal fold for contact with the reconstructed thyroid wall. In four patients, stroboscopy showed the vibrating edge of the remaining vocal fold to be "rough and irregular" although minimal reductions in amplitude of vibration relative to a normal vocal fold was noted.

Information presented in Table 5–1 shows frequency, intensity, and trans-glottal airflow data obtained from the seven

TABLE 5–1.
Vertical Hemilaryngectomy: Mean and Range Values for Fundamental Frequency (F$_0$), Intensity (I), Transglottal Airflow (TGA), and Duration Obtained During a Maximum Phonation Time (MPT) Task.

	Vowel Context		
	/i/	/a/	/u/
	F$_0$ (in Hz)		
M	191.3	168.2	206.9
Range	79.2–274	60–241.4	71.1–300
	I (in dBSPL)		
M	74.1	72.7	75.7
Range	67.8–86.7	66.1–83	67.3–84.3
	TGA (in cc/sec)		
M	204.8	201.0	210.5
Range	110–403	61.5–271	141.5–330
	MPT		
M	9.9	9.9	8.2
Range	4–19.5	3.8–15.2	3.5–14.1

Source: Adapted from Leeper et al. (1990), Vocal function following vertical hemilaryngectomy: A preliminary investigation, *Journal of Otolaryngology, 19,* 62–67. Reprinted with permission.

patients. The fundamental frequency values generated exceed the anticipated values for adult males of similar age (see Baken, 1987); however, intensity levels were generally within the normal range for age-equivalent speakers. Mean airflow values were found to be within the expected range for adult males, although these values are at the upper end of that range. Durational values obtained are substantially reduced on average from those reported for older males.

Thus, data presented by Leeper et al. (1990) suggest that although intensity and transglottal airflow rates do not differ substantially from those of individuals with normal laryngeal mechanisms, frequency and durational characteristics were generally increased and decreased from normal expectations, respectively. Supraglottic constriction (ventricular vocal folds and epiglottis) noted in five of the patients is consistent with a functional compensation for the loss of laryngeal tissue. This compensation is also believed to result in irregular, and perhaps nonsynchronous vibration of the remaining vocal fold and the supraglottic tissues. As such, the perceptual features that were observed, namely, "rough, breathy, and constricted" are consistent with these visual observations. However, the perception of low pitch as a characteristic feature in five of the seven subjects is inconsistent with the acoustic information gathered from a variety of tasks. This suggests that additional aspects of vibration may carry substantial weight for the listener in judging the voice quality in those who undergo vertical hemilaryngectomy.

Treatment: Vertical Partial Laryngectomy

Anatomical differences associated with vertical partial laryngectomy procedures are substantial. Consequently, voice differences associated with this form of conservation laryngeal surgery must be viewed as a function of two primary factors: (1) those related to the extent of laryngeal ablation, and (2) those related to the requisite reconstruction of the mechanism following removal of the tumor. Thus, a balance between tissue which is sacrificed and residual tissue that remains may vary considerably across patients. This fact alone contributes significantly to the range of vocal capabilities that are demonstrated by patients who receive this type of surgical treatment (Leeper et al., 1990; Leeper, Doyle, Heeneman, Martin, Hoesjoe, & Wong, 1993) and the perceptual judgments of postsurgical voice quality (Doyle, Leeper, Houghton, Heeneman, & Martin, 1992).

Because of this variability in postsurgical structural integrity vocal difficulties may be anatomical and/or physiologic in origin. However, changes observed and which prove problematic to patients are usually a function of both factors. Alteration in glottic sufficiency may play a key role in many compensatory behaviors. Specifically, a more open postsurgical glottis will result in a more breathy vocal quality as opposed to changes where the conduit exhibits improved anatomical approximation.

Although rough voices in those who receive vertical partial laryngectomy may not be judged as "normal" it may be preferable for many patients when compared to a breathy quality. This is particularly important to many adult males. As a result, voluntary adjustments by the patient may be observed to overcome a weak and breathy voice. Although this compensation may not be ideal from a variety of speech production perspectives, it may carry substantial social value to the patient.

Many patients who undergo vertical partial laryngectomy have the capacity to exhibit unique primary or secondary sources of laryngeal vibration. As noted, supraglottic activity may be quite common (Leeper et al., 1990). If possible, the speech-language pathologist should determine the "source" of vibration. This can be easily accomplished with nasoendoscopy and may provide a valuable feedback mechanism to the patient. Attempts at decreasing constriction of the laryngeal valve, particularly if supraglottal contributions are observed may be extremely valuable. However, if the remaining true vocal fold is incapable of achieving adequate glottal approximation with the reconstructed region, supraglottal activity may serve a valuable communicative purpose.

The contributions of supraglottal activity must be viewed in the context of finding the optimal degree of laryngeal approximation. Thus, similar goals to those discussed under cordectomy are appropriate in vertical partial laryngectomy. The extent of "normal" voice quality achieved will be highly individualized as a direct result of surgery. A therapeutic format that uses a continuum-based comparison for the patient to assess his or her own vocal quality during a sustained vowel production task may be useful. This involves working with the patient to determine the end points of his or her ability to reliably control glottal and/or supraglottal closure. Successful attempts will result in extremely turbulent voice at one end and excessively "squeezed" vibrational voice at the other. If the patient can achieve a reasonable range of performance he or she can identify (along with input from the speech-language pathologist) the best compromise in voice quality. This task can then be expanded to involve short phrase or sentence length materials that are comprised of all voiced components (vowels and voiced consonants). This will, hopefully, afford the patient an opportunity to mimic performance obtained in the more artificial sustained phonation task in one that is more realistic.

Finally, a clinical focus on easy voice production and controlling utterance length is frequently helpful to the patient. Regarding utterance length, the goal is to teach the patient to avoid speaking in excessively long utterances. This may limit the patient from exerting increased levels of laryngeal constriction in circumstances

of a decreasing pulmonary driving source. The goal is to train the patient to speak in shorter bursts, thereby producing voice and speech at more optimal levels of respiratory support. Such durational tasks may be facilitated through use of visual feedback (e.g., Visi-Pitch).

Antero-frontal and Extended Fronto-lateral Partial Laryngectomy

These procedures are much more extensive than resections that fall in the category of vertical partial laryngectomy. As a result, not only is the amount of tissue resected often increased, but concomitant reconstruction is required. The laryngeal mechanism is, therefore, altered considerably during these types of laryngectomy. Voice changes that are observed may be viewed to exist on the more extreme end of the abnormality continuum. Yet variability is once again considerable across patients. There are limited data on vocal performance capabilities in those who undergo this subtype of conservation surgery.

Reconstruction frequently involves procedures that may result in a rather tortuous postsurgical laryngeal conduit. While this is not always true, changes in the anatomical configuration of the lower vocal tract may exert considerable influences of voice production. Many of the procedures outlined previously for cordectomy and vertical partial laryngectomy are applicable in this subgroup of patients.

Treatment: Antero-frontal and Extended Fronto-lateral Partial Laryngectomy

One particular therapeutic focus in this group may seek to address voice production that is characterized by less vocal noise. A frequent complaint by this subgroup is that the level of voice abnormality may be more pronounced than other procedures described previously. Thus, clinical attempts to reduce the presence of attributes that impact negatively on the listener's judgment may be valuable goals in treatment.

Vocal noise is almost always found in association with increased pulmonary effort in patients who complain of voice difficulties. Attempts must then be made to reduce excessive respiratory effort; however, increased aerodynamic effort may be necessary to drive a tight or somewhat noncompliant postsurgical laryngeal source. In some patients, slight changes in head position may result in a decreased desire for the patient to "push" and subsequently result in reduced levels of vocal noise.

The clinician should also monitor the depth of inhalation prior to voice production. In patients with increased approximation of the reconstructed larynx, they may attempt to compensate by inspiring at greater levels. Thus, the larynx will be required to impede higher airflows via increased laryngeal constriction. Clinicians should then observe the relationship of vocal tract squeeze and respiratory support. Again, a balance must be found between the pulmonary support and the characteristics of the conduit in which it will be regulated. Finally, clinical efforts that seek to identify the best overall voice possible should always be the emphasis with patients who undergo these more extensive resections.

Near-Total Laryngectomy

Near-total or subtotal laryngectomy is an extensive resection of the laryngeal valve. Because of the rationale for the application of such procedures, considerable variability across patients is quite common with regard to reconstruction (DeSanto, Pearson, & Olsen, 1989; Pearson, 1981; Pearson, Woods, & Hartman, 1980). This observation (Pearson, 1981) is consistent with the acoustic and perceptual attributes that

characterize voice production in this population (Doyle et al., 1992; Leeper et al., 1993; Hoasjoe, et al, 1992; Keith & Pearson, 1987; Keith et al., 1988). Variability is evident across numerous vocal components and parameters. However, in contrast to the previously described categories of surgical treatment, near-total and subtotal laryngectomy require the clinician to focus on additional nonspeech features associated with voice and speech production. This includes the patient's ability to monitor closure of the tracheostoma to divert air through the reconstructed laryngeal conduit. As such, numerous nonspeech behaviors must be carefully observed and should problems be noted they should be targeted immediately.

Treatment: Near-Total Laryngectomy

Because of the need for patients who undergo near-total laryngectomy to volitionally close their airway for speech production, issues regarding their ability to obtain a good airway seal, as well as extraneous noise due to incomplete closure, and so forth are common concerns. Although initial sessions of treatment will focus on the generation of voice and its expansion, nonspeech behaviors must be closely monitored as they may prove to be negative to overall communication. Treatment in these patient is a twofold process. Prior to direct therapy, each patient should be informed about the structural changes that have occurred and what the impact is on the voice and speech production mechanism. Although this information has ideally been presented in the preoperative period, reiteration is recommended to ensure at least a cursory understanding of what has occurred.

The speech-language pathologist should then begin to direct the patient in how to effectively and completely seal the tracheostoma prior to exhalation for voicing purposes. Mirror work is invaluable for many patients. Aspects of digital pressure must also be addressed; specifically, the patient must be taught to avoid excessive pressure that may make voice production more effortful. Many procedures used for tracheoesophageal speech may be applicable in training this behavior. In cases of digital closure, care must be taken so that closure is always complete. Incomplete closure will result in air leaks that provide extraneous, competing, and often bothersome noise during communicative interactions. However, some patients may be successfully fitted with a tracheostoma breathing type valve that will eliminate the need for digital closure.

Due to a potential for increased levels of effort to produce voice, the clinician should be aware of the development of facial grimaces or unusual head postures. These behaviors may not be apparent to the patient who is attempting to adjust to rather significant anatomical changes. Patients may also exhibit relatively substantial degrees of muscular tension in the upper chest region, the neck, and the face during attempts at speech production. If these types of concerns can be acknowledged early in therapy, patients may be successful in reducing, if not entirely eliminating, their occurrence.

Although nonspeech behaviors must be addressed early in therapy, they can be merged with voice rehabilitation efforts. Unfortunately, many patients may exhibit sufficient levels of abnormality in their voice quality and many vocal behaviors may not be modified substantially. However, aggressive early efforts that emphasize the patient's ability in maintaining control and continuity of voice production, as well as efforts to refine overall aspects of voice quality, are essential. Fundamental frequency and maximum phonational frequency range have been shown to be extremely variable in near-total speakers

(Hoasjoe et al., 1992; Leeper et al., 1993). Vocal fundamental frequency may span over two octaves (Leeper et al., 1993). Acoustic and perceptual data from near-total speakers have shown that vocal control may vary from voice that is entirely turbulent in nature to that which is continually voiced (Doyle et al., 1992; Keith, Leeper, & Doyle, 1993; Leeper et al., 1992). Use of a "percent voicing" measure obtained from the Visi-Pitch may be used to monitor a given patient's control of voicing. During production of a sustained vowel a normal patient should exhibit 100% voicing; thus, a relative performance index may be gathered over the course of therapy. This procedure can also quantify intermittent stoppage of voice in a sustained vowel task through the measure termed "percent pause time."[2]

Because vocal behaviors must be coordinated with additional requirements (i.e., closure of the airway), progress may be somewhat slow. Eliminating negative behaviors before they emerge is absolutely essential in those who undergo near-total or subtotal laryngectomy. Further, many patients may struggle with their attempts in producing voice in the immediate postoperative period. Similar to the total laryngectomized patient who struggles to acquire esophageal speech, the near-total laryngectomized patient must be encouraged to relax and not become overly anxious during voicing attempts. These patients are now attempting to cope with a variety of anatomical and physiologic changes in addition to the reduction of loss of speech capabilities. Encouragement and support are, therefore, essential components of the clinical process.

In summary, therapeutic efforts with patients who receive near-total or subtotal laryngectomy must focus on both nonspeech and speech behaviors. Nonspeech efforts are usually directed at

---

[2]The reader is encouraged to consult the operations manual for the Visi-Pitch for a complete description of this particular analysis routine.

achieving complete airway closure and reducing extraneous noise and physical tension. Speech production goals should focus on eliminating compensatory behaviors before they become firmly established with a primary emphasis on seeking the most efficient and best voice possible.

Supraglottic Laryngectomy

Unfortunately, limited data on aspects of voice following supraglottic laryngectomy appear in the literature. This primarily is because, in its classic form, supraglottic laryngectomy does not generally interfere with function of the true vocal folds from a voice production point of view. Such information would be beneficial to determine if any substantial vocal change is evidenced following supraglottic laryngectomy. This type of surgical resection does disrupt the integrity of the laryngeal valve from a biological perspective. Hence, the most salient postsurgical concerns related to supraglottic laryngectomy pertain to aspiration. Maintaining a safe airway is paramount to the success of this procedure (Silver, 1981).

Treatment: Supraglottic Laryngectomy

As a result of changes in the valving capacity of the larynx following supraglottic laryngectomy and the associated possibility of aspiration, speech-language pathologists may often be called on to assess swallowing abilities in this group of patients. Although the clinician will clearly focus attention on the patient's performance in the domain of aspiration, he or she should also pay close attention to the patient's voice. Changes in voice quality should be monitored closely for signs of hypo- or hyperfunctional behavior. Some patient's may adopt a rather closed laryn-

geal posture, particularly in instances where aspiration has been experienced. This will result in changes that might be best described as strained, strangled, harsh. If such behaviors are observed, the clinician should bring this to the surgeon's attention. If a referral for formal voice evaluation is made, the speech-language pathologist should perform a standard voice evaluation. If problems are noted, they can often be managed directly through facilitating techniques common to other voice disorders. Excessive hyperfunctional behaviors may be viewed as almost entirely compensatory and can often be addressed through explanation and attempts to reduce squeezing of the lower vocal tract and effortful voice production. Again, many methods outlined for other conservation procedures may be appropriate for the reduction of such behaviors.

Summary

This chapter has addressed aspects of treatment for patients who undergo conservation laryngectomy. Generally, the more tissue resected the greater the chance that more significant changes in voice will be observed. However, considerable variability exists among each specific subtype of conservation laryngeal surgery. This requires that the speech-language pathologist accept the individualized performance patterns for each patient. Similar to intervention with other voice-disordered populations, the clinician should seek information on whether problems noted are primarily related to changes in anatomy, physiology, or a combination of the two. Dependent on whether changes observed are hypo- or hyperfunctional, treatment protocols can be developed to either increase or decrease glottic closure and concomitant changes in the acoustic signal. In many instances, clinicians must address reduction of compensatory behaviors that may prove to be detrimental to communication effectiveness.

Although a focus on issues specific to voice characterize treatment with many conservation laryngectomy procedures, those who undergo near-total or subtotal laryngectomy must also have nonspeech behaviors observed and monitored. The ultimate goal with all who receive conservation laryngectomy is to attempt to facilitate the best possible voice quality with the least amount of effort. Extraneous and negative nonspeech behaviors should be targeted at the earliest possible convenience to ensure the best overall communication.

The Preoperative Counseling Session: Issues and Answers

Counseling patients who have been diagnosed with laryngeal cancer, as well as family members is widely accepted as an essential responsibility of the speech-language pathologist. Counseling entails many facets for those working with the communicatively impaired (Rollin, 1987). Yet for the most part counseling by the speech-language pathologist primarily involves the simple act of providing information to the patient, or simply offering to listen to what the patient has to say. The importance of these two basic areas cannot be understated as they form the foundation from which the patient will embark on his or her course of postsurgical rehabilitation. The purpose of this chapter is to discuss these issues in detail and provide a foundation for preoperative counseling of patients and members of their family.

Challenges for the Speech-Language Pathologist

In spite of the very real challenge that speech-language pathologists confront when providing preoperative counseling to an individual with laryngeal cancer, this meeting will most likely provide the framework from which a strong, cooperative relationship will develop with a majority of patients. Few patients are truly uninterested in their plight.

It is what transpires in this initial meeting that ultimately sets the tone for the postoperative visitation and counseling, as well as that which may occur during the entire course of rehabilitation and long-term follow-up. This first meeting provides an opportunity for the patient to understand what the speech-language pathologist's role is in the rehabilitative process, in addition to receiving information on the potential loss of verbal communication and the anatomical and psychological changes they will encounter in the postoperative period. This information forms the basic elements of what the patient will need to know almost immediately.

Although it has seldom been identified as such, this initial meeting between the patient and the clinician may offer the first opportunity for addressing broadly defined psychological concerns of the patient. In fact, Diedrich and Youngstrom (1966, p. 125) have stated that "The psychological adjustments which the person sustains as a result of laryngectomy are not given adequate consideration." Issues related to potential psychological changes are not frequently noted in the literature except as afterthoughts. Additionally, some members of the rehabilitation team may be reluctant to address certain concerns that may have explicit psychological consequences (Berkowitz & Lucente, 1985). There is, however, an implied impression that psychological factors that may impact on the patient and his or her family occur in the later stages of the rehabilitation after treatment has already been provided and completed.

There is no question that the gravity of total laryngectomy is typically not realized by the patient until well after the primary treatment has been completed. Gates, Ryan, Cooper, Lawlis, et al. (1982) have reported that denial may be present in a large percentage of individuals who are laryngectomized, even at 6 months postsurgery. However, psychological changes most likely begin when the patient first hears the word "cancer"; this "trauma" may persist for the remainder of the patient's life. Thus, the speech-language pathologist may be provided with a golden opportunity to begin the true process of comprehensive rehabilitation at the time of preoperative counseling.

It is important to point out that "counseling" offered by the speech-language pathologist may not be conducted in the traditional sense of the word. The term counseling frequently carries with it a rather narrow interpretation, one which implies that the patient's psychological status is under some form of scrutiny by the clinician. However, counseling involves a wide spectrum of responsibilities and objectives. One of the most important aspects of counseling focuses on providing information in a prudent and *unbiased fashion*. Many clinicians are not necessarily comfortable or competent in addressing psychological issues that emerge from aspects of the disease process itself, the related disfigurement associated with some surgical treatment procedures, or the general consequences of treatment. Yet, the speech-language pathologist should understand the psychological impact of partial or total laryngectomy on the patient from a communication perspective. Rollin (1987) has stated:

By definition, the communicative interaction we have with our clients is the essence of what the field of communicative disorders is all about and at the core of the counseling process. (p. 24)

Simply stated, the interaction among the clinician, patient, and the patient's spouse or partner forms an intangible foundation for what will come in the months ahead. Loss of verbal communication may relegate the individual who undergoes total laryngectomy to a communicative purgatory that has a significant potential to affect the patient over the long term of the rehabilitative process. Preoperative counseling should, therefore, focus on the development of a clinical partnership and the presentation of basic information about anatomical and physiological changes postoperatively and specifically to changes in communication status in the immediate postoperative period.

What Constitutes Good Patient Counseling?

Unfortunately, essential elements of successful counseling in general, and for laryngeal cancer patients in particular, are frequently unknown or unrecognized by speech-language pathologists. Although speech-language pathologists have a variety of resources available on "what" information must be provided, the "unstated" elements of counseling may be the most critical factors to the rehabilitative relationship between the speech-language pathologist and the patient. This includes establishing credibility with patients so that they develop confidence in those professionals with whom they will work. This is particularly important for those confronting a life-threatening illness such as cancer.

Although providing information is primary in a majority of counseling endeavors, provision of information alone is insufficient. Consideration of issues related to how the information is presented may lead to more effective and more personalized counseling. The manner in which counseling is pursued will affect the patient's receptiveness to future information and assistance.

If these concerns become integral to the preoperative counseling process there is an increased likelihood that counseling will successfully meet objectives of any given session (e.g., preoperative or postoperative). This is a significant issue for the patient who will undergo total laryngectomy as the speech-language pathologist will often become the primary contact and liaison with other professionals.

Is Preoperative Counseling Necessary?

Even though disagreement exists among clinicians who serve patients with laryngeal cancer, differences of opinion are particularly evident across different disciplines (e.g., speech-language pathology, medicine, nursing, social work, etc.) relative to the manner in which counseling takes place (Reed, 1983a; Salmon, 1986a, 1986b). Regardless of such disagreement, counseling is acknowledged as a cornerstone to the rehabilitation process (Square, 1986a). Preoperative counseling is an essential component of a patient's recovery and rehabilitation. Despite widespread clinical acknowledgment of the importance of preoperative counseling, however, a void continues to be perceived if not fully experienced in this area by patients and members of their family (Gates, Ryan, Cantu, & Hearne, 1982; Gates, Ryan, & Lauder, 1982; Blanchard, 1982; Salmon, 1986a). This is disturbing in that one single professional source cannot possibly provide all the information that is necessary; thus, it might appear that the rehabilitation team is failing the patient.

At a minimum, it appears that all potential members of the team may share some portion of the responsibility for this void. Although the surgeon may adequately present information on cancer as a disease process, the types and extent of treatment options and the concomitant loss of speech postsurgically, and other areas such as those addressing important psychosocial issues (e.g., effect of surgery on family relationships) may be overlooked (Berkowitz & Lucente, 1985). Thus, a multidisciplinary approach is needed to meet the needs of the patient.

Responsibilities Associated with Patient Counseling

Because of the need for input from a variety of sources, a team approach to counseling is most effective. Therefore, it is important that specific responsibilities be defined for each member of the rehabilitation team. Ongoing communication between team members is essential to ensure that necessary information is provided to the patient. Defining roles and responsibilities does not need to be standard across settings. In smaller centers, certain team members may accept more responsibility in comparison to centers that have substantial professional resources. Nevertheless, all areas of importance to the patient cannot be adequately addressed by a single source.

In an effort to reduce the chance that inadequate preoperative preparation of the patient and spouse or partner occurs, discipline-specific issues must be addressed (i.e., medical, nursing, speech-language pathology, social services, etc.). Members of many different disciplines have the expertise and opportunity to provide much needed information to the patient and members of his or her family. This is critical following surgery. However, if essential issues are addressed in an organized and cohesive manner preoperatively, rehabilitation "roadblocks" will be eliminated before they emerge postoperatively.

Counseling the Patient and Family Members

Insufficient preparation in the preoperative period may not be exclusive to the patient (Berkowitz & Lucente, 1985; Blanchard, 1982; Duguay, 1966; Gilmore 1986; Salmon, 1986a). Preoperative counseling should generally include members of the patient's family in early and later periods of rehabilitation. Inclusion of family members at this difficult time is essential in that they form the foundation of the patient's support system during postsurgical convalescence and recovery. Similar to that noted directly for the patient, a void in preparation of the patient's family via counseling in the preoperative period may be sufficiently pronounced. If adequate

counseling is not provided to family members, the consequences for both the patient and his or her loved ones may provide a formidable obstacle in the postoperative period (Kommers & Sullivan, 1979).

Concerns of Significant Others

Most individuals would agree that "family" members (spouse, siblings, longtime companion, etc.) provide an invaluable source of strength in times of a crisis. Individuals in the patient's social network may also serve as a valuable support system. This is particularly evident in those who are diagnosed with cancer of the larynx. When one considers the rapid and dramatic changes resulting from laryngectomy, the importance of family becomes even more pronounced (Gonnella et al., 1978). Excluding family members from the preoperative counseling process may eliminate the most important resource the patient has available to him or her. Similarly, providing members of the patient's family with inadequate, incomplete, or incorrect information (Salmon, 1986a) in the preoperative period may result in many interpersonal difficulties in the early postoperative period. This may in turn affect the patient's progress during rehabilitation.

Spouses of those who are to undergo laryngectomy often appear neglected in regard to counseling efforts by members of the rehabilitation team (Blanchard, 1982; Salmon, 1979, 1986a). The spouse or partner needs to clearly understand the consequences of the surgery that lies ahead. However, they too are often dealing concomitantly with their own sense of shock and fear. The potential loss of a loved one due to cancer, not to mention the unravelling of financial and family structures (Ranney, 1975; Salmon, 1986a, 1986b) may provide a significant source of stress for the patient and family members. The patient's spouse or partner may also experience stress and anxiety due to their loved one's impending surgery. Family members must cope with and adjust to a variety of changes, many of which will be permanent, in the postsurgical period (Gates, Ryan, & Lauder, 1982).

Salmon (1979) has noted that a spouse's most immediate concerns relate to whether the patient will survive surgery and whether the cancer can be "cured." Information regarding the patient's medical condition and the treatment he or she will undergo falls within the domain of the physician. More specific consequences pertaining to information the physician provides may then be offered and reiterated, reinforced and repeated by other team members (i.e., nursing staff). Collectively, these concerns may be addressed most effectively by including significant others at the outset of the counseling process.

Concerns about postsurgical communication were noted by spouses to be a secondary concern beyond the disease and its direct sequelae (Blanchard, 1982; Salmon, 1986a). The speech-language pathologist serves as a facilitator for both the patient and members of his or her family. This will help to ensure that adequate information is provided by the most appropriate source. Thus, concerns of family members must be sought and addressed by the speech-langauge pathologist during preoperative counseling. The speech-language pathologist may also provide substantial information on other related areas, such as postoperative expectations, and so forth.

Are Counseling Needs Being Met Sufficiently?

Based on data obtained from a survey of 115 laryngectomized individuals and their spouses, Blanchard (1982) reported that 12% of those surveyed had no contact with a speech-langauge pathologist prior to or following surgery. Regardless of who was identified by the patient or spouse as being the primary provider of information

(surgeon, speech-language pathologist, esophageal speaker, nurse, etc.), on the whole sufficient pre- and postoperative counseling was not provided. Blanchard (1982) noted that 16% of the spouses surveyed indicated that counseling by a speech-language pathologist was lacking. Overall, speech-language pathologists were judged to be the second most "significant source" of information either pre- or postoperatively. These data raise two important concerns that must be addressed and hopefully rectified in the future.

Although Salmon (1979) reported higher percentages in regard to preoperative contacts by speech-language pathologists (29%), this percentage is still quite low. Considering the myriad of speech and nonspeech changes that patients will encounter in the postoperative period, counseling would appear to be insufficient. Based on his findings, Blanchard (1982) suggested that a "greater coordination of efforts" was needed from those professionals involved in the rehabilitative team. This need appeared most pronounced in the area of preoperative counseling for both patients and spouses. Blanchard (1982) concluded that "once the laryngectomee leaves the hospital, he also leaves the support of a multidisciplinary counseling team" (p. 240). Obviously, some patients cannot be seen preoperatively for a number of reasons (e.g., urgency for surgery due to obstructive tumors, etc.). However, other than a patient's outright refusal, there is no reasonable excuse to withhold preoperative counseling, in the hospital prior to surgery. Preoperative counseling facilitates the initial step in the patient's rehabilitation journey; hence, coordination of efforts is mandatory if the best care is to be offered to the patient and members of his or her family.

Counseling as a Process

Counseling of individuals who undergo partial or total laryngectomy is a process that continues to evolve along many dimensions over the rehabilitative period. This evolution frequently involves changes in the professional relationship between the patient, and family members, and the clinician. Specifically, counseling sessions may vary from early sessions which address the basic consequences of laryngeal cancer and its treatment, to those that become more detailed and global in nature (e.g., changes in spousal dynamics). Thus, counseling of those individuals diagnosed with laryngeal cancer comprises a variety of goals which are often overlaid on a process the patient transcends over the course of rehabilitation.

Counseling ideally addresses pertinent issues from the period immediately following diagnosis of laryngeal carcinoma (Williams, 1961) to that which may take place many months (and even years) after the patient is discharged from formal therapy. This counseling process begins with the simple goal of providing essential, basic information to the patient and family members (e.g., anatomical and physiologic changes). It often expands to more precise problem-solving sessions that are specific to an individual patient and which may be necessary many months following surgery (e.g., difficulty communicating in noisy environments). It may also be directed toward specific needs of not only the patient, but members of his or her family or perhaps even close friends (Square, 1986a). If undertaken correctly, this type of counseling provided by the speech-language pathologist is truly evolutionary. Such counseling is clear, well-organized, and sequential and moves from preoperative sessions that are informative to postoperative sessions that are educational.

The Patient's Response to Preoperative Counseling

One of the most difficult and challenging encounters a speech-language pathologist confronts in clinical practice is the preoper-

ative counseling of an individual diagnosed with laryngeal cancer. Counseling those who have heard the word "cancer" and are now attempting to deal with potential consequences of the disease may result in a variety of responses and/or reactions (Sanchez-Salazar & Stark; 1972; Stoll, 1958). Clinicians may encounter patient responses that range dramatically from complete ambivalence to emotional outbursts and anger. The speech-language pathologist may be uncomfortable interacting with these patients because he or she fears not knowing what to say or what may be observed when information is presented. This concern is not unusual and, quite frankly, should always remain to some degree in the speech-language pathologist's mind as it ensures that the clinician is not complacent about what is to occur. Yet the clinician should not be reticent of these fears for in some respects they may serve to facilitate the bond between clinician and patient.

Flexibility in Counseling

Although the importance of preoperative counseling has been stated by numerous authors and clinicians for many years, the role and scope of counseling has changed considerably in recent years with the advent of viable surgical-prosthetic methods of voice restoration (Reed, 1983a). With increasing numbers of women being diagnosed with laryngeal cancer and with the age of diagnosis decreasing (Kommers, Sullivan, & Yonkers, 1977), new issues have emerged that must be considered along the entire continuum of counseling for the laryngectomized patient (Gardner, 1966; Stack, 1986).

Even when one has the opportunity to provide preoperative counseling, the process undertaken does not become easier with each new encounter. In fact, it may become more complex for the speech-language pathologist attempting to address individual needs. Experience offers the speech-language pathologist a capacity to "fine tune" preoperative counseling to be consistent with his or her own clinical philosophy. The clinician must, however, present and discuss several key components in all sessions.

The speech-language pathologist's ability to perceive what the patient must absorb during this time of crisis is imperative. Consider the immediate consequences of the diagnosis that the patient has recently received from his or her physician. The diagnosis itself may, in essence, disable the patient from fully appreciating what he or she can expect in the postoperative period (Reed, 1983a). Whether the surgical treatment recommended is a partial laryngectomy or a total laryngectomy, the majority of patients will still be focused on a single, primary issue—that a cancer has been detected! According to Evans (1990, p. 15), "Fear of the unknown can be a major cause of anxiety." The consequences of treatment are usually of lesser concern. Nevertheless, it is at this point in the clinical course that they must be provided with basic, introductory information on the *anatomical, physiological*, and *communicative consequences* of whichever surgical procedure they are to undergo.

Preliminary Goals of Preoperative Counseling

From the perspective of the speech-language pathologist, preoperative counseling is essential in that it may eliminate misconceptions about postoperative speech capabilities (Duguay, 1966). This is an area where problems continue to be observed (Blanchard, 1982; Salmon, 1986a). It is important to note, however, that the preoperative meeting *must not* be viewed as an educational session; it is not. Preoperative counseling is not undertaken to educate the patient, but to *inform* the patient and significant others. Despair should not

be exacerbated, but hope should be instilled, even in the presence of such a harsh reality as the diagnosis of cancer. If care is taken in the preoperative counseling session, the individual and his or her spouse or partner may become less fearful at this important time of crisis (Sanchez-Salazar & Stark, 1972).

Components To Be Addressed During Preoperative Counseling

Several authors have provided information that is to be covered during preoperative counseling (Reed, 1983a; Salmon, 1986a; and others). Information gleaned from the literature, professional meetings, and workshops varies according to clinician bias; however, there are several areas common to all. In essence, this may be the only stage of counseling for these patients that subscribes to a generally invariant set of goals. Once counseling moves to the postoperative period, there is greater potential that information presented will become more individualized to the patient and family.

Salmon (1986a) has stated that the emphasis of counseling with patients and their spouse should not be on who provides information, or when it is provided, but more importantly that the information presented is "accurate and complete." The degree of completeness, however, must be based on each patient's ability to absorb the information presented. The speech-language pathologist must also have an awareness of both the amount and overall detail of information to be provided. This awareness permits the speech-language pathologist to adjust such components of the session "on-line" so that the patient can cope with this new information (Evans, 1990). The patient's ability to cope with new information at such a difficult time will affect the degree to which essential information will be comprehended. Given the option, it is better to provide less information and ensure its comprehension, than to provide more information with less understanding and/or retention. Counseling about communication should always be provided by the speech-language pathologist because the broad concerns, as well as concerns unique to the patient and his or her communication needs and conditions (e.g., hearing loss, employment demands, etc.) and impact on communication, are best understood by this member of the rehabilitation team. Based on survey information (Salmon, 1986a), spouses identified "speech communication" as the greatest problem area following total laryngectomy. Although communication is one segment of information that needs to be provided in the preoperative counseling protocol, its importance is equal to that of other primary areas.

According to Salmon (1986a), the speech-language pathologist has four primary areas that need to be covered preoperatively: (1) basic anatomical changes and physiologic effects of the surgery, (2) what to expect in the immediate postoperative period, (3) postsurgical speech options, and (4) availability of speech-language pathology staff members. The specific details from each of these areas that Salmon reports as being essential for the patient (and spouse or partner) are provided in Table 6–1.

Reed (1983a) has suggested that preoperative counseling involves three primary goals: (1) to emphasize support from the speech-language pathologist, as well as other members of the rehabilitation team; (2) to provide information to the patient and his or her spouse or partner; and (3) to answer appropriate questions. Two other broad areas may be served in the preoperative session, namely, an opportunity to establish a relationship with the patient and the opportunity to gather a history and assess the patient's current communicative status (Murrills, 1983). Case history information beyond that considered "basic" (e.g., medical status, family, employment, etc.), may often be obtained directly from medical records and, thus, need only to be confirmed during preoperative counseling. Some a priori knowledge about the patient may also serve the speech-language pathologist so that the counseling session may be initiated in a more informed manner. A detailed summary of areas to be addressed and their objectives is provided in Table 6–2.

TABLE 6–1.
Essential Information That Must Be Provided To Each Individual Who Is To Undergo Total Laryngectomy.

Anatomical and Physiological

The larynx will be removed and the individual will be required to breathe through a permanent tracheostoma; normal laryngeal voice will be lost.

Immediate Postoperative Expectations

Neck and face tissues will be swollen, may be bandaged in the area of the incision, a nasogastric (NG) tube will be in place, the airway and tracheostoma will require cleaning and suctioning.

Postsurgical Speech Options

There are several options for postsurgical alaryngeal communication.

Availability of Speech-Language Pathologist

The clinician will be available soon after surgery and will consult the patient regarding the first postoperative visit several days following surgery.

Source: Adapted from Reed (1983a) and Salmon (1986a)

TABLE 6–2.
Areas That May Be Covered During The Preoperative
Evaluation and Counseling Session.

1. Review patient's medical chart or record
   Objective: To gather pertinent information on medical history, scheduled date of surgery, procedure outlined by the surgeon, presurgical radiotherapy, general health problems which may influence recovery and/or rehabilitation.

2. Provision of basic information
   Objective: To provide information or clarification on the procedures they are to undergo, anatomical changes in the airway and aspects of neck breathing, the loss of voice postsurgically, alterations in coughing and sneezing, general aspects of the postoperative course (i.e., presence of intravenous and nasogastric tubes, monitors, etc.), and immediate postsurgical changes in eating and drinking.

3. Examination of oral mechanism
   Objectives: To gather information on the structure and function of the speech mechanism. This includes evaluation of lips, tongue, hard palate, and velum, jaw movement, changes in neck tissue as a result of radiation therapy (e.g., fibrosis, edema), the status of dentition or presence of partial or complete dental plates. Additionally, observations of speech rate, vocal intensity, and intelligibility should be undertaken, including potential influences of regional or second-language accents, and spoken language preference.[a]

4. Social and family history
   Objectives: To obtain general information on family members and relationships, and the potential support system that may be available to the patient. Further information on vocational and avocational interests should be noted, with particular emphasis on employment. Educational level and literacy should be noted.

5. Visit by a laryngectomized patient
   Objective: To provide the patient with an example of an individual who has returned to as near-normal a lifestyle postsurgically. However, this area is controversial and should not be implemented in a de facto manner (see further discussion in this chapter).

6. Counseling of spouse or partner
   Objectives: To provide a spouse or partner sufficient information about the consequences of surgery. This includes issues related to postoperative changes in appearance and basic anatomical and physiological changes that will occur. Information related to what one can "expect" in regard to surgical time, immediate postoperative appearance, and so forth should be presented.

7. Postoperative communication options
   Objective: To provide initial exposure to the concept of postlaryngectomy communication options. The emphasis should be placed on the likelihood that the patient will obtain some form of functional alaryngeal speech following surgery. It should be stressed, however, that written communication or the use of a communication booklet will be necessary in the early postoperative period.

8. General information on postoperative changes
   Objectives: To provide general information on aspects of becoming a permanent neck breather, care of the tracheostoma, alteration in the mechanism of coughing and blowing the nose, changes in olfaction and taste.

9. Determination of the next visit
   Objective: To inform and reassure the patient that the clinician will maintain contact with them in the postoperative period.

10. Written documentation of information presented
    Objective: To provide a record of information provided to the patient for review by medical and/or nursing staff.

Source: Adapted from Evans (1990), Reed (1983a), and Salmon (1986a).
[a]This issue is gaining increased importance across North America as patterns of foreign emigration are increasing substantially.

Requirements Prior to Counseling

Prior to initiating preoperative counseling, a single critical requirement falls to the speech-language pathologist. The speech-language pathologist *must confirm* that the patient has been informed by the physician that he or she has cancer and will undergo surgery to remove all (total laryngectomy) or part (conservation laryngectomy) of the larynx. Several options exist to ensure that the patient has indeed been informed. It is important to stress that the speech-language pathologist *cannot* assume that (1) the patient has been informed of his or her condition (cancer) and the extent of anticipated treatment (surgery), or (2) that the patient fully understands the *consequences* of this information. First, if the patient is an inpatient, the speech-language pathologist can frequently obtain this information directly from the physician or the nursing staff (Reed, 1983a). Second, if the patient has not been admitted to the hospital, the speech-language pathologist will need to contact the otolaryngologist directly.

Two questions must then be asked of the physician: (1) Has the patient been informed that he or she has cancer? and (2) Has the patient been informed that he or she will undergo a (partial or total) laryngectomy. Once confirmed by the physician, the speech-language pathologist reduces the chance that he or she will raise issues related to diagnosis and treatment of the disease that are unknown to the patient. In most settings, the speech-language pathologist may know the physician due to previous referrals and, thus, confirming that the appropriate information has been presented to the patient prior to arranging the preoperative counseling session is not a problem. In cases where a professional relationship is not yet established the speech-language pathologist must ensure that these two important questions have been addressed by the physician (Berkowitz & Lucente, 1985). If they are not, the patient should be referred back to the otolaryngologist. The speech-language pathologist should also speak to the surgeon regarding concerns about the apparent lack of preparatory information indicated by the patient.

Regardless of how the speech-language pathologist obtains confirmation for the two important questions noted, the essential portion of the preoperative counseling session should always begin with two additional succinct and straightforward questions: (1) What has your doctor told you about the problem you have? and (2) What has your doctor told you about the treatment you will receive?[1] These questions will hopefully provide direct confirmation that the patient has heard the term "cancer" and that surgery to remove all or part of the larynx is to be performed.

It is important for the speech-language pathologist to realize that the "trauma" or "shock" incurred when the patient heard of the malignancy may have also affected his or her ability to process and comprehend subsequent information provided by the physician. In this situation a spouse or a loved one may provide confirmation regarding the diagnosis and recommended surgical treatment. Once the speech-language pathologist is assured that both areas have been addressed by the physician more specific aspects of the preoperative counseling can begin.

---

[1]Some physicians routinely require that patients sign a statement confirming that the physician has discussed specific issues related to diagnosis and treatment or have patients write in the medical chart that they have been informed of this information.

The Structure of Preoperative Counseling

Once information on diagnosis and treatment is confirmed, the session should always begin with a general inquiry about the patient's marital and family status to determine whether the patient has a family support network. Information is then obtained about whether the patient is employed and if he or she desires to return to work postoperatively. Finally, information about the patient's (and spouse or partner) social and recreational activities is obtained (Reed, 1983a). Reed (1983a) then suggests that the patient be asked about specific concerns he or she has and, subsequently, to place them in order of importance. Although some of these concerns may be addressed briefly during preoperative counseling, detailed discussion of some issues raised may be pursued postopera-

tively. Reed (1983a) is careful to note that initial questions vary from patient to patient depending on their relative appropriateness. Specific questions may be raised based on the speech-language pathologist's review of the patient's medical chart. Once these introductory questions are completed, the counseling session progresses to providing information regarding the proposed surgery. A summary of Reed's (1983a) recommendations in relation to fundamental information in this area is provided in Table 6–3.

The preoperative counseling session should always be completed by reiterating key points with a particular emphasis on the following issues. When completed, the patient must know that: (1) he or she can live an essentially normal life following laryngectomy, (2) in the immediate postoperative period he or she will not be able to speak due to the loss of the "voice

TABLE 6–3.
Format for Presentation of Fundamental Preoperative Counseling Information.

1. Briefly review preoperative and postoperative anatomy and physiology with emphasis on postsurgical communication changes.
2. Review "normal" breathing and that associated with postsurgical anatomy (separation of oral and nasal system from primary airway).
3. Provide physical analog related to speech: power source (lungs), vibrating source (larynx), and valves and filters (articulation).
4. Specify that larynx will be removed, thus, vibratory source will be lost.
5. Emphasize that patient will not be able to speak in a normal manner postsurgically; the patient *must know* that his or her voice will be lost.
6. Provide preliminary information on postsurgical verbal communication options (artificial laryngeal, esophageal, and tracheoesophageal speech) and specify that one of these methods has a "very high probability" of resulting in successful communication.
7. Indicate that a speech-language pathologist will stay in contact with them postoperatively and follow them once medical clearance is obtained.
8. Specify that communication in the immediate postoperative period will require writing.
9. Provide information on postsurgical need for intravenous (IV) and nasogastric (NG) tubes, a humidification and oxygenation mask will be placed over the stoma. Emphasize that these are "normal" postoperative procedures.
10. Briefly discuss the tracheostoma, increased production of mucous, and hygiene during coughing.
11. Briefly discuss related changes such as loss of taste and smell, difficulty impounding air in the thorax for lifting, and so forth.

Source: Adapted from Reed, C.G. (1983a).

box," and (3) although there are no guarantees, the patient has a high probability of learning to effectively use one of the alaryngeal methods noted (Reed, 1983a).

Although some overlap is clearly apparent in the protocols used during preoperative counseling of the patient who is to undergo laryngectomy, many commonalities exist. All areas addressed (see Tables 6–1, 6–2, and 6–3) may not be of equal importance; hence, the clinician may need to develop a hierarchy of what can be covered *effectively and completely*. It is suggested that areas common across the work of Salmon (1986a), Murrills (1983), and Reed (1983a) would appear to be essential components of preoperative counseling. Therefore, essential information includes: (1) presenting anatomic and basic physiologic changes postoperatively and a limited overview of immediate postsurgical expectations, (2) discussing postoperative speech rehabilitation (alaryngeal) options, and (3) offering assurance to the patient and indicating when further contacts will take place following surgery. Although this direct contact with the patient is important, the dissemination of essential information can also be facilitated through the use of diagrams, handouts, and patient-oriented handbooks such as *Looking Forward* (Keith, Shane, Coates, & Devine, 1984) or several other guidebooks.

Improving the Preoperative Session: Issues in Content and Form

To facilitate the patient's understanding of information provided, two particular recommendations are suggested. First, the speech-language pathologist should avoid using "jargon" and opt for the use of more generic terms (e.g., windpipe for trachea). Although more formal terminology should be acquired by the patient at a later time to facilitate communication with other members of the rehabilitation team, the speech-language pathologist should use simple lay terminology at this critical point in the rehabilitative process. The use of jargon frequently serves as a barrier to effective communication. This may be a twofold function; first, new terminology may not be adequately explained to the patient by the clinician, and thus, critical information may be missed. At this point, few patients are likely to ask for clarification of terms that are new and with which they are unfamiliar. The clinician must remember that the patient is confronting a potentially life-threatening illness; therefore, *simplifying the preoperative session in both its content and form* is highly recommended. Simple explanations and redundancy serve to facilitate the patient's comprehension. As stated by Salmon (1986a, p. 289), the speech-language pathologist is most often "reiterating what has already been said at least twice before," and "each time it is said the patient and spouse have an opportunity to understand a little bit more of what they are about to undergo." Thus, redundancy provides a valuable communication vehicle in those confronting a serious disease (Reed, 1983a; Salmon, 1986a). Carefully organized, carefully worded, and simple communication is the key to success in preoperative counseling endeavors with those who have laryngeal cancer.

The second area of concern relates to "how" the patient and clinician communicate. The use of jargon is pedantic, and parading one's knowledge can only decelerate the development of the clinician-patient relationship. The use of jargon may distance the patient from the clinician because it provides a vehicle for establishing status in this relationship. Darley (1978) has suggested that successful clinical encounters with patients are achieved when "mutual respect" between the patient and clinician occur. For any counseling to be successful, a hierarchy among the participants cannot exist. Thus, the provision of information in preoperative counseling to those diagnosed with laryngeal cancer and awaiting surgery, must be provided in a nonjudgmental, clear and precise, yet compassionate manner. One only needs to see the fear on a single patient's face to understand the importance of equalizing the communicative process and initiating a cooperative relationship that will need to be maintained over the course of rehabilitation. If the speech-langauge pathologist is able to accomplish this goal, the chance of a successful outcome for the patient may be enhanced considerably.

Preoperative Visitations by Laryngectomized Individuals

Significant controversy surrounds the issue of whether a preoperative visit by an individual who has previously undergone the same procedure should be recommended. Historically, it was believed that by exposing the patient to an individual who had been successfully rehabilitated, the patient would be provided with hope that he or she too could be successfully rehabilitated (Stoll, 1958). It was also believed that the rehabilitated patient could provide a "model" for the individual who was to receive the same surgical procedure. Diedrich and Youngstrom (1966) reported that a majority of patients who had received a *postoperative* visit by a laryngectomized individual would also have desired a preoperative visit. Diedrich and Youngstrom were careful to point out that "most" of these patients were esophageal speakers, hence, this factor may have been influential in their desire to have such a visit in the preoperative stages. It may be quite safe to say that visitations by a laryngectomized individual have most commonly involved esophageal speakers. Thus, professional bias may be presented inadvertently.

In contrast, however, some have suggested that patients may establish unrealistic expectations based on the model to whom they were exposed (Gates, Ryan, & Lauder, 1982). This suggestion emanates from the fact that typically, individuals who have been utilized in the preoperative counseling capacity have been good-to-excellent alaryngeal speakers (usually esophageal speakers), who had apparently "re-entered" society without difficulty. Thus, laryngectomized individuals who conduct preoperative visitations are, in essence, idealized representatives of those who have undergone laryngectomy. It may be safe to say that the average or typical former patient is seldom used in this counseling capacity. There may be some merit, therefore, to the argument that such visitors may provide an unrealistic image to the patient, particularly in the preoperative period. Diedrich and Youngstrom (1966) also have suggested that the "psychological acceptance of esophageal speech" as an alaryngeal method of communication may be more prominent in the postoperative period as opposed to its acceptance in the preoperative period (Diedrich & Youngstrom, 1966). However, the disagreement among professions and their respective dogma should cease, and professional opinions should be viewed in the context of patient choice.

Specifically, the option to meet with an individual who has already confronted what the patient is now encountering should be the patient's choice. Consequently, the patient and family members should always be asked if they desire such a visit. Contrary to popular belief, patients who actively participate in decisions regarding their care may be more apt to adapt over the long term (McNeil, Weichselbaum, & Pauker, 1981). Should the patient decline, this does not exclude the option to receive a laryngectomized visitor in the postsurgical period. It must again be stressed that this choice *rests solely with the patient*, and this choice should be fully respected by all members of the rehabilitation team. If the answer is in the affirmative, a visitation should be arranged with an individual who has been trained by the speech-language pathologist specifically for this purpose.

Problems Associated with Visitations by Laryngectomized Individuals

The fact that better-than-average, if not excellent, laryngectomized individuals usually perform this service at either the patient's or clinician's request may in itself carry some unique yet subtle disadvantages. Beyond the argument that a given laryngectomized individual may not provide a representative example of one's postlaryngectomy potential, the visitation may generate two negative reactions in the patient. First, early in the rehabilitative period it is not unusual to see some patients working quite vigorously at the "physical" level. These patients expend considerable effort and energy attempting to acquire their initial esophageal sound. This effort is perceived by the patient to be an explicit example that he or she is doing everything possible to achieve esophageal voice. This increase in effort may often culminate in poor performance (i.e., output of esophageal sound) because of muscle tension and associated fatigue.

Discussions with some patients who experienced difficulty early in the rehabilitative process have indicated that their effort level may have been driven by the performance of the preoperative laryngectomized visitor. That is, the excellent model that was provided set an expected level of performance for the patient. This expectation subsequently may have been the underlying reason for increased effort in therapy; specifically, "If I work harder, I will learn more quickly." However, the net result of "working harder" was disruptive

to the esophageal voice acquisition process in that too much effort decreases the potential utility of the pharyngoesophgeal segment for alaryngeal voice production (Damste, 1958; Diedrich & Youngstrom, 1966; Salmon, 1979, 1986d; Winans, Reichback, & Waldrop, 1974).

The second factor that must be considered in relation to preoperative visitations by a laryngectomized individual also pertains to patient expectation. Desire by the patient to become as proficient a speaker as the visitor may culminate in unrealized expectations. Data in the literature indicate that much variability exists relative to what percentage of patients can truly acquire functional levels of esophageal speech (Gates & Hearne, 1982; Gates, Ryan, Cantu, & Hearne, 1982; Ryan, Gates, Cantu, & Hearne, 1982). Estimates have been as low as 25% (Schaefer & Johns, 1982). This suggests that even in the best case scenario the chance of being laryngectomized and achieving excellent esophageal speech may in actuality be very low.

If the patient is not as proficient a speaker as that of the laryngectomized visitor, or if he or she cannot master esophageal speech, the patient may feel a distinct sense of failure. This failure may have carryover effects to other methods of alaryngeal communication, such as the use of the artificial larynx. It may now be apparent that extreme care must be taken to not represent the artificial larynx as a secondary option. This may further influence the patient's perception that he or she has failed in the attempt to acquire the "best" method of alaryngeal communication. Obviously, the speech-language pathologist desires to see patients achieve the best level of success regardless of the alaryngeal method pursued. However, a preoperative visitation carries with it some potential for direct comparisons by the patient in relation to the model that is observed. Care must be taken to ensure that expectations are not presented in an unrealistic manner and to attempt to reduce perceptions of failure by the patient.

A third potential consequence that may be associated with use of a preoperative visit by a laryngectomized individual involves unrealistic self-perceptions by the patient regarding his or her level of proficiency. That is, some patients may view the visitor's speech in a rather discrete fashion. In doing so, these patients see only the verbal output of speech as the model, rather than other aspects (vocal) that may result in a more favorable postsurgical voice for the listener. Although there is nothing wrong with a focus on successful vocal output without regard to fine details inherent in voice and speech production (e.g., pitch, loudness, effort, etc.), this view is inadequate. These patients may request discharge from therapy before refinements in acoustic-perceptual parameters of voice, as well as other features in their alaryngeal speech (e.g., rate control, pause time, etc.) can be taught, achieved, and mastered (Amster, 1986). This may be of significant concern to the speech-language pathologist whose patients are females (Shanks, 1986b) and require comprehensive efforts to refine voice quality. The speech-language pathologist must carefully consider these issues and their potential impact on ultimate effectiveness of treatment.

Unfortunately, no consensus among clinicians exists regarding whether it is appropriate to use the services of a past patient in a counseling role. Additionally, no clear data exist to either support or refute their effectiveness in this capacity. Obviously, proponents of using laryngectomized patients in a counseling role are just as opinionated as those who share a contrary opinion. There is clear merit in the comment by Stoll (1958, p. 552) that "the presence of an intelligent, psychologically astute person who has experienced a laryngectomy and has learned to use good esophageal speech can be of great support to the patient" in the preoperative period. However, three potential rehabilitative options now exist for patients who undergo total laryngectomy (esophageal, artificial laryngeal, and tracheoesophageal speech).

This necessitates that a more global, and perhaps more tolerant, view of what constitutes a "good visitor" is implemented.

What is the best advice to the clinician for assessing the potential value of a preoperative visitation by a laryngectomized individual? The answer is not clear; however, it does appear that well-rehabilitated laryngectomized individuals *may in some cases provide a valuable service* from a preoperative perspective (Greene & Mathieson, 1989; Salmon, 1986c). In fact, the individual who has successfully undergone laryngectomy can provide "a real and unique contribution" and provide and example of "what can be accomplished" (Murrills, 1983, p. 68). However, the term "well-rehabilitated" implies a much broader definition than that of just speech, and this service may be of greater value postoperatively.

The controversy about whether preoperative visits are recommended, therefore, may center around issues of who provides the counseling and *what* the focus of such counseling is directed toward. It may indeed be the case that such factors serve as differentiating features for whether a preoperative visitation is "good" for the patient. It is clear then that some important considerations must be undertaken by the clinician and that guidelines must be followed to increase the chance that the visitation is successful in meeting important objectives in a subtle fashion.

Salmon (1986c) has provided a detailed description of the "do's and don't's" of preoperative or postoperative visitations by laryngectomized individuals. It is recommended that these guidelines be carefully adhered to in a comprehensive and consistent manner. A summary of these recommendations is provided in Table 6–4. Despite the provision of such guidelines, the essential aspect of what constitutes a successful patient visitation ultimately rests with who provides the visit and how it is conducted (Gates, Ryan, & Lauder, 1982; Salmon, 1986c).

TABLE 6–4.
Recommended Guidelines for Pre- and Postoperative Visitations
of Patients by Laryngectomized Individuals.

1. Do not violate the physician's responsibility for determining who has contact with their patient.
   Rationale: The physician has both a legal and ethical responsibility to his or her patient. Thus, a "referral" must be received from the physician prior to visitation. This referral can come in "proxy" form from the speech-language pathologist *provided* the physician has been notified and approved the visit.
2. Do not visit a patient prior to contacting nursing staff.
   Rationale: This will ensure that the visit is noted in the patient's chart. Further, the nurse may provide details on whether it is an appropriate time for visitation (e.g., patient is not feeling well, surgeon is conferring with patient, etc.).
3. Always present a "name card" for the patient to keep with the visitor's name, address, and phone number. Provide written information on local Laryngectomees' Club, location, and meeting schedules. Finally, always complete a name and address card for the patient.
   Rationale: Patient is provided with a resource in the community, and additional contacts can be made if requested. Patient's name and address care can be used to request information from the International Association of Laryngectomees.
4. Meet with or arrange to meet with the patient's spouse or partner.
   Rationale: Spouses and partners have not typically been involved in counseling. This will serve to eliminate feelings of being "omitted" and will serve overall rehabilitation of the patient.
5. Use the best and most effective communication skills.
   Rationale: The patient and/or spouse or partner may exhibit some degree of hearing loss. When combined with decrements in various parameters of alaryngeal speech, attempts must be made to ensure the best overall communicative interaction.
6. Be aware of physical proximity during communication exchange.
   Rationale: Optimizes ability of patient and/or spouse to hear what is being said (see #5 above).
7. Facilitate speechreading.
   Rationale: By allowing patient to observe face and mouth, intelligibility may be enhanced. Remember that alaryngeal speech is "new" to most individuals and some orientation to enhance listening may be required.
8. Be aware of ambient noise levels.
   Rationale: If extraneous sources of noise are eliminated, communication between parties will be improved. Turn off radios or TVs, close doors, and so forth in an attempt to provide a quiet communication environment.
9. Use good judgment in what topics are discussed.
   Rationale: The visitor should not answer questions that are within the purview of professional members of the rehabilitation team. Be honest in answering appropriate questions posed by the patient, and do not hesitate to indicate when you are unable to respond to some questions, or simply do not know the answer.

Source: Adapted from Salmon (1986c).

The speech-language pathologist must work directly with potential laryngectomized visitors before a visitation occurs. Early on, the speech-language pathologist might even wish to "follow along" and provide constructive feedback to the visitor. This will facilitate independence in later visits that the visitor may perform alone. Clinicians who have used the services of one or two laryngectomized individuals over extended periods of time know the value of such people in the rehabilitative process. The time spent developing pre- and postoperative visitation (counseling) skills in these invaluable human resources cannot be stressed enough, and the potential service and support they may provide to a patient must be fully recognized by the speech-language pathologist.

In reviewing the broad guidelines for preoperative visitations by a laryngectomized individual, the speech-language pathologist can see that some degree of "training" is required. Responsibility for training always falls to the speech-language pathologist. No visitation should take place without proper discussions taking place between the speech-language pathologist and the potential visitor. One method of training that may prove to be of value takes the form of role-playing between an experienced visitor and one who desires to do the same. Obviously, the experienced visitor is usually able to ask a variety of questions that fall within "appropriate-to-answer" or "not-appropriate-to-answer" categories. This format for preparing a laryngectomized visitor may prove fruitful, particularly in settings where many laryngectomies are performed each year. This role-playing situation must also be monitored by the speech-language pathologist to assure that correct and appropriate information and responses are being provided. A well-prepared visitor whom the clinician can rely on to function within a specific nonprofessional domain and provide empathetic information to the patient is a valuable adjunct to the rehabilitation team.

Preoperative Counseling Associated with Conservation Laryngeal Surgery

Given the lack of data to the contrary, it may be assumed that counseling in any substantial form beyond that presented by the surgeon may be nonexistent for patients who are to undergo partial laryngectomy. Individuals who undergo partial laryngectomy procedures will have some postsurgical change, albeit relatively minor in many cases, in their vocal communication. These changes may persist beyond the immediate postoperative period in most cases and may not be amenable to therapeutic intervention and change. However, behavioral compensations that may be detrimental to voice production may be fruitful areas to address clinically. Speech-language pathologists are clearly those who will be called on for voice and speech rehabilitation purposes, yet they may not be actively involved in the rehabilitation process until surgery is completed. Efforts by speech-language pathologists must be expanded to effect changes and meet the increasing need in this important area of management for laryngeal cancer. Thus, the education of team members may provide improved opportunities for such patient referrals.

Summary

This chapter reviewed several broad issues pertaining to preoperative counseling in patients diagnosed with laryngeal cancer. Preoperative counseling is perhaps the most important single service that may be provided to the patient. Although disagreement exists among professional as to who is best able to provide preoperative counseling, a team approach is required to meet the basic needs of this type of counseling. A successful preoperative counseling session is not viewed as an educational session, but rather one which seeks to provide basic information to the patient. The speech-language pathologist can certainly fill this requirement, particularly as it is related to changes in anatomy and physiology and the postsurgical communicative consequences of laryngectomy. Additionally, preoperative counseling serves to initiate the patient-clinician relationship that will follow in the postoperative period. Any preoperative counseling must, however, involve the patient's spouse or partner and, therefore, must always consider the impact of surgery on both the patient and members of his or her family.

Postoperative Considerations

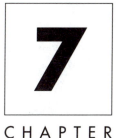

7

CHAPTER

Postoperative counseling of patients who have undergone surgical treatment for laryngeal cancer may be viewed as an extension of preoperative efforts. Much of the information provided to the patient and family members preoperatively will no doubt be addressed again following surgery. Information presented in the postoperative period must focus on (1) the changes that have occurred and (2) on the patient's ability to adapt to these changes.

Because of the myriad of changes that the patient will encounter postoperatively, the rehabilitation team serves a critical role in establishing the basis of postsurgical recovery and rehabilitation. The purpose of this chapter, therefore, focuses on several issues that will be addressed following surgery. While the speech-language pathologist should accept the primary responsibility in the area of communication rehabilitation, he or she will often also need to serve as a mediator between some

members of the rehabilitation team. Thus, the speech-language pathologist may provide an essential link among a variety of professionals in the postoperative period.

The Postoperative Period

Postsurgical counseling is most often guided by specific concerns which evolve from the patient's experiences and observations outside of the speech clinic. Counseling that occurs during the patient's inpatient stay, however, evolves from information presented preoperatively. This may be viewed as an elaboration and expansion of information provided. As Williams (1961) stated more than 30 years ago regarding those who are diagnosed with laryngeal cancer, "rehabilitation of the laryngectomy patient should start before surgery" (p. 127). More recently, Evans (1990) has stated that "inadequate preparation for the surgery can result in a post-operative reaction which can effect rehabilitation" (p. 15). If preoperative counseling has been sufficient, transition to the presentation of issues in the postoperative period is significantly enhanced.

Preliminary Considerations

In most instances, preoperative counseling will be provided within several days of the patient's diagnosis. Although the focus of preoperative counseling centers on primary changes that will occur following surgery (Reed, 1983a; Salmon, 1986a), complete understanding of such information by the patient or loved ones is infrequently observed prior to surgery. Thus, the postoperative period allows the speech-language pathologist to again address those issues discussed previously. The reiteration of almost all areas covered in the preoperative session(s) is of value to the patient. This reiteration of information, however, is now done in the "first person" as the patient is now aware of changes that have occurred subsequent to surgical treatment for cancer management.

During the early days following surgery, the patient must rapidly adapt to the consequences of surgery. Specific components of surgery and the subsequent postoperative changes that were discussed preoperatively can now be more accurately described and discussed with the patient (e.g., discussion of the tracheostoma). This may, therefore, require more of a "hands on" approach to the provision and explanation in a variety of topics. The clinician must, however, acknowledge that the patient's "shock" from having heard a diagnosis of cancer is now compounded by the shock of dramatic and significant physical changes (Dropkin, 1989). The patient's emotional well-being is challenged at this early period of recovery; thus, support systems (both from loved ones and professionals) must be offered and encouraged.

Although the clinician's responsibility at this point in the rehabilitative process is to begin educating the patient about the effects of surgery, the patient must not be overwhelmed by the information presented; good judgment will most certainly lead to more successful postoperative encounters with the patient. The presentation and discussion of either too much information or a discussion that is overly detailed must be avoided in the early postoperative period. The clinician must also be sensitive to how the new information is being received by the patient and members of his or her family. Determining how receptive the patient is to the information presented is critical to the success of future clinical interactions.

The First Postoperative Visit

Once surgery is completed, the speech-language pathologist should maintain direct and regular contact with either the surgeon or members of the nursing staff on the patient's ward. General inquiries should seek to determine if any complications were encountered either during surgery or in the early postoperative course. Additionally, information on the patient's general health should be obtained.

It is not unusual to find that by the third day postoperatively many patient's become more alert and active relative to the immediate postsurgical period. It is at this time that the speech-language pathologist should make the first visit to see the patient. The purpose of this visit is ostensibly to maintain the link with the patient that was promised in the preoperative session. If the patient has been informed by the speech-language pathologist that he or she will be seen several days following their surgery (Reed, 1983a; Salmon, 1986a), all attempts should be made to ensure that such a visit is conducted. A simple greeting and a promise for a daily visit is most appropriate. The patient should, however, know that the speech-language pathologist will monitor the patient's recovery and most likely will be able to initiate some alaryngeal training (i.e., use of the intraoral electrolarynx) at bedside over the next several days. This contact and introduction to alaryngeal communication can then be expanded during the patient's first visit to the speech clinic as an inpatient.

During this initial visit, the patient should be asked if he or she would like to have paper and pencil for writing (frequently, nursing staff will have already provided these items to the patient). An additional option is a "magic slate"; however, the slate should be removed from any child-oriented mounting (e.g., cartoon characters, etc.) as this may be viewed negatively by the patient and communicative partner alike. For patients who are unable to write, simple communication booklets with either pictures or written words, names, and so forth can be provided. Core vocabulary and basic needs (e.g., bathroom, medication, pain, etc.) are usually sufficient in the early period.

At the termination of this first visit, a promise of a daily visit should be made. The clinician should inform the patient that should he or she have any questions, to let the nursing staff know so that the speech clinic can be contacted. On completion of the first postoperative visit, the clinician should provide a brief summary of this encounter in the patient's medical chart. This will ensure that other professionals are aware that an initial visit was conducted. In most instances, this initial contact may establish the speech-language pathologist as the *primary contact and liaison* to other services and professionals.

Adapting the Clinical Interaction to Maximize the Provision of Information

Two particular considerations must always occur during the course of postoperative contacts with the patient. It is critically important for the clinician to subjectively assess the patient's postoperative status for "absorbing" information that the speech-language pathologist wishes to provide. This assessment is also required for family members or loved ones who are actively involved in the recovery and rehabilitation process. Thus, the speech-language pathologist will need to assess each patient's ability to comprehend information presented and make the necessary adjustments in what and how information is provided. This involves impressions of each patient's general cognitive status, as well as aspects of general level of health postsurgically (e.g., degree of physical pain or discomfort). The second area of consideration must address phases of recovery in a somewhat global manner.

Basic Considerations Related to Recovery Status

The first 7 to 10 days postoperative may be loosely segmented into two distinct periods. The first 3 to 4 days postoperatively may be best defined as the *immediate postoperative period*, and the fourth or fifth through the days until formal discharge may be arbitrarily defined as the *transitional postoperative period*. Although provision of health care is changing dramatically in the United States (Conley, 1984), as well as in Canada, it is not unreasonable to assume that despite any complications a patient who undergoes total laryngectomy will be discharged from the hospital somewhere between 10 and 14 days postoperative at the maximum. Obviously, complications will delay this process dependent on the severity of the problem(s). Thus, use of the terms *immediate* and *transitional* may be viewed to correspond to the patient's recovery within a broad physical and psychological context.

The *immediate* postoperative period is characterized by the patient's inability for the most part to act on his or her environment. At this time, the patient is not likely to be ambulatory, is likely to be connected to a variety of equipment and instrumentation (monitoring, humidification, feeding), and is often experiencing some level of discomfort as a result of the surgery and healing process. In contrast, however, the *transitional* postoperative period may find the patient making his or her *first active progress* toward recovery. The patient is now acknowledging the gravity of the surgery, may be up and around for short periods, may be able to use the bathroom with assistance, may be increasing oral nutritional intake (Tait & Aisner, 1989), and may also be more responsive and oriented to information that is presented.

This increase in the patient's responsiveness is likely related to early phases of adapting to the consequences of surgery. Additionally, increased responsiveness may relate to the diminishing effects of general anesthesia. Thus, clinical interactions with patients during their postoperative stay may be more productive if the level of presentation and the demand for their direct participation is adjusted accordingly. A patient's desire for independence is a positive step toward rehabilitation.

Establishing a Clinical Partnership with the Patient

The postoperative period provides challenges for both the patient and the speech-language pathologist. It is at this time that the patient fully begins to appreciate the dramatic effects that surgery will have on their return to the social milieu. These effects are evident for patients who undergo both conservation laryngectomy procedures and total laryngectomy, although the effects are more apparent in patients who undergo the latter.

Postoperative counseling is truly an open-ended process relative to preoperative counseling. Postoperative counseling frequently continues for many months,

albeit in a less formal manner. For each patient, different and often unique concerns and questions about their surgery and its sequelae will arise. This requires coordinated efforts across many professional domains. Similar to preoperative roles, the speech-language pathologist can serve a critical role in this phase of rehabilitation. Even brief, initial postoperative meetings with the patient are essential in establishing the patient's confidence in the clinician and the services he or she will provide.

Patients may exhibit a variety of postoperative behaviors that may appear negative to the rehabilitative process; however, many such behavioral changes are likely related to a normal grieving process. Depression is not uncommon at this stage and, hence, professional assistance may be warranted. In clinical settings where the patient has access to external services from a counselor or psychologist, such a service may be recommended and utilized.

In settings where services may not be available, the responsibility for counseling frequently falls on the shoulders of individuals who are involved directly with the patient. Thus, nurses, physicians, social workers, physical therapists, and the speech-language pathologist may be called on to provide some degree of counseling. Such counseling is best and certainly appropriate if it remains within a given professional's realm of expertise unless he or she has more formal training.

The appropriateness of "counseling" interactions is best determined on an individual basis. Each patient is different, comes with unique experiences, and, fortunately, many patients come with considerable resourcefulness at this time of emotional distress. It is essential for the speech-language pathologist to realize that early postoperative contacts with the patient should be directed at providing general support rather than specifically focusing on the patient's loss of speech. Issues related to speech rehabilitation will occur once the patient is fully ambulatory.

Although the loss of the patient's ability to verbally convey his or her concern and fear may culminate in feelings of isolation and loss, it may also serve as the catalyst that the speech-language pathologist may seize on. Specifically, the speech-language pathologist has the opportunity to facilitate communication between the patient and others.

Avoiding Barriers to Communication

Interactions between health care providers and patients are frequently disrupted because of a language barrier. Professionals may present themselves in a manner that isolates them from their patients. This is often a result of overuse of technical terminology. This may not only result in poor comprehension of information provided, but perhaps more importantly, it may separate the clinician and the patient by implying differences in status. For effective counseling to occur, those who engage in the interchange must be equal, as equality permits successful communicative interaction. Darley (1978) has clearly stated the importance of acknowledging this issue for the speech-language pathologist during the clinical interchange:

> You and the informant are by no means on equal grounds, for he or she has come for help which you are in a position to give . . . yet you as the interviewer cannot afford to be aloof, superior, critical, moralistic, rigid, intolerant, disdainful, or amused. (p. 42)

Aspects of terminology may also impact on the patient's future well-being. If communication in the early, formative stages of patient counseling and management can be facilitated, long-term success may be enhanced commensurately. Cousins (1983) has elegantly stated the importance of communication with those who are ill:

> Words . . . can be gate-openers or gate-slammers. They can open the way to recovery, or they can make a patient dependent, tremulous, fearful, resistant. The right words can potentiate a patient, mobilize the will to live, and provide a congenial environment for heroic response. The wrong words can produce despair and defeat or hinder the usefulness of whatever treatment is prescribed. The wrong words can complicate the healing environment, which is no less central in the care of patients." (Cousins, 1983, p. 131)

Thus, care must always be taken in presenting information in a manner that facilitates its comprehension by the patient and significant others. This will also serve to reduce the distinctions between the clinician and patient that may threaten the clinical process later in rehabilitation.

Postsurgical Issues

Anatomical and Physiological Changes

The anatomical and physiological changes associated with total laryngectomy are significant in and of themselves. It is not uncommon to find the individual who has undergone total laryngectomy to be inundated in information that, quite frankly, is too voluminous to comprehend. When this is coupled with the patient's lack of verbal communication, the potential for increased depression, and insulation from others, their sense of being overwhelmed is increased. Changes that occur in relation to surgical removal of the larynx and associated reconstruction following neck dissection must be addressed early on with each individual patient. This usually requires the clear presentation of information without the confounds of teaching a new lexicon. Although the more widely used terms in the professional community are important, they really serve no early purpose to the patient. The individual is often more concerned with "the hole in my neck" than with the tracheostoma at this point in recovery. Each patient should be provided with a review of information related to the separation of the airway and the oral-pharyngeal structures. Issues related to airway protection (stoma coverings, external threat from water or other foreign substances, etc.) and hygienic concerns (coughing, stoma care, etc.) need to be discussed (Keith et al., 1984; Lauder, 1989). If they have not already been given to the patient, written materials should be provided.[1]

Effects of Multimodality Treatment

Anticipated changes associated with post-surgical radiotherapy should be discussed with the patient prior to the initiation of such treatment. The radiologist will often address these issues with the patient; however, some additional clarification may be necessary. In cases where teeth have been extracted, a consultation with the dental surgeon may be beneficial to the patient. Although this list of areas is not exhaustive, it points out that several basic areas associated with multimodality treatment will need to be considered by members of the rehabilitation team. Nevertheless, each patient will require individualized postsurgical counseling based on his or her own needs. As with preoperative counseling, family members should be included in postoperative counseling from the outset. This will afford the patient and his or her family the maximum opportunity to address primary needs in the postoperative period, as well as providing information specific to each patient.

Communication Between Members of the Rehabilitation Team

Ongoing communication between members of the rehabilitation team is essential during the postoperative period. As noted previously, the roles of each member of the team must be clearly specified. This establishes who will be responsible for what information as it arises. While the preoperative period is filled with anticipation, the postoperative period requires the patient to begin accepting what has occurred. Thus, combined efforts of the speech-language pathologist, laryngologist, oncology nurse, social worker, dentist, as well as others may be required.

Information on anatomical changes in the airway (care and protection of the tracheostoma and airway) may be covered by several professionals; this may aid in the patient's ability to understand a variety of issues surrounding this important topic area. Additionally, questions regarding supplies that may be required (stoma bibs, humidifier, etc.) will need to be addressed by someone on the team. Issues related to secondary treatment for the malignancy such as radiotherapy will also need to be covered.

Postsurgical Communication Options

It is during the postoperative period that more detailed discussion of alaryngeal speech options will typically be provided. Each patient should be introduced to the three primary alaryngeal options: artificial laryngeal, esophageal, and tracheoesophageal speech. Although some introductory information may have been provided

---

[1]It is advised that information on each patient's literacy be obtained during the preoperative period. If a patient is unable to read, a member of the family or a friend may be provided with written information for reference purposes.

preoperatively, further details must now be provided to the patient.

Once the patient is ambulatory, a visit to the speech clinic may offer the most suitable setting for a more advanced presentation and discussion of these communication options. Videotaped examples offer an excellent vehicle for this type of introduction. Clear information should be provided regarding the relative advantages and disadvantages of each method (Reed, 1983b). It also provides the ideal opportunity to introduce the patient to the artificial larynx in a more formal manner.

Following the presentation of this information, patient's should be encouraged to evaluate each method and make a choice that is best for their particular needs. Patient's need to be informed that several methods may be used in combination should they desire (e.g., esophageal speech and the artificial larynx). Despite the relative limitations of each method, it is essential that the patient fully understands that one of these methods has a high probability of providing a means of verbal communication.

Although the patient ideally needs to make an independent decision on which approach to pursue, the speech-language pathologist should acknowledge that use of an artificial larynx is an excellent method of communication at this point in their recovery (i.e., esophageal speech training cannot begin at this time, and those who have received primary tracheoesophageal puncture are not typically using a prosthesis for several weeks). Following this discussion, a formal therapy appointment should be made with the patient so that additional counseling and direct voice and speech rehabilitation can commence. Finally, a general framework for how therapy will be structured (i.e., number of sessions per week, etc.) should be provided to the patient and family members.

Postoperative Visitations

Visitations by a laryngectomized patient may be requested by some patients in the postoperative period. As noted for preoperative visitations, the speech-language pathologist needs to carefully select who will perform this visitation. In contrast to preoperative visitations, the postoperative visitation may involve the communication of more than the potential for speech reacquisition. It might not be unreasonable to view the laryngectomized visitor from a perspective that excludes his speech effectiveness as a *primary* factor.

The postoperative visitor may provide a model for the patient that stresses the fact that patients recover and re-enter their world to live as normal a life as possible (Reed, 1983a). Further, postoperative visitations demonstrate that (1) the physical changes and aesthetic effects of surgery can be "covered up" so as to not draw attention, (2) a support system of others who have undergone the same is available to the patient as a resource, (3) relationships with family members and friends can be maintained, and (4) a return to a productive life is possible. Although these topics may not be discussed directly in many visits, they may emerge as subtle issues that are conveyed in a nonverbal manner. What is unspoken is often quite powerful in many of the meetings between a patient who has recently undergone laryngectomy and an individual who has previously gone through the same. What transpires in such visitations can be seen to have great potential as a first stepping stone to the patient's rehabilitation.

Summary

This chapter has addressed several issues related to postoperative counseling with laryngectomized patients. Clinicians must acknowledge numerous factors during this period that impact on recovery and the capacity for a successful rehabilitation program. This involves more global consideration of the patient's well-being at this difficult stage in the recovery process. Although the speech-language pathologist is the patient's single best source of information related to communication disruption and associated changes that will occur postsurgically, their early role may be seen as a supportive one. The speech-language pathologist may also provide an essential link between the patient and other professionals on the team. Finally, issues that seek to familiarize and orient the patient to postsurgical communication options and the general process of speech and voice rehabilitation will be presented by the speech-language pathologist.

Alaryngeal Voice and Speech Options

Speech pathologists have the responsibility of providing the best means of communication for the laryngectomee at any given period after his operation. . . . The question is not which method is better, but which methods are best, not only for a given patient, but also for any given time. (Diedrich & Youngstrom, 1966, p. 148)

Information presented in previous chapters of this text has explicitly indicated that once a total laryngectomy is performed on a patient, the essential anatomical structure for the generation of voice is lost permanently. This loss of a primary vibratory (voice) source requires that a new, *alaryngeal* voice source is either developed by or provided to the patient. This new alaryngeal voice source will be achieved through the use of either an extrinsic electronic artificial laryngeal device (also known as an electrolarynx), or through intrinsic alaryngeal methods (i.e., esophageal or tracheoesophageal voice).

For the patient to make the most appropriate alaryngeal choice for his or her communicative needs, information must be provided on relative strengths and weaknesses of each method. No alaryngeal option is free of communicative liabilities. These strengths and weaknesses must also be viewed within the context of the patient's physical, psychological, and cognitive capabilities. However, patients should be able to assess their own needs and make an informed decision about which method will best meet their particular communication requirements.

Once a decision is made by the patient on which method will be pursued, the process of *speech production* can be developed and refined for verbal communicative purposes. The purpose of this chapter is to provide an overview of the three primary alaryngeal options that are currently available for patients who undergo laryngectomy. Additionally, general advantages and disadvantages associated with each specific alaryngeal option will be outlined. Further details on each of the three specific alaryngeal methods are provided in subsequent chapters.

Postlaryngectomy Alaryngeal Communication

The speech-language pathologist should be the patient's single best source of information of postsurgical communicative options. Although the speech-language pathologist is responsible for providing clear and concise information regarding each method of alaryngeal speech, an effort should be made to avoid any explicit or implicit "bias" for or against a particular method of alaryngeal speech (Duguay, 1978; Rothman, 1982). Such bias historically has been most notable as it is associated with the use of artificial laryngeal speech approaches (Lauder, 1968, 1970). Thus, the presentation of comprehensive and unbiased information on postoperative speech options is a prerequisite of good patient care.

An Informed Choice of Alaryngeal Communication

In preoperative counseling the patient and members of his or her family are generally presented with information that several methods of postlaryngectomy communication exist. Patients are also informed that there exists a high probability that one method of communication will meet their communicative needs and that they will be able to speak again. Postoperatively, patients are introduced to these methods more formally through viewing of videotaped examples of speakers using each method of alaryngeal speech. This exposure, along with discussion of the relative merits of each method, will hopefully lead the patient to decide which rehabilitative option to pursue. This does not, however, imply that the clinician should avoid suggesting the use of or instructing the patient in more than a single method of alaryngeal communication.

Pursuing Multiple Alaryngeal Options

Substantial advantages may be offered to the patient in cases where two alaryngeal methods (e.g., artificial laryngeal speech and esophageal speech) are trained concurrently (Duguay, 1983). Specifically, Duguay has pointed out that if the clinician is successful in teaching the patient to use more than a single method of alaryngeal speech, the chance of communicating more effectively in a variety of situations may be improved (Lauder, 1970; Rothman, 1982). When intrinsic and extrinsic methods of alaryngeal speech are compared, intrinsic methods may be susceptible to both physiologic and psychologic influences (Duguay, 1979, 1983; Lauder, 1970).

Certain situations at times may render even functional esophageal communication ineffective (Miller, 1958). Lauder (1970) provided several compelling reasons why an individual who has been laryngectomized should be trained in the use of the artificial larynx. Without an alternative source of verbal communication, the individual is essentially helpless, particularly in times of a crisis (Lauder, 1970). Other factors can also occasionally disrupt the effectiveness of intrinsic methods of alaryngeal speech (e.g., esophageal speech) even in highly proficient speakers. As stated by Duguay (1983):

> Fatigue, illness, extreme tension, or a high ambient noise level could be overcome by the use of an artificial larynx device, and "normal" conversational situations could be managed by esophageal voice. (p. 127)

While Duguay's (1983) comments were directed at potential limitations of esophageal speech, tracheoesophageal speech may be similarly affected in some situations. Regardless of method, teaching two options of alaryngeal speech is certainly ideal in that the patient is provided alternative methods of communication dependent on the needs of any given communicative situation. The advantage of the patient's access to more than a single mode of alaryngeal speech is likely to have widespread effects on the patient's ability to interact in varied communicative environments and settings (Blood & Blood, 1982; Byles, Forner, & Stemple, 1985).

If facilitating effective *communication* is the goal of postsurgical speech rehabilitation, then clinicians must demonstrate a tolerance for all alaryngeal options. Although some patients may desire to use a specific alaryngeal method based on features generally unrelated to communication effectiveness (e.g., a method that requires less or no maintenance relative to other methods), many patients are quite practical. In regard to this clinical dilemma for some patients, Duguay (1983) stated that:

> For some, good artificial larynx speech is more desirable than poor esophageal speech even for those "normal" conversational situations. (p. 127)

Regardless of which method a patient chooses, no data exist to confirm that a patient's use of one alaryngeal method will retard or diminish the ability to successfully acquire another alaryngeal method. Thus, clinical consideration of multiple alaryngeal options is recommended.

Is There a Perfect Method of Alaryngeal Speech?

It may be safe to say that for any given patient, there is not one "perfect" method of alaryngeal speech; each method may have unique limitations for that particular patient. From the perceptual standpoint

listeners may judge features inherent in alaryngeal speech in an inconsistent manner (Green & Hults, 1982). That is, although one perceptual parameter (e.g., pitch) may be judged as "better" for one alaryngeal method relative to another, this may not necessarily result in improved global judgments of speech effectiveness or acceptability for that method. If provided adequate information about each alaryngeal method, the patient can develop a hierarchy of what method will best suit his or her communicative needs.

Alaryngeal Speech Options

From a speech pathology perspective, two categories of alaryngeal speech exist. These categories are best described as *intrinsic* or *extrinsic* methods of alaryngeal voice production (Weinberg, 1982). The essential difference relates to whether the patient is able to generate his or her own alaryngeal source by developing use of a vicarious voicing mechanism (intrinsic), or whether the alaryngeal vocal source must be generated through the use of a nonsystemic mechanical source of vibration (extrinsic). Thus, *esophageal speech* and *tracheoesophageal speech*[1] (TE) are intrinsic methods of alaryngeal voice because they rely on the patient's use of residual anatomical structures as the source of voice production. In contrast, the use of an *artificial larynx* (electronic or aeromechanical) is an extrinsic method of alaryngeal speech.

Although two additional types of intrinsic alaryngeal speech exist, *buccal* and *pharyngeal* speech, these methods are not desirable (Scripture, 1916; Weinberg & Westerhouse, 1971, 1973) and should be

---

[1]Even though the method of tracheoesophageal voice and speech uses a prosthesis, the prosthesis does not serve in a source capacity, but rather is used as an air shunt to directly facilitate insufflation of the esophageal reservoir for the purpose of alaryngeal voice production.

discouraged. Buccal speech is the result of compressing air between the cheek and the teeth, or between the tongue and the alveolar ridge (Diedrich & Youngstrom, 1966). Buccal speech is, therefore, produced in the oral cavity proper. In contrast, pharyngeal speech is a result of compressing the tongue against oral or pharyngeal structures; this may involve contact of the tongue with the posterior pharyngeal wall, faucial pillars, or the hard palate or velum (Diedrich & Youngstrom, 1966; Finkbeiner, 1978; Weinberg & Westerhouse, 1973).

Advantages and Disadvantages of Esophageal Speech

Because of the source of vibration associated with esophageal speech, its acoustic characteristics differ substantially from that of normal speakers (Snidecor, 1978a). This includes aspects of fundamental frequency, intensity, and speech rate, as well as other internal features of these parameters. Fundamental frequency of esophageal speech has been demonstrated to be about half that of a normal male adult (Curry & Snidecor, 1961; Diedrich, 1968; Snidecor & Curry, 1959, 1960). Although this may pose minimal difficulties for a male, it has significant effects for a female who has been laryngectomized (Gardner, 1966; Weinberg & Bennett, 1972) despite reliable gender identification (Weinberg & Bennett, 1971). That is, the fundamental frequency of esophageal voice is relatively consistent regardless of the patient's gender. Hence, females will exhibit vocal pitch levels that are about two octaves lower than expected. Speech intensity is also reduced from that of normal speakers (Blood, 1981; Robbins, Fisher, Blom, & Singer, 1984; Weinberg, Horii, & Smith, 1980). Finally, because of the need to frequently insufflate the limited capacity of the esophageal reservoir (Diedrich, 1968), speech rate is reduced commensurately with consequential effects on speech

prosody. Additional details regarding characteristics of esophageal speech are provided in Chapter 13.

Several advantages of esophageal speech have been reported in the literature (Diedrich & Youngstrom, 1966; Gardner, 1971; Reed, 1983a, 1983b; Snidecor, 1978a). The primary advantage is that no external devices are required for esophageal voice production. Because of this feature, the speaker's hands are free for other purposes. Although clear and distinct acoustic differences exist for esophageal speech, this alaryngeal method is not characterized by a mechanical voice quality found with electronic devices. This is seen to have advantages in that esophageal speech may be less noticeable than artificial laryngeal speech (Bennett & Weinberg, 1973). Proficient esophageal speakers have also been found to exhibit the capacity for coding linguistic aspects (i.e., lexical stress, intonation, and juncture) of the speech code (Gandour & Weinberg, 1982; Gandour, Weinberg, & Garzione, 1983; Gandour, Weinberg, & Petty, 1985; McHenry, Reich, & Minifie, 1982; Scarpino & Weinberg, 1981).

The disadvantages of esophageal speech are primarily related to poor rates of acquisition (Gates, Ryan, Cooper, Lawlis et al., 1982; Ryan et al., 1982; Schaefer & Johns, 1982). Most estimates suggest that successful acquisition is demonstrated by less than half of all who attempt to learn esophageal speech. This figure, however, may be much lower. Another disadvantage of esophageal speech is that its acquisition may require a substantial commitment of time in treatment. This may become a particular liability relative to changes in the health care system. Although early progress in skill acquisition may signal a high probability of long-term success with esophageal speech (Berlin, 1963, 1965), the process for refinement may require substantial allotments of time.

As noted previously, the greatest liabilities associated with esophageal speech generally pertain to alterations in acoustic and temporal characteristic. Decreased pitch and loudness and alterations in speech rate and prosodic features may be viewed as negative factors by some patients. Esophageal speakers also lack proficiency in effecting and controlling changes in the voicing source (Angermeire & Weinberg, 1981). Esophageal speech has, however, been shown to be preferred to artificial laryngeal speech (Bennett & Weinberg, 1973). Decreased speech intensity is also a liability for esophageal speakers, particularly in relation to competing noise situations (Hoops & Noll, 1969; Horii & Weinberg, 1975; Weinberg, Horii, & Smith, 1980). Esophageal speakers appear to exhibit intensity levels that are about 10 dB SPL less than normal speakers (Weinberg et al., 1980). This degree of reduction in intensity has also been reported for specific phonetic contexts (Blood, 1981). A decreased speech rate associated with esophageal speech may also be viewed negatively by the listener (Hoops & Noll, 1969; Shipp, 1967). Although speech intelligibility may be quite good in some speakers, the nature of the voicing source offers the potential for increased perceptual confusions (Doyle, Danhauer, & Reed, 1988; Sacco, Mann, & Schultz, 1967). Finally, esophageal speech production may result in secondary behaviors (facial grimacing, lip-smacking, etc.) that may detract from communication interactions.

Advantages and Disadvantages of Tracheoesophageal Speech

Tracheoesophageal (TE) speech is best viewed as pulmonary powered esophageal speech. TE speech requires that a fistula is surgically created to allow communication between the trachea and the esophagus. Once this TE "puncture" is completed, a one-way voice prosthesis is placed in the puncture site. The voice prosthesis permits the flow of tracheal (pulmonary) air from the airway into the esophageal reservoir when the airway is sealed. Thus, insufflation of the esophageal reservoir *does not* require the injection of oral air. While TE speech shares an esophageal sound source, the access to pulmonary air provides several advantages relative to that alaryngeal method. Additional details on TE speech are provided in Chapter 13.

The primary advantages of TE speech are directly related to the speaker's access to pulmonary air. Pulmonary air permits a substantially increased capacity for more lengthy excitation of the PE segment. Thus, phrase length and consequently, overall speech rate are improved and closely mimic those of a normal speaker (Robbins, 1984; Robbins et al., 1984). This also allows the speaker to exhibit more natural speech prosody and the ability to systematically effect associated linguistic changes (Gandour et al., 1985; Gandour & Weinberg, 1985a, 1985b).

A secondary advantage of the speaker's access to pulmonary air is related to frequency and intensity of voice production. The increased amounts of air available for speech production permits increased *transpseudoglottal* airflow which results in increased PE segment duty cycle (Robbins et al., 1984). Thus, an increase in voice fundamental frequency is observed with TE speakers when compared to esophageal speakers. Increased flows, as well as the speaker's ability to voluntary control pulmonary expiration also allows the speaker to generate greater intensity. In fact, TE speakers have been shown to generate vocal intensity levels that are about 10 dB SPL greater than normal speakers (Robbins, 1984; Robbins, et al., 1984). This is viewed as advantageous to the TE speaker, particularly in situations of competing noise. Although data are varied, overall speech intelligibility appears to compare favorably with other methods of proficient alaryngeal speech (Blom, Singer, & Hamaker, 1986; Tardy-Mitzell, Andrews, & Bowman, 1985; Williams & Watson, 1985). At the phonemic level, TE speech appears superior to that of esophageal speech (Doyle, Danhauer, & Lucks Mendel, 1990; Doyle, Danhauer, & Reed, 1988; Doyle & Haaf, 1989; Haaf & Doyle, 1986).

The final advantages associated with TE speech center around the fact that this method can be acquired quickly following surgery. However, careful evaluation of patients who are considering TE puncture is essential. Although acquisition of TE speech may be more rapid compared to esophageal speech, both speech and nonspeech skills must be learned. Specifically, each patient must fully understand aspects of the TE puncture site, function of the voice prosthesis, prosthesis insertion, care, and maintenance.

The disadvantages of TE speech relate to issues of prosthesis care and maintenance. Although substantial changes in TE puncture voice prostheses have occurred, a variety of skills must be learned in order to maximize the utility of TE speech. These demands are expanded if related prosthetic devices such as the tracheostoma breathing valve are use in conjunction with the voice prosthesis. If patients use only a voice prosthesis, one hand is required for digital closure of the tracheostoma in order to produce voice. Patients who have poor eyesight or manual dexterity, cognitive deficits, and so forth, or who are in generally poor health are not ideal candidates. Additional disadvantages relate to prosthesis cost (which varies dependent upon manufacturer and prosthesis type) and in some locales, access to necessary supplies.

Finally, TE puncture does require additional surgery in some instances. With any surgical procedure some risk is involved, and complications may occur. While TE puncture is gaining acceptance as a primary surgical procedure (i.e., at time of laryngectomy), secondary procedures require additional surgery post-laryngectomy. Many patients are fearful of additional surgery, and thus, this factor must always be considered. If the procedure is done as a primary procedure, patients will need to not only adapt to changes related to total laryngectomy, but acquire necessary skills specific to use, maintenance, and care of the voice prosthesis. Thus, patients must be fully prepared for this inevitability prior to primary TE puncture procedures.

Advantages and Disadvantages of Artificial Laryngeal Speech

The artificial larynx provides the speaker with an external voice source. Two general types of devices exist, *intraoral* and *transcervical* devices. Intraoral devices permit the speaker to introduce an electronic voice source directly into the oral cavity where speech is then articulated. Transcervical devices require placement on tissues of the neck or check, and the signal is then passed into the vocal tract/oral cavity where speech is articulated. Each type of device has its own relative merits.

Artificial laryngeal speech has the distinct advantage over other alaryngeal methods in that it can be acquired quite quickly by the majority of patients. Although some physical factors may preclude use of certain types of artificial laryngeal devices (e.g., neck type devices may not be appropriate in patients with radiation-induced fibrosis), other options are available (i.e., intraoral devices). The artificial larynx is, therefore, an extremely viable option particularly in the early post-operative period.

Overall, intelligibility may be quite good if speakers are trained effectively. Intelligibility may, however, vary by the type of alaryngeal device (Stalker, Hawk, & Smaldino, 1982). As with other alaryngeal methods, intelligibility difficulties associated with effecting voicing contrasts has been reported (Weiss & Basili, 1985; Weiss, Yemi-Komshian, & Heinz, 1979).

Loudness using the artificial larynx also appears to be better than that of esophageal speech (Hyman, 1955). This appears to offer the patient an advantage in noisy environments, and this may be further enhanced with amplification (Verdolini, Skinner, Patton, & Walker, 1985). Many modern devices also permit the speaker to manually adjust output intensity, thus allowing adjustment for specific situations. It may also be an important feature for communicative partners who exhibit some degree of hearing loss.

The major disadvantages of artificial laryngeal speech have been attributed to the mechanical voice quality it produces. Although some modifications in the artificial laryngeal source have been undertaken in recent years, problems associated with mechanical quality persist. The artificial laryngeal speaker may also have difficulty signaling linguistic components of the spoken code (Gandour & Weinberg, 1982, 1983, 1984; Gandour et al., 1985; Gandour, Weinberg, & Kosowsky, 1982). Despite the speaker's ability to communicate effectively with an artificial larynx, its level of acceptability for both the patient and listener appears to be reduced relative to other methods (Bennett & Weinberg, 1973). The artificial laryngeal device also requires the use of one hand and is clearly visible to others, which may cause the speaker concern. This disadvantage should be offset in many instances by the overall effectiveness of artificial laryngeal communication. Finally, some devices that offer unique features such as rechargeable batteries, volume and pitch controls, and so forth, may be rather expensive and, thus, are cost-prohibitive for some patients.

Summary

This chapter has addressed issues related to postsurgical speech rehabilitation options following total laryngectomy. The relative advantages and disadvantages of each method, esophageal, tracheoesophageal, and artificial laryngeal speech, have been outlined for comparative purposes. Issues related to the use of more than one method of alaryngeal communication has also been discussed.

If living as normal a life possible postlaryngectomy is the paramount purpose in rehabilitation (Reed, 1983a, 1983b),

information regarding disadvantages of each option are provided, the likelihood that each patient will make the best choice possible will be improved.

Esophageal Function

It is without question that numerous factors are involved in any given patient's eventual postoperative speech rehabilitation outcome. These factors are believed to influence a patient's ability to acquire functional and serviceable esophageal voice. The majority of information in the literature suggests that the basis of this outcome derives from general issues of structure and function of the upper esophageal region (Diedrich & Youngstrom 1966; Gardner, 1971; Kallen, 1934; Singer & Blom, 1981). Thus, the influence of anatomy and physiology of the esophageal sphincter on the acquisition or nonacquisition of serviceable esophageal voice remains of interest.

To provide a basis from which particular approaches to speech treatment emerge, information related to both normal and postsurgical function of the region is necessary. To develop this understanding, the purpose of this chapter is to elucidate general components of both volitional and reflexive components of function within the anatomical region. Issues related to normal and postsurgical esophageal structure and function, continuing areas of controversy, and the relationship between successful or failed attempts to acquire esophageal voice are addressed. To reduce confusion associated with nomenclature, the general terms esophagus, pharynx, and pharyngoesophageal (PE) junction will be used as primary terminology. However, generally synonymous terms such as esophageal sphincter may be used with specific caveats identified for their usage.

Structure and Function of the Esophagus

Normal Esophageal Function

Questions related to esophageal function have long been of interest to those involved in voice and speech rehabilitation following total laryngectomy. This is because esophageal speech provided the only viable method of alaryngeal voice postlaryngectomy (Keith & Shanks, 1983, 1986) before the development of a mechanical artificial larynx or introduction of the contemporary tracheoesophageal puncture technique and use of an associated voice prosthesis (Singer & Blom, 1980). Extensive information centered on the normal structure and function of the human esophagus and related structures of the digestive path may be found primarily in the gastroenterologic and laryngologic literature. Briefly, the esophagus is a soft tissue muscular tube that extends from the bottom of the pharynx to the entrance of the stomach. At both transitional regions (i.e., pharynx-esophagus and esophagus-stomach) a *tonic zone of high pressure* (Henderson, 1983; Zaino et al., 1967) can be found. These two zones of high pressure, or sphincters, have been termed the *upper esophageal sphincter* (UES) and *lower esophageal sphincter* (LES), respectively. Biologically, these sphincters help to restrict the abnormal flow (reflux) of contents from the stomach or esophagus into more superior regions of the aerodigestive path. It is the upper esophageal sphincter that is most important from the perspective of esophageal voice production.[1] It has been suggested, however, that a balance of muscular forces between the upper and lower esophageal sphincters is a prerequisite for the acquisition of esophageal voice (Shanks, 1986a; Wolfe et al., 1971).

Although some degree of controversy exists regarding which muscular components comprise the upper esophageal sphincter, the *cricopharyngeus* muscle is most commonly identified as the primary muscle of this sphincter. The cricopharyngeus is closely associated with muscular fibers that emerge from the lower pharyngeal region (i.e., inferior pharyngeal constrictor muscle) and is quite complex in both form and function. The cricopharyngeus muscle essentially "rings" the upper esophagus, covering a region of approximately 2 to 4 centimeters (cm) in length (Christensen, 1981; Fyke & Code, 1955; Henderson, 1983). The muscle is noted to have attachments on the posterior aspect of the cricoid cartilage of the larynx (Henderson, 1983).

Tonicity of the Upper Esophageal Segment

The maximum constant or resting pressure of the normal upper esophageal sphincter has been reported to range from approximately 18 to 60 cm above that of atmospheric pressure (Ellis, 1971). Contractile pressures associated with deglutition may vary from approximately 70 to 100 cm H_2O, but these pressures are short in their duration (2–4 seconds) prior to returning to levels consistent with resting pressures (Ellis, 1971).

The intraluminal resting pressure profiles of the upper esophagus (cricopharyngeus) may differ substantially when directionality of the pressure sensor is assessed. In fact, Winans (1972) has shown that anterior and posterior pressures differ considerably from those exhibited by the lateral portions of the sphincter when assessed using manometry. Thus, association of the cricopharyngeus with a cartilaginous structure (cricoid) in the normal system, as well as its possible interdigitation with slinglike fibers from the inferior pharyngeal constrictor muscles, may provide more variable, directional measures of resting pressure within the lumen of the upper esophagus.

Viewing such anatomical structures, specifically the cricopharyngeus and

---

[1]It should be noted, however, that Wolfe, Olsen, and Goldenberg (1971) have provided fluoroscopic data from 13 laryngectomized patients and have suggested that those patients who failed speech rehabilitation demonstrated an incompetent *distal* (lower) *esophageal sphincter.*

inferior constrictor muscles in their collective form, has a distinct advantage. A combined, systemic view of the upper esophageal sphincter is perhaps most representative of what occurs on a physiologic level. This system acts in a synergistic fashion during normal function, although the sequence of temporal relationships must always be considered (Henderson, 1983; Logemann, 1983; Young & Adams, 1980). In contrast, it does limit (at least to some degree) what might be discerned about the functional response of the cricopharyngeus as an "isolated sphincter" (Lund & Ardran, 1964). Although considerable interest about the cricopharyngeus exists, the reality of assessing its function in isolation is difficult if not impossible. The relative merit of both views (i.e., isolated muscle function versus multiple muscle system response) is obvious from a physiologic point of view.

Based on our understanding of the upper esophageal sphincter, the information leads one to conclude that esophageal function of individuals who have undergone laryngectomy will differ substantially from that of *nonlaryngectomized* subjects (Doyle, 1985; McGarvey & Weinberg, 1984). Further, it might be anticipated that function will be quite individualized across the population of laryngectomized individuals. These individual patterns of performance are likely to be represented by substantial intersubject variability. This assumption appears consistent with data reported in the literature across a variety of laryngeal behaviors.

From a functional perspective, physiology of the normal upper esophagus is quite complex in the normal human system and must be viewed within an anatomic, physiologic, and neurophysiologic context (Doyle, 1985). The relationship between muscles of the inferior pharynx and those of the cricopharyngeus and the relative neurologic control mechanisms associated with each add to the complexity of this system (Chodosh, Giancarlo, & Goldstein, 1984; Code, 1981; Lund & Ardran, 1964; Dey & Kirchner, 1961). Additionally, the UES appears to respond differentially depending on which element (e.g., air versus fluid distention) interacts within the system (Creamer & Schlagel, 1957). Esophageal distention via the introduction of air may result in a unique functional response and adjustment when compared to the introduction of fluid (Henderson, 1983). This response is a direct result of innervation influences.

Innervation of the Pharyngoesophageal Segment

Both the pharynx and the cricopharyngeus receive innervation from parasympathetic and sympathetic fibers (Henderson, 1983). Parasympathetic fibers to the region emerge from several cranial nerves including the glossopharyngeal (IX), vagus (X), and spinal accessory (XI). Sympathetic influence is provided via branches from the cervical sympathetic ganglia (Henderson, 1983). Normal relaxation of the cricopharyngeal sphincter occurs via mediation from the sympathetic system, with the sphincter responding to changes in internal pressure via proprioceptive fibers. Thus, normal tonicity of the upper esophagus is mediated through input from the cervical sympathetic chain (Henderson, 1983). The motor response of the upper esophageal sphincter is primarily accomplished through direct input from the vagus nerve, as well as from branches of the recurrent laryngeal nerve (Henderson, 1983; Henderson, Boszko, & van Nostrand, 1974) and possibly branches from the trigeminal nerve (Chodosh et al., 1984).

Palmer (1976) has suggested that separate systems of neural innervation may exist for the cricopharyngeus muscle and those of the pharyngeal muscles. Thus, normal function of the upper esophageal sphincter, that region comprised by the cricopharyngeus and inferior pharyngeal constrictor muscles, requires complex interaction of both *afferent and efferent components* of the nervous system. Therefore, disturbance to either the afferent or efferent control mechanism(s) can result in cricopharyngeal or PE segment dysfunction.

Variability Associated with Physical Structure and Orientation

Because of the physical relationship that exists between muscular components of the sphincter and those of more dense structures (e.g., cartilage) the resting pressures within specific regions or locations in the esophageal lumen may differ. It has been demonstrated that pressure in the anterior and posterior regions may be almost three times greater than that observed in lateral regions of the esophageal lumen (Gerhardt, et al., 1978; Winans, 1972). Consequently, consideration of normal structural relationships within the sphincter, as well as those pertaining to the rather significant alterations in anatomy which occur postlaryngectomy would result in disruption of the underlying control of the cricopharyngeal region. Additional concerns related to pre- and postlaryngectomy function would also appear to have the potential to influence esophageal function for alaryngeal voice production purposes.

Considerations Following Total Laryngectomy

Postlaryngectomy Esophageal Function

Function of the upper esophageal sphincter following laryngectomy has been shown to be altered considerably from that observed in the normal human system. This alteration in function appears to be a primary consequence of anatomical reconstruction following laryngectomy (Dey & Kirchner, 1961; Kallen, 1934). Reference to the potential contributions of muscle reconstruction concomitant with laryngectomy and associated radical surgical procedures for head and neck cancers have been raised by many researchers (Conley, 1964; Gates, 1980; Robe, Moore, Andrews, & Holinger, 1956; Simpson, Smith, & Gordon, 1972; Singer, 1988; Singer & Blom, 1980, 1981; Singer, Blom, & Hamaker, 1986).

It is essential, however, to note that anatomical reconstruction carries with it the potential for alteration of the neural innervation to the structures of this sphincter. This observation may then play a significant role in postsurgical function of the PE segment (Conley, 1964). Welch, Gates, Luckmann, Ricks, and Drake (1979) have noted that "partial sensory denervation due to section of the superior laryngeal nerves may impair the coordination of sphincter relaxation" (p. 808). All of the muscles that will ultimately form the reconstructed upper esophageal region were once attached in some manner to the laryngeal mechanism. These structures also share some common sources of innervation; therefore, the disruption of normal control as a consequence of surgery can be appreciated along with general anatomical changes across several dimensions.

Although the superior border of the esophagus itself is a contiguous band of muscular tissue (smooth and striated muscle fibers), the cricopharygeus and inferior constrictor muscles are slinglike, each having lateral attachments to laryngeal cartilage (McMinn et al., 1981). During total laryngectomy, the pharyngeal constrictor muscles are detached from the cartilage and then reconstructed via midline approximation (Kirchner, Scatliff, Dey, & Shedd, 1963; Silver, 1981). This reconstruction necessarily requires that the ends of each muscle be opposed to one another to close the existing surgical defect left by removal of the larynx.

The method used to surgically close the postlaryngectomy hypopharynx has been raised as a potential variable which influences postoperative function of the upper esophageal sphincter (Davis, Vincent, Shapshay, & Strong, 1982). Hence, surgical resection and subsequent closure ostensibly creates an entirely new anatomical zone at the inferior border of the pharynx and the superior border of the esophagus. The remaining two pharyngeal constrictor muscles may also be approximated during surgical reconstruction and closure.

As a result of surgical resection associated with total laryngectomy, it is possible that discrete areas of constriction that correspond with particular muscles (i.e., the cricopharyngeus) may not be clearly evident. That is, an isolated response by the cricopharyngeal muscle or the inferior pharyngeal constrictor may not be easily discerned (Henderson, 1983; Lund & Ardran, 1964). Therefore, what may be more appropriate in attempting to understand function of the reconstructed upper esophageal region is to view this region in its collective sphincteric form (Damste, 1986; Diedrich & Youngstrom, 1966; Zwitman, 1986). Dey and Kirchner (1961) have suggested that when contraction and relaxation of the upper esophagus, cricopharyngeus, and lower pharynx are observed in laryngectomized individuals via manometric procedures, "these three areas appeared to contract as a whole" (p. 108).

Because of the historical controversy that exists regarding what constitutes anatomical components that form the upper esophageal region, Welch, Gates et al. (1979) have used the term "pharyngoesophageal high pressure zone" or PE-HPZ. This more global view of the postlaryngectomy "esophageal" mechanism may prove valuable in interpreting physiologic data (Shipp, 1970). This suggestion may also correspond to several earlier reports in the literature that indicate that the location of the "pseudoglottis" is variable (Damste, 1986; Diedrich & Youngstrom 1966; Welch, Gates et al., 1979). Additionally, others have suggested that variability in the location or number of postsurgical vibratory source(s) may exist (Brewer, Gould, & Casper, 1974; Damste & Lerman, 1969; Daou, Shultz, Remy, Chan, & Attia, 1984).

Pharyngoesophageal Function Following Laryngectomy

Several investigations have sought to obtain detailed information on the comparative function of the upper esophageal sphincter in normal individuals and those who have undergone total laryngectomy. Kirchner et al. (1963) conducted an investigation which sought answers to two specific questions in those who had undergone total laryngectomy: (1) How do postoperative changes in the pharynx influence esophageal voice? and (2) What effect has laryngectomy on the upper esophageal sphincter? Thirty-five patients were assessed using cinefluorography, and 23 patients were assessed using intrapharyngeal and intraesophageal pressure measures (20 patients underwent both assessments).

Based on the cineflorographic data gathered, Kirchner et al. (1963) concluded that no significant relationship could be identified between good esophageal speakers and anatomical morphology in the postlaryngectomy pharynx. They also noted that size of the "hypopharyngeal lumen" appeared to offer a minimal contribution to an individual's speech ability. Similar to other studies, Kirchner et al.'s (1963) work did indicate that variable or multiple sources of pseudoglottal vibration may exist in some patients (Brewer et al., 1974; Damste, 1979, 1986; Damste & Lerman, 1969; Daou et al., 1984). Intraesophageal pressure data provided by Kirchner et al. (1963) indicated that pressure stages or resting pressures were absent or weakened relative to the normal system. These combined findings led Kirchner et al. (1963) to suggest that characteristics of the postlaryngectomy pharynx did not appear to affect esophageal voice production. Further, in the case of an absent intraesophageal resting pressure, these authors did not believe that this would be detrimental to esophageal speech.

Winans et al. (1974) evaluated 20 patients who had undergone laryngectomy and 20 control speakers using intraliminal (esophageal) manometry. These investigators found reduced resting pressures in the cricopharyngeal sphincter of laryngectomized patients who had acquired fluent, sustained esophageal voicing relative to those who were unable to acquire esophageal voice. Fluent esophageal speakers exhibited mean pressure values of 13 mm Hg, whereas those who could not produce esophageal voicing exhibited a mean value of 30 mm Hg.

In contrast, normal speakers studied by Winans et al. (1974) demonstrated mean esophageal pressures of 39 mm Hg. Although Winans et al. indicated that fluent esophageal speakers could be differentiated from those who were unable to use this intrinsic alaryngeal speech method, they were also careful to note that there was "considerable scatter and overlap of values" (p. 220). Therefore, Winans and his colleagues suggested that other factors needed to be considered in relation to their influence on esophageal function in the laryngectomized population and the apparent influence on esophageal speech. Winans et al. (1974) indicated that patient age and time of assessment could be important factors. Based on the collective results of their study, Winans et al. (1974, p. 14) stated the following:

> The results of our study invite the surgeon to cautiously alter his laryngectomy technique in favor a looser reconstruction of the cricopharyngeus or to utilize other techniques, such as myotomy, whereby the postoperative constricting function of this muscle can be reduced.

Thus, the basis for use of selective myotomy which appeared in the alaryngeal

speech literature in the 1980s (Chodosh et al., 1984; Singer, 1988; Singer & Blom, 1981; Singer, Blom, & Hamaker, 1981, 1986) found its impetus in the work of Winans et al. (1974). Ten years later, Chodosh et al. (1984) offered a similar suggestion based on their concerns about postlaryngectomy alteration in anatomy, physiology, and neural innervation. The functional significance of this postsurgical change has been clearly outlined by Chodosh and his colleagues (1984, p. 55):

> It would appear that laryngectomy repair subsequently can interfere with the orderly contraction and relaxation of the constrictors as well as the cricopharyngeus. This may produce a functional block to inspired and regurgitated air interfering with esophageal speech.

Welch, Luckmann, Ricks, Drake, and Gates (1979) assessed resting pressures of the upper esophageal sphincter in a group of normal and laryngectomized individuals. Based on comparison of these groups, Welch, Luckman, et al. (1979) found those who had been laryngectomized exhibited mean peak resting pressures that were reduced by more than half from those observed for normal individuals (51 ± 8 versus 121 ± 14 mm Hg). These data appear consistent with differences in the function of the upper esophageal sphincter that have also been reported by other investigators based on comparisons of pre- and postlaryngectomy physiologic performance (Shipp, Deatsch, & Robertson, 1970; Welch, Gates, et al., 1979).

In a companion study Welch, Gates, et al. (1979) also evaluated sphincter pressures in a group of patients both pre- and postlaryngectomy. Although Welch, Gates, et al. (1979) found postlaryngectomy sphincter pressure measures to decline from those observed preoperatively (130 ± 24 mm Hg vs. 66 ± 9 mm Hg), they noted little difference between *mean postlaryngectomy pressures* for individuals who acquired esophageal speech (70 ± 10 mm Hg) and those who did not (59 ± 18 mm Hg).

Viewing the individual subject data presented by Welch, Gates, et al. (1979), the range of performance was also similar (27 ± 2 to 130 ± 18 mm Hg for esophageal speakers, 15 ± 2 to 158 ± 11 mm Hg for nonspeakers). Therefore, questions about the potential impact of pharyngoesophageal-high pressure zone (PE-HPZ) pressure measures on the ability of the laryngectomized to acquire esophageal voice were once again raised. As such, resting pressure does not appear to be a sole determinant of esophageal voice acquisition or overall voice and speech proficiency (Shanks, 1986a).

Welch, Gates, et al. (1979) also pointed out the importance of differences in the "radially situated pressure" (p. 804) that exists within the sphincter. This refers to variation in tonic pressure relative to positional orientation in the sphincter (i.e., posterior-anterior, lateral). This is observed in both normal subjects and those who have been laryngectomized (Welch, Gates, et al., 1979). However, it appears that radial pressure asymmetries decrease with removal of laryngeal cartilage associated with total laryngectomy. Welch, Gates, et al. (1979) were also careful to specify that while their measures (Welch, Gates, et al., 1979; Welch, Luckmann, et al., 1979) were noted to be approximately twice that noted by Winans et al. (1974) this difference was most likely best related to methodological issues. Based on their findings and in contrast to others, Welch, Gates, et al. (1979, p. 808) stated:

> It appears that residual sphincter tension after laryngectomy plays no role in the acquisition of esophageal speech. Unfortunately, this makes it unlikely that a simple procedure such as myotomy of the sphincter muscle would be of benefit for patients with high pressures who were unable to master esophageal air charging.

Thus, controversy continued to exist regarding the potential effects of a hypertonic or hypotonic UES.

Another manometric study conducted by Bozymski and Pharr (1972) suggested

that lower manometric pressures were always associated with good as opposed to poor esophageal speakers as judged through a closed-set multiple choice intelligibility test. Pressure measures between "good" and "poor" speakers were found to differ by 27%. Unfortunately, clear operational definitions of how speakers were classified by proficiency level were not provided.

In a prospective study of 10 subjects diagnosed with laryngeal carcinoma and who eventually underwent total laryngectomy, Hanks et al. (1981) evaluated esophageal motility using manometry. Measures were obtained from subjects preoperatively, at 2 weeks postlaryngectomy, and at 6 months postsurgery. Based on data obtained, upper esophageal sphincter resting pressures decreased by almost half from measures obtained preoperatively and 2 weeks postoperatively (24.5 ± 4 versus 13.5 ± 2 mm Hg). Hanks et al. (1981) also noted that this change was maintained at six months postlaryngectomy. This trend of pressure reduction between the pre- and postlaryngectomy measures was also noted for measures of mean peak upper esophageal sphincter pressures (37.5 ± 5.9 versus 21.7 ± 2.7 mm Hg).

The combined data presented by Hanks et al. (1981) suggest that changes in esophageal motility will be evidenced immediately in the postlaryngectomy period. Further changes in the status of the esophageal sphincter apparently are not, however, evidenced at more lengthy periods postoperatively. It seems, therefore, that there is some merit to the interpretation offered by Sandberg (1970). Specifically, Sandberg (1970) suggested that for those patients who do not experience any complications in wound healing, the "early" training of esophageal voice may be beneficial. Sandberg (1970, p. 127) posits this suggestion based on his belief that:

> Early training exposes the wound area to function (tension and strain) at a time when function improves the appropriate

differentiation of the newly formed healing tissue.

Others have suggested that, in general, function of the reconstructed upper esophageal region is markedly different from that noted for normal individuals (Davis, Vincent, Shapshay, & Strong, 1982; Kirchner et al., 1963; Sandberg, 1970). Sandberg (1970) has shown that intraluminal pressure measures obtained from individuals who have been laryngectomized are altered substantially from normal individuals. This includes relaxation and contraction pressures, as well as the overall resting tone of the PE sphincter (Sandberg, 1970). Again, substantial individual variability in patient performance seems to be characteristic of postlaryngectomy esophageal sphincter function.

In summary, although the literature does convey the presence of a consistent trend in manometric data relative to postsurgical changes in function of the upper esophageal region, no clear unifying patterns appear to exist or can be discerned from the data. Careful consideration of these data in a more temporal manner would seem to have important clinical implications for the speech-language pathologist. Further, manometric data obtained and reported by numerous researchers may be susceptible to the influences of particular methodological variables (e.g., directional orientation of the pressure sensing probe, fidelity of recording equipment, structural inconsistencies within the upper esophageal sphincter, etc.).

Influence of Esophageal Function on Esophageal Voice Production

Interest in Postlaryngectomy Esophageal Function

A considerable body of information on the functional capability of the esophagus and related structures (i.e., cricopharyngeus, inferior constrictor muscles, etc.) for use as a vicarious voicing source can be found in the literature across several disciplines. Inquiry has led to discussions of success and failure rates associated with the acquisition of esophageal speech as a mode of alaryngeal communication. As information related to the comparative percentages of success and failure in acquiring esophageal voice emerged, esophageal function generated even greater interest (Diedrich, 1968; Diedrich & Youngstrom, 1966; Gates, Ryan, & Cantu, 1982; Snidecor, 1978). This interest almost always led to questions of why some laryngectomized individuals could not produce the "first" esophageal sound, or for some of those who could, why this ability could not be expanded to meet functional communicative needs (Berlin, 1963; Diedrich & Youngstrom, 1966; Shanks, 1986a; Snidecor, 1978a). However, contradictory information exists concerning esophageal function in those who are laryngectomized.

Shipp (1970) evaluated electromyographic (EMG) activity of the *cricopharyngeus* muscle and the *inferior pharyngeal constrictor* in 18 male laryngectomized speakers to assess patterns of motoric activity associated with esophageal speech. Data indicated that 17 of the 18 speakers demonstrated a similar pattern of muscular activity associated with insufflation of the esophagus. This pattern involved activity in one or both of the muscles under study. In contrast, no specific pattern of activity was found to exist during the phonatory stage (i.e., air expulsion) of the esophageal voicing process. Regarding the variability in EMG activity that was observed, Shipp (1970, pp. 191–192) suggested that:

> Each individual utilizes a method of alaryngeal phonation that is most efficient for him consistent with his postoperative anatomy and physiology.

Shipp (1970) suggested that a given speaker's ability to volitionally "control" these muscles (particularly the cricopharygeus) may serve to differentiate proficiency level. That is, Shipp (1970) believed that adequate speakers may exhibit greater control over both the "velocity and magnitude of pharyngoesophageal muscle contraction" (p. 192) when compared to less proficient speakers. This may then culminate in a poorer speaker's inability to provide sufficient contractile resistance to air insufflated into the esophageal reservoir (Diedrich & Youngstrom, 1966; Shanks, 1986a).

Clearly, the smooth temporal transition across the various stages of esophageal phonation (i.e., injection, prephonatory, phonatory) would appear to influence durational aspects of voice production. It would, therefore, not be unreasonable to assume that these influences would have direct effects on the continuity or "fluency" associated with alaryngeal voice and speech production. Data provided by Shipp (1970) would support unique and individualized patterns of pharyngoesophageal function, at least in the eggressive (phonatory) stage of esophageal function, for individuals who have been laryngectomized.

Differences of opinion regarding what the postsurgical pharyngoesophageal (PE) segment should look like morphologically (Damste, 1979, 1986) and how it must function in order to permit the acquisition and use of esophageal speech is a prominent area of disagreement. For example, Dey and Kirchner (1961) characterized the basis of these differences of opinion regarding the PE segment quite well by stating:

It is believed that the more normal the sphincter, the better the speech. The emphasis has been to reconstruct a tight sphincter in the laryngectomized patient at the time of surgery. (p. 100)

Based on their review of the literature, Dey and Kirchner (1961) observed and reported

that "normal" function of the upper esophageal sphincter was thought to be conducive to the production of esophageal sound. However, these authors observed inconsistencies in this opinion. Specifically, Dey and Kirchner (1961, p. 100) contended that:

The most difficult feature in mastering esophageal speech, however, is not in forming sound, but rather in acquiring the ability to swallow and regurgitate air. It appeared to us (Dey and Kirchner) that a tight sphincter would make this procedure more difficult.[2]

The importance of (Dey & Kirchner, 1961) these statements appear to carry considerable importance in how both surgeons and speech-language pathologists have traditionally viewed the postsurgical *pharyngoesophageal* (PE) system (Diedrich & Youngstrom, 1966; Lindsay, Morgan, & Wepman, 1944).

From a clinical perspective, credence was given to the possibility that lack of motivation or desire might not account for all "failed" esophageal speakers (Shanks, 1979, 1986a). Rather, an anatomical and physiological basis may provide a more plausible explanation. Contrary to the opinion expressed by Hunt (1964), not all laryngectomized individuals can easily acquire functional esophageal speech if they only have the "will to learn" (p. 393). Although desire and motivation which emanates from the "psyche" certainly play a critical role in development of esophageal voice, changes in the "soma" (e.g., function of the upper esophageal sphincter) also contribute substantially to a patient's final outcome (Shanks, 1986a).

Snidecor (1978) clearly pointed to the importance of physiologically manipulating the sphincter to charge the esophageal reservoir for esophageal voice production by stating:

---

[2]The term "swallow" is implied to refer to any method of air injection into the esophageal reservoir. For a brief discussion of the controversy surrounding the use of this term, the reader is referred to Keith and Shanks (1983, pp. 129–130).

The fundamental act in learning esophageal speech is the charging and releasing of air from the esophagus, and the most difficult aspect of this two-sided problem for most patients is that of getting air into the esophagus. (p. 159)

It is, therefore, essential that the surgeon and speech-language pathologist consider potential anatomical and physiological reasons that might underlie failure to acquire esophageal voice. All patients who fail to acquire esophageal voice *may not* be casualties of a lack of motivation.

Failure to Acquire Serviceable Esophageal Voice

Regardless of the underlying reason for a patient's failure to acquire esophageal voice, many laryngectomized individuals are unable to acquire "serviceable" esophageal speech for basic communication purposes. Although "voice" per se may be obtained, it either cannot be generated in a consistent and reliable manner (Berlin, 1963) or cannot be extended temporally to functionally serve the patient. Multiple factors may, therefore, influence a patient's success or failure (Damste, 1986; Diedrich & Youngstrom, 1966; Duguay, 1977; Gardner, 1971; Zwitman, 1986). What is clear is that the following proposition offered by Hunt (1964) may be overly simplistic. Hunt (1964, p. 391) wrote that:

It would seem that all that is necessary for production of speech is an air reservoir, the esophagus, and unknown vibrating structures; possibly the mouth of the esophagus and hypopharynx.[3]

Although Hunt's (1964) comment forms the foundation for "alaryngeal" speech, a rather complex set of events ultimately constitutes whether a given patient can produce "esophageal" sound and develop it for communicative purposes. In essence, esophageal voice and speech may be viewed as the patient's Holy Grail when contrasted to buccal and/or pharyngeal speech (Weinberg & Westerhouse, 1971, 1973).

It is the integrity of anatomical structures and their complex physiologic function and interplay that underlie success in acquiring esophageal speech. This relationship would appear to influence and contribute (at least to some degree) to the level of success and/or proficiency that a given speaker is able to achieve with his or her esophageal speech production. This includes a variety of attributes that may constitute intelligibility, as well as acceptability features that underlie esophageal "voice quality" (Smith, Weinberg, Feth, & Horii, 1978).

Does Normal Esophageal Function Influence Acquisition of Esophageal Voice?

Questions about differences between the normal esophageal system and its function and that exhibited by the individual who undergoes total laryngectomy have been discussed frequently in relation to the success or failure to acquire esophageal voice. This concern has been extended to include a variety of issues evolving from postsurgical changes in esophageal anatomy, and hence, the physiology of the esophageal mechanism (Damste, 1986; Diedrich & Youngstrom, 1966; Zwitman, 1986). A classic statement offered by Kallen (1934) has been frequently referenced in regard to the postsurgical status of the esophageal sphincter or pseudoglottis.

---

[3]The suggestion by Hunt (1964) would also appear to indicate that any alternative voicing source would be sufficient for communicative purposes. However, in the case of intrinsic methods of laryngeal speech, the PE segment is the only acceptable vicarious generation site. Buccal and pharyngeal speech (as alluded to by Hunt) have been shown to be characterized by "distinct vocal liabilities" (Weinberg & Westerhouse, 1971) and undesirable as an alaryngeal method of speech production (Weinberg & Westerhouse, 1973).

Kallen's comments explicitly focused on the potential relationship between the care with which postlaryngectomy reconstruction was undertaken and the functioning of the postsurgical esophageal voicing mechanism. Kallen (1934) suggested that if the surgeon were to maintain the maximum amount of tissue permitted in the presence of adequate oncologic safety margins, the possibility of utilizing the postsurgical system as a vicarious voicing source could be enhanced. Specifically, Kallen (1934, p. 502) stated:

> Every muscle, or muscle remnant, may serve as the basis of the development of a pseudoglottis. Many a striking case of pseudovoice owes its development to the hand of the watchful surgeon.

Thus, the postoperative *structural and functional consequences of surgical reconstruction* may be viewed as an important determinant of esophageal speech potential. Although the potential contribution(s) of psychological factors may play a significant role in some patients, structure has historically been accepted to play a fundamental role in the success or failure of postlaryngectomy voice acquisition.

Continuing Controversies Regarding Esophageal Function

The structure and function of the normal and postsurgical esophageal sphincter remains of interest to speech-language pathologists who work with individuals who have undergone a total laryngectomy. Despite considerable information on esophageal function in normal and laryngectomized individuals, controversy continues to exist on what form of physiologic behavior facilitates esophageal voice production. There is no consensus whether it is the "normal" or "abnormal" functioning of the esophageal sphincter that facilitates or disrupts its utility for the acquisition and

production of serviceable esophageal voice. The re-emergence of such anatomical-physiological questions in the "modern era" of postlaryngectomy voice rehabilitation was certainly enhanced by the development and use of the tracheoesophageal puncture technique and voice prosthesis (Singer & Blom, 1980).

Observations relative to this pulmonary powered method of "esophageal" voice production (i.e., *tracheoesophageal voice*) have offered new insights into the function and dysfunction of the esophageal sphincter (Chodosh et al., 1984; Doyle, 1985; McGarvey & Weinberg, 1984; Singer & Blom, 1981; Singer et al., 1986; Weinberg, Horii, Blom, & Singer, 1982). Specifically, the observation of what Singer and Blom (1981) termed "pharyngoesophageal spasm" has led to medically based interventions to eliminate the apparent "spasm" (Chodosh et al., 1984; Singer, 1988; Singer et al., 1986). However, questions persist regarding whether a normal or abnormal functional response by the PE segment creates this problem.

Summary

This chapter has presented information on normal esophageal function, as well as that which occurs postlaryngectomy. Additionally, continuing controversies surrounding the potential relationship between esophageal function and postsurgical esophageal voice acquisition have been discussed. It is felt that the clinician must have an appreciation of the basic function of the normal and postsurgical esophageal region. What is often lost is an appreciation for the number of variables that may affect its function. That is, when one views a "system" he or she must consider not only the "parts" which comprise it, but also the interactive contributions of each component within the system (Moon & Weinberg, 1987). Clinicians may also neglect nonstructural variables (e.g., age, effort level, stress, etc.) that influence esophageal function (Shanks, 1986a; Simpson et al., 1972). The speech-language pathologist should also avoid broad assumptions that "high pressure" or "low pressure" in the upper esophageal sphincter or particular methods of surgical reconstruction will subsequently result in specific patterns of change that affect (either negatively or positively) esophageal voice production (Robe et al., 1956; Simpson et al., 1972).

Suggestions which emphasize that factors such as the specific length, shape, or level of the postsurgical "pseudoglottis" may coincide with successful acquisition of esophageal speech must be examined through additional research (Daou et al., 1984). More detailed evaluations are mandatory given the rather considerable heterogeneity that exists among individuals who undergo total laryngectomy.

Conclusion

Esophageal Speech

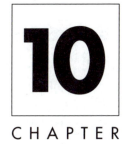

10

CHAPTER

Historically, considerable attention has been directed toward use of an intrinsic postsurgical pseudoglottis for alaryngeal voicing in those who undergo laryngectomy. The term *intrinsic* refers to the fact that the speaker is able to utilize some internal, anatomical structure as an alaryngeal voice source. Although several intrinsic sources of postsurgical alaryngeal voicing have been reported (Finkbeiner, 1978), buccal and pharyngeal speech being the most notable (Weinberg & Westerhouse, 1971, 1973), only the upper esophageal sphincter appears to meet basic requirements for this purpose. That is, use of this system provides greater utility to the speaker as opposed to other intrinsic sources.

As noted in the previous chapter, the term *esophageal* may be a misnomer. While the esophagus serves as the air reservoir, it is the tissue that forms the upper esophageal sphincter that serves as the vicarious voicing source for esophageal speakers (Damste, 1986; Diedrich & Youngstrom, 1966; Gardner, 1971; Singer, 1988). Thus, a more regionally centered terminology evolved, one that includes components of both the pharynx and esophagus. Since the early reports of Negus (1929) and Jackson and Jackson (1939) use of the term *pharyngoesophgeal* (PE) segment has gained widespread usage in the literature on postsurgical voice for those who undergo laryngectomy (Diedrich & Youngstrom, 1966; Gardner, 1971; Singer, 1988). The purpose of this chapter is to address issues related to esophageal speech and esophageal speech training. This includes a discussion of the PE segment, as well as a variety of factors that influence its structure and function. This chapter also provides detailed information of the mechanism of esophageal speech and protocol for teaching this method of alaryngeal speech.

The Pharyngoesophageal Segment

In his excellent review on the mechanism of esophageal speech, Diedrich (1968) used the term "pharyngoesophageal" to describe the anatomical region used for the generation of a postlaryngectomy voicing source. The term pharyngoesophageal appears to have considerable merit in that it specifies a region or zone of function. By adopting this broader anatomical description, it is implied that one particular structure or area may not be used consistently across speakers. Further, by referencing general regions of the postsurgical conduit one is not biased to assume that only a single muscular or tissue structure provides the alaryngeal voice source. It is, however, essential to realize that alaryngeal voice generation may be a product of multiple sources of vibration (Diedrich & Youngstrom, 1966) and that the structures involved may vary somewhat between individuals. This is particularly helpful given the long standing assumption that the source for alaryngeal voice, the *neoglottis*, is the cricopharyngeus muscle.

The cricopharyngeus muscle is best described as the band of muscle located in the transitional region between the lower pharynx and the upper esophagus. It has been suggested that the source of esophageal phonation is primarily derived through response of the cricopharyngeus muscle (Damste, 1958; Levin, 1962; Robe et al., 1956; van den Berg & Moolenaar-Bijl, 1959; Vrticka & Svoboda, 1961). Although some controversy exists regarding whether the cricopharyngeus is a distinct muscular structure, as opposed to a structurally distinct segment of another muscular structure (e.g., the inferior pharyngeal constrictor muscle), it is clear that muscular fibers are present in this transitional anatomical region (Singer, 1988; Weinberg, 1982; Zwitman, 1986). Muscular fibers from the inferior constrictor muscle are, however, also closely associated with the cricopharyngeus (Zemlin, 1988, p. 274). Therefore, the potential source of the intrinsic alaryngeal voice method that has traditionally be called esophageal speech may be best identified and described as the *pharyngoesophageal* (PE) segment. Consequently, the variability of the postlaryngectomy voicing source across speakers may be related to the fact that the alaryngeal voice source may emanate from a reconstructed region that differs substantially from individual to individual. Several researchers have attempted to measure the diversity of this postsurgical region.

The Relationship of Surgery to the Acquisition of Esophageal Voice

Information provided previously in this text has outlined the substantial degree of alteration in anatomy following total laryngectomy. Because of the type and extent of surgical resection that is required for management of laryngeal carcinoma, considerable reconstruction takes place even in procedures referred to as "simple laryngectomy" (Silver, 1981). This is particulary true in extended laryngectomy (Silver, 1981). Once the larynx is removed and the primary airway (i.e., the trachea) repositioned in the anterior midline of the neck, reconstruction of the pharynx and upper esophageal regions are undertaken. This requires that usually discontinuous tissues that comprise this anatomical region (e.g., the pharyngeal constrictor muscles) be opposed and sutured together. Altered anatomical structures and mucosa that are a result of surgery, in additional to other aspects of the pharyngeal anatomy, must also be reconstructed to provide continuity in the pharynx proper. The reconstruction is maintained as contiguous with the superior aspect of the esophagus. Thus, the extent of the surgical defect once the larynx is removed dictates that a reconstructed pharyngeal and esophageal conduit be created.

Consequences of Reconstruction

Reconstruction undoubtedly results in considerable variability in both residual anatomical structures, and perhaps most importantly, their postsurgical physiologic function. The literature does not, however, appear to address this potential relationship sufficiently. Consideration of this issue may offer important insights into numerous problems that may be encountered by the laryngectomized patient and rehabilitation specialists who provide treatment. The maintenance and retention of anatomic structures that may ultimately be used as a pseudoglottis has been described frequently in the literature. Care in the preservation of essential tissues, those which may serve as an intrinsic alaryngeal voicing source, has been both implied and explicitly outlined by many (Damste, 1979; Finkbeiner, 1978, p. 67; Kallen 1934; Negus, 1929; Singer, 1988).

Surgical removal of the larynx necessitates reconstruction of the residual tissues of the pharynx and upper esophagus in a highly individualized manner. Careful review of case summaries appearing in the clinical literature support the notion that no two individuals who undergo laryngectomy are left with the same structural or functional integrity. This has considerable importance from a clinical perspective as it relates to postlaryngectomy voice and speech rehabilitation. Although unique aspects of postsurgical anatomy, physiology, and neurophysiology have an obvious influence on the individual's rehabilitative potential and progress (Berlin, 1963; Weinberg, 1982),

other factors (e.g., age, general health, etc.) may further confound these more clinically "salient" aspects of laryngectomy. However, careful consideration of anatomic, physiologic, and neurophysiologic substrates that are precursors to the successful acquisition of esophageal voice deserve serious attention.

Esophageal Voice and Speech

Variability of the PE Segment

Despite substantial information to the contrary, it is at times implied that the successful acquisition of esophageal voice and speech postlaryngectomy is a result of (1) at least near-normal functioning of the upper esophageal sphincter, and (2) the individual's ability to access and utilize a vicarious, postsurgical anatomical structure that is relatively invariant from individual to individual. Attempts to explain the mechanism of esophageal voicing is often fraught with this simplicity. Yet there are many reports in the literature that suggest that the postsurgical esophageal voicing source is indeed extremely variable. This variability is manifested in form, function, and location. Some investigations have even suggested that this voicing source may migrate with increased practice and, possibly, that more than one "alaryngeal" site of voicing may exist.

Damste and Lerman (1969) have noted that observations on the "different forms of the pharyngo-esophageal junction" (p. 347) may be accounted for by multiple variables. The most intriguing variable is that which may occur over time with practice, and which may result in "selective activation" of the musculature associated with esophageal voice. Specifically, Damste and Lerman (1969, p. 348) state:

The fact that pharyngeal voice can be re-educated into esophageal voice is proof that individuals can learn to differentiate constriction at various levels.

Although this statement may be true (Torgerson & Martin, 1976), it assumes that afferent (sensory) feedback from structures that comprise the intrinsic alaryngeal source is available to the patient. Unfortunately, confirmation of this assumption is lacking. Further, several reports have also suggested that nonanatomical structures such as mucus may form the essential element which underlies the creation of pseudoglottal voice production (Brewer, Gould, & Casper, 1974; Daou et al., 1984). Thus, it is only natural to ask questions about variability and the essence of the postsurgical sound source in esophageal speakers.

Damste (1979) has addressed questions pertaining to postsurgical anatomical differences and their potential relationship to problems in acquisition of esophageal voice. He specifically notes that the outcome of voice rehabilitation may hinge on both the extent of surgical reconstruction and the "woundhealing" process. Regarding the extent of surgical reconstruction, Damste (1979) was quite explicit about the anatomical form of the pseudoglottis stating that the vibratory segment "can vary from wide to narrow, from long to short, and its shape can be flat, round, and prominent" (Damste, 1979, p. 55).

Diedrich and Youngstrom (1966) also noted that "tremendous individual differences" (p. 21) are found to exist in the *morphology* of the pseudoglottis. They suggested further that these individual differences were not only observed between different speakers who participated in their investigation (Diedrich & Youngstrom, 1966), but also may be observed in association with specific tasks (e.g., swallowing, phonating, blowing, etc.). Thus, morphological structure and function cannot be viewed in a discrete or static fashion. This has direct implications for the clinical rehabilitative process and may

account for discrepancies in the successful acquisition of esophageal speech (Berlin, 1963; Gardner, 1971; Weinberg, 1985).

The literature also suggests that the vibratory (i.e., PE) segment may be found in a variety of anatomical locations. The majority of information indicates that its location is typically identified between the landmarks of cervical vertebrae 4 and 6 (i.e., C4-C6). Diedrich and Youngstrom (1966) reported a location in their subjects that ranged from C3 to C7, although most were found in the C5-C6 region. These findings indicate that the intrinsic alaryngeal voice source associated with esophageal speech may vary across a variety of internal structural dimensions, namely size, length, and configuration. It may also vary in relation to *where the primary structure exists* anatomically, as well as anatomical structures or regions with which it is most closely associated. For example, one individual may exhibit a postsurgical alaryngeal voice source that is wide, short, and flat (Damste, 1979), and which is located relatively lower in the reconstructed area in association with mostly esophageal fibers. Another individual may exhibit very different structural morphology which is located in a very different area and, as such, related to very different muscular or tissue structures.

Diedrich and Youngstrom (1966) assessed the length of the pharyngoesophageal (PE) segment during phonation using a cinefluorographic method and found the average length to be 21 mm. The average length of the PE segment was found to be 29 mm when assessed by these same investigators using a "spot film" x-ray analysis method. This suggests that the potential area used for alaryngeal voice production may be quite variable; it also suggests that areas of greater or lesser constriction within the segment may vary. One would assume that reconstructed areas of the pharyngoesophageal region would often be characterized by various degrees of tissue continuity, opposition, compliance and/or tension. Many summaries of surgical resection and reconstruction note that the reconstructed areas postlaryngectomy are not smooth and continuous, but quite tortuous. This type of inconsistency increases the possibility that the location and form of the pseudoglottis will vary, in addition to the possibility that more than a single anatomical site will be utilized for alaryngeal voicing purposes. Thus, variability both within and across speakers is likely to be observed.

Finkbeiner (1978) addressed issues pertaining to the site of the postlaryngectomy pseudoglottis and acknowledged the general lack of agreement that exists on this topic. While Finkbeiner noted that a consensus opinion seemed to indicate that the cricopharyngeus muscle was the most typical source of intrinsic alaryngeal voice production, she also pointed out that many anatomic structures may serve this postlaryngectomy function. Sensitivity to individual differences in structural integrity and function is, therefore, not a new concept in relation to individuals who undergo laryngectomy.

Damste (1979, 1986) has considered the evolving nature of the reconstructed upper aerodigestive pathway from the point of laryngectomy until healing is complete. Not only may variance be noted in regard to structural remnants which exist postsurgically, but these remnants may change in the early postoperative period. This information should be contemplated collectively with information on the rate of acquisition for esophageal voice and speech skills (Berlin, 1963). Does the possibility exist that changes in the development and/or refinement of particular esophageal speech skills are influenced by aspects of tissue healing over the early postoperative period (e.g., the development of scar tissue, etc.)? If so, such changes may not be amenable to change even with extensive esophageal voice treatment regimens.

Clinical Implications of PE Segment Variability

Based on information from the literature, some degree of inconsistency exists with regard to what structure(s) form the pseudoglottis in individuals who undergo laryngectomy. Although this inconsistency may result in confusion for some, it most definitely exemplifies the need for a more open-minded view of the postlaryngectomy system. Variability in the structure and function of the postlaryngectomy voice source provides an interesting view of this remarkable compensatory voicing source. Yet, clinical methods cannot and should not necessarily be dictated by the morphological details of the vibratory source. This is based on two primary factors.

The first deals directly with the simple notion that each patient will most certainly have unique postsurgical anatomy and physiology (Duguay, 1979; Shipp, 1970; Zwitman, 1986). As such, it should make no difference whether the individual uses the cricopharyngeus, portions of the inferior constrictor muscle, or any other related muscular structure for generation of an intrinsic alaryngeal voice.[1] If the clinician can clearly distinguish that the sound being heard *is not* buccal or pharyngeal in nature, the only question need rest with further facilitation, development, and refinement of the alaryngeal source (Amster, 1986; Gardner, 1971). The second factor deals with voice and speech rehabilitation as a process. This process will likely ebb and flow as healing progresses and the individual demonstrates what he or she can and cannot do (Damste, 1979, 1986).

---

[1]Excluding buccal and pharyngeal sources.

Although information in the literature does suggest that acquisition patterns for those who will likely learn serviceable esophageal speech may be quite rapid (Berlin, 1963; Gates, Ryan, Cantu, & Hearne, 1982; Gates, Ryan, Cooper, Lawlis et al., 1982), there is also information to suggest that esophageal skills may continue to develop over time (Palmer, 1970; Snidecor, 1978a).

The Mechanism of Esophageal Speech

Methods of Air Insufflation

Information on esophageal voice and speech indicates that two general classes of air insufflation for alaryngeal voicing purposes may be used. These two classes of esophageal air insufflation are defined by the primary physical principle that underlies the insufflation process. Using this classification system, the processes are best classed as (1) *positive pressure approaches* and (2) a *negative pressure approach* (Diedrich, 1968; Diedrich & Youngstrom, 1966; Gardner, 1971; Snidecor, 1978; Weinberg, 1983a). Regardless of which method of insufflation is utilized, the speaker must effect a change in pressure between the oropharyngeal cavity and that of the esophageal reservoir. By accomplishing this goal, natural physical principles come into play in an attempt to equalize relative differences in disparate air pressures.

For one to produce esophageal voice using a positive pressure approach, several prerequisite capacities must be met. Using a sequential model, the individual must (1) be able to trap air within the oral cavity, (2) be able to volitionally create an increase in air pressure above the pseudoglottal sphincter, (3) be able to create an increase in oral-pharyngeal pressure which is sufficient to overcome the resistance of the pseudoglottal (PE) sphincter, (4) be able to volitionally compress the contents of the esophageal reservoir, and (5) be able to overcome the resistance of the esophageal reservoir in an egressive (outflowing) fashion (Diedrich & Youngstrom, 1966; Gardner, 1971; Snidecor, 1978).

Although this simplified sequence of events captures the basic elements necessary to achieve intrinsic alaryngeal (esophageal) voice production, this sequence is not invariant. Further, aspects related to what occurs between each successive stage, particularly in respect to temporal intervals, will offer substantial benefit to the speaker and the listener. Rapid insufflation and expulsion of air provides the most basic element of esophageal speech fluency (Duguay, 1977; Snidecor, 1978). Again, the above sequence of events assumes an *active maneuver* by the individual to increase oral-pharyngeal air pressure as an initial step in the sequence. The sequence may, however, change if other methods of esophageal reservoir air insufflation are used by the speaker.

The primary methods of esophageal air insufflation based on positive pressure manipulations between the oropharynx and esophagus include the glossal or glossopharyngeal press (Weinberg & Bosma, 1970), stop consonant injection (Moolenaar-Bijl, 1953; van den Berg, Moolenaar-Bijl, & Damste, 1958) and what may be best described as a modified swallow maneuver (Diedrich & Youngstrom, 1966). Additionally, several "variations on a theme" (i.e., combined methods) have been observed clinically with some provided in the literature (c.f., Gately, 1976; Lauder, 1989).

Difficulties in Esophageal Voice Acquisition

Duguay (1979) suggested that inability by the patient to successful acquire postlaryngectomy oral communication may be due to numerous factors. This includes anatomic, physiologic, psychologic, and sociologic factors (Aronson, 1980). Ultimately, however, the inability to acquire functional esophageal voice and speech is the result of the individual's difficulty with achieving several critical behaviors. Although Duguay (1979) has identified four specific behavioral inabilities which may impact the patient's success in acquiring esophageal voice, all fully center around the functional capacity and control of the PE sphincter and the esophageal reservoir (Shanks, 1986a).

To learn esophageal speech, the patient must be able to inject air into the esophageal reservoir; must be able to maintain this injected air for at least a brief period of time; must be able to eject air from the esophagus; and, finally, the individual must be able to exert *some volitional control* over the PE segment. While many might view these four behaviors as "physiologic" in nature, the combined act of injecting and ejecting air into and from the esophagus is clearly influenced by factors other than anatomy and physiology (Shanks, 1986a; Snidecor, 1978a). Duguay (1979) has explicitly stated what many other clinicians have noted intuitively, namely, that psychological and sociological factors may be more important to the acquisition of esophageal voice and speech

than the postsurgical anatomy and physiology of the pseudoglottis. Thus, both physiologic, psychologic, and sociologic influences must be considered.

Stages of Esophageal Voice Acquisition and Monitoring Progress

Snidecor (1978a) suggested that nine distinct stages of speech reacquisition exist. These stages were deemed by Snidecor to represent "levels of achievement rather than lessons as such" (Snidecor, 1978a, p. 183). However, the elements which comprise the nine levels have direct consequences on how the patient progresses through therapy and what their proficiency level will be. A summary of these stages is presented in Table 10–1.

Monitoring Patient Progress

Berlin (1963) carefully addressed the importance of measuring a patient's progress during early esophageal speech training. The emphasis of Berlin's system of measurement was directed at four essential skills that were required in the introductory

TABLE 10–1.
Stages of Esophageal Speech Development.

1. Get air in—get air out.
2. Produce plosive consonants, vowels and diphthongs.
3. Voice simple, useful, monosyllabic words.
4. Voice two-syllable words.
   a. initially with one air charge per syllable.
   b. terminally with both syllables on a single air charge.
5. Voice simple phrases with a single air charge.
6. Practice articulation and connected speech with emphasis on vowels, diphthongs, and consonants.
7. Stress is achieved by changes in loudness, pitch, quality, and time.
8. Use "active" conversation.
9. The achievement of satisfactory rate usually results along with the mastery of the previous eight stages.

Source: From Snidecor, J.C. (1978). *Speech rehabilitation of the laryngectomized* (pp. 183–193), Springfield, IL, Charles C. Thomas, reprinted with permission.

stages of esophageal speech acquisition. According to Berlin, the underlying rationale for the four areas of measurement sought to "quantify, rather than describe qualitatively" (p. 42) the patient's ability to attain foundation behaviors that could then be used to further develop more refined esophageal speech capabilities.

Specifically, quantitative measures of the following four behaviors were gathered from individuals who attempted to learn esophageal speech as a method of alaryngeal communication: (1) the ability to phonate reliably on demand, (2) maintenance of a short latency between inflation of the esophagus and vocalization, (3) maintenance of an adequate duration of phonation, and (4) the ability to sustain phonation during articulation.

Teaching the Patient to Insufflate the Esophageal Reservoir for Alaryngeal Voice Production

The acquisition of the first esophageal sound for the laryngectomized patient finds its foundation in a single origin—the ability to "charge" the esophagus with air (Snidecor, 1978a). This air supply then becomes the power source for egressive flow of air through the PE segment. Without air injection, the generation of an esophageal tone is not possible. Successful air injection requires that two distinct components can be manipulated by the patient. The components are (1) the ability to increase pressure within the oropharyngeal cavity in a consistent and reliable manner, and (2) the ability to decrease the mechanical (muscular) resistance in the tonically closed PE segment (Shanks, 1986a). It is hoped that these two components can be coordinated in some fashion as insufficient air pressure and/or an inadequate capacity to relax the PE segment can prove deleterious to injection of air into the esophagus. Hence, the ability to produce esophageal voice is decreased.

Methods of Air Injection

Although some disagreement regarding how many methods of air intake exist, Snidecor (1978a) has stated that several methods may be used in combination. Some of the best esophageal speakers have been shown to be both "injectors" and "inhalers" (Diedrich & Youngstrom 1966; Snidecor, 1978). Regardless of what method(s) is/are used in the early stages of voice reacquisition, it is imperative that the clinician conduct sessions in a highly structured manner. Sessions need not be lengthy; however, they must be full regardless of their duration.

One of the most frequently used vehicles for determining if the patient has a sense of what he or she is trying to achieve during esophageal speech training is to ask if he or she has ever voluntarily produced a "belch" (Keith, 1977; Lauder, 1989). If the patient is able to achieve this goal without direction, the potential for developing this preliminary skill into a more advanced and refined one is good. In patients who do not recall ever having done this, or who are unable to replicate this behavior, several methods of instruction should be undertaken (Keith, 1977). Instruction must be tailored to meet the needs of a particular patient and, thus, may vary from very indirect instruction to that which is quite direct (Duguay, 1977).

Esophageal Air Insufflation: Methods of Instruction

As mentioned earlier, two general approaches can be used to insufflate the esophagus, positive and negative pressure maneuvers. For the purposes of teaching esophageal insufflation and the first esophageal sound, use of *positive pressure* approaches may be best. This does not imply that the clinician should disregard consideration of the negative pressure approaches (the inhalation method). Yet use of positive pressure maneuvers is recommended because three specific facilitation techniques may be utilized and because it is frequently a more "salient" method for the patient to appreciate from a mechanical standpoint. Snidecor (1978a) posited that three distinct methods of injection were used by esophageal speakers: (1) "the suction breathing or inhalation method" (p. 159), (2) "air injection by tongue and related structures," and (3) "the gloss-opharyngeal press or plosive-injection method." Regardless of method, one injection method may serve as a facilitator of other methods, and, therefore, more comprehensive skill in insufflating the esophagus may be acquired with practice. Thus, use of the plosive consonant, glossopharyngeal press, or modified swallow techniques are recommended in the early training stages.

Plosive Consonant Injection

The *plosive consonant injection* (Damste, 1958; Moolenaar-Bijl, 1953; Moolenaar-Bijl et al., 1958) technique is a relatively easy approach to teach the patient. This method of esophageal insufflation also provides flexibility in training in that a variety of stimulus items may be used. By varying the phonetic construction of the "target sound" repeated trials of the same task can be avoided. Trials are always initiated by using a consonant-vowel (CV) context.

The simple principle that underlies the plosive consonant injection method is based on the fact that plosive sound production requires a build up of intraoral pressure. This is particularly true in contexts were a voiceless plosive is present (Warren, 1982), particularly in the syllable-initial position (Diedrich, 1968; Diedrich & Youngstrom, 1966). If sufficient intraoral pressure can be achieved in an "air tight"

system (i.e., no leakage through the velopharyngeal port or lips),[2] this pressure has the capacity to overcome the muscular resistance offered by the tonically closed PE segment. As Diedrich and Youngstrom (1966, p. 37) have noted, the injection of air in such a positive pressure approach "implies a hermetic seal, and velopharyngeal closure must be made." Thus, if intraoral air pressure can exceed that of PE segment resistance, oral air will transgress the sphincter and move into the esophageal reservoir.

Stimulus Consideration When Using the Consonant Injection Method of Injection

From a strict methodological perspective consonant injection methods have stressed use of voiceless stop-plosives (Moolenaar-Bijl, 1953) in what appears to be a somewhat isolated form. Pairing of the plosive with a vowel can be beneficial. That is, it may permit syllabic production of esophageal sound as opposed to sound production as an isolated event following the production of the consonant. Use of the plosive in the initial consonant position may also be the best starting point in the training program because of its high potential of "evoking" voice (Shanks, 1986a). It may also have direct effects on a given patient's ability to produce voicing contrasts in that the temporal sequence of events can be controlled (Connor, Hamlet, & Joyce, 1985; Doyle, Danhauer, & Reed, 1988; Doyle & Danhauer, 1986; Doyle & Haaf, 1989; Haaf & Doyle, 1986; Sacco, Mann, & Schultz, 1967; Shanks, 1986a).

In addition to plosives, clinical experience has shown that use of other phonemic elements such as affricatives (/tʃ/ and /dʒ/), and potentially even some sibilants

---

[2]Berlin (1964) has suggested that palatal function may be impaired following laryngectomy, hence, the ability to produce and sustained adequate intraoral pressure levels for esophageal insufflation may be limited in some patients.

and or consonant blends, can facilitate esophageal insufflation (Shanks, 1986a). A variety of stimulus constructions can and should be used in attempting to train the patient to generate his or her first esophageal sound.

The speech-language pathologist should also carefully consider the vowel contained in the consonant-vowel (CV) pairing. To maintain the focus of early therapy on the patient's ability to successfully inject air into the esophagus, one simple approach involves a structured shift from simple CV syllables (/puh/, /tuh/, /kuh/, into symmetrical CVC stimuli such as "pop," "tot," and so forth.

One issue seldom discussed in an explicit manner relative to consonant injection involves contributions of the tongue musculature to this process. Specifically, pressure build-up within the oropharyngeal cavity requires more than just the entrapment of air (Diedrich, 1968; Duguay, 1977; Snidecor, 1978a). Once air can be trapped and maintained in the sealed (oral) system, some degree of volitional compression must then take place. This compression of the oropharyngeal cavity will result in increasing intraoral pressure levels. Increased pressure is mandatory to overcome PE segment resistance (Diedrich, 1968; Duguay, 1977; Salmon, 1986d, 1986e; Shanks, 1986a) prior to PE segment excitation for voicing.

Stimulus Influence

One of the best methods for meeting the requirement of increased intraoral pressure is a function of the structure itself. For example, consider the following three CV pairings: /pʌ/, /tʌ/, and /kʌ/. In the /p/ stimulus, compression required for injection is primarily accomplished through compression of the lips and cheeks, for /t/ movement of the tongue to the alveolar ridge provides compression, and finally for /k/ compression again may be a primary result of lingual movement and contact

with posterior regions of the oral cavity. From a mechanical perspective, each of these consonant pairs may provide unique advantages and disadvantages for a particular patient.

Duguay (1977) has likened use of the phonemes /p/, /t/, and /k/ to specific methods of air injection. He states that use of /p/ mimics "oral-pharyngeal contraction," /t/ mimics the "glossal press", and finally, /k/ mimics the "glossopharyngeal press" method of injection. Duguay's (1977) suggestion offers an important area of consideration for speech-language pathologists. The production of particular phonemic elements may be facilitated more easily by some methods of injection. Thus, while we may train the patient to use a particular insufflation procedure, the clinician ultimately realizes that the patient has adapted his or her productive system so that injection, and consequently, voice and speech production is increased in its efficiency. This information is consistent with the statement made by Shanks (1986a) that "voicing and articulation are not dichotomous." Shanks (1986a) goes on to say that the clinician must clearly acknowledge the link between articulatory units and esophageal voice production. In fact, the patient's ability to volitionally increase intraoral air pressure influences both articulatory accuracy, as well as providing an added dividend of reinjecting air into the esophagus (Shanks, 1986a).

Nevertheless, the speech clinician is faced with a single discrete goal at this early point of esophageal speech training—namely, the patient must insufflate the esophagus (Snidecor, 1978). Careful clinical consideration of what stimulus constructions might offer the best chance of achieving esophageal insufflation is warranted. This consideration should involve two specific questions: (1) What stimulus is likely to result in the greatest compression of air (i.e., best chance of increasing oropharyngeal pressure)? and (2) What stimulus item can provide the best "feedback" to the patient?

Using the three stop-plosive examples noted earlier, the speech-language pathologist might come to the conclusion that /pʌ/ has the best chance for achieving the greatest degree of compression. However, this phoneme requires considerable strength of associated orofacial musculature and dictates that no leaks exist in the system (Berlin, 1964; Diedrich, 1968). In contrast, /tʌ/ has the potential advantage of providing good sensory feedback to the patient; yet tongue mobility and strength must be intact. Finally, /kʌ/ requires a relatively smaller cavity that needs to be compressed, however, sensory feedback is a limiting factor and velopharyngeal adequacy is again essential (Diedrich & Youngstrom, 1966). What is important about stimulus considerations is that the clinician must explore which phonetic contexts are most appropriate (i.e., successful) for a given patient. Further, an important element of these pairings is related to what vowel is used. Higher vowels may permit increased levels of compression in most instances, and thus, must be explored as possible facilitators of injection.

Other Factors Influencing the Ability to Insufflate the Esophagus

In addition to stimulus considerations, the speech-language pathologist must also be sensitive to nonspeech consequences of training esophageal insufflation. This implies that care must be taken when requesting patients to perform particular tasks designed to increase the possibility of esophageal insufflation. For example, excessive physical effort by the patient during attempt(s) to produce adequate levels of compression may result in the development of extraneous behaviors (Gardner, 1971; Weinberg, 1983a) that will be problematic later on in therapy (e.g., stoma noise, grimacing, abnormal oral posturing, etc.).

Use of excess effort has the potential to affect the tonicity of the PE segment. The patient must exert some control over the PE segment in an effort to relax excessive tonicity, thus, facilitating air insufflation and voice production. This will optimize the response of the PE segment so that air can move through the sphincter into the esophageal reservoir (Diedrich, 1968; Shanks, 1986a). In some patients, it is not unusual to see the initial impetus for development of facial grimaces and other detrimental nonspeech behaviors to have its roots in an overly aggressive therapy program. The speech-language pathologist will, therefore, need to carefully observe the performance of the patient beyond those aspects that are most germane to the therapy protocol (i.e., facilitating esophageal insufflation).

Gardner (1971) has provided one of the most detailed and systematic programs related to the use of plosive consonant injection. He suggested that a sequence of production moving from bilabial, to alveolar, to velar plosives be followed. One of the best methods that can be easily performed involves production of the consonant paired with various vowel entities. It is important that the clinician keep on-line data on whether esophageal insufflation has occurred for any given pairing. Collection of such data permits the clinician to identify the presence of "easy" versus more difficult phonetic contexts. This concern should not be judged as unimportant as each laryngectomized patient exhibits slightly different articulatory physiology postsurgically (Diedrich & Youngstrom 1966). Attention must, therefore, be directed toward identifying the most favorable contexts; this is extremely valuable in early phases of the training program.

Essentially, Gardner (1971) recommends a rather rapid transition from production of the isolated phoneme to its production in a CV pairing and then to single syllable CVCs. Use of CVC stimuli where the final consonant is a plosive may also be structured in a manner so that reinsufflation may occur with production of that consonant. This may then aid patients in the subsequent production they attempt.[3]

Gardner's (1971) program is well-structured and capitalizes on rapid progression through multiple trials of productions. This is perhaps one of the keys to successful esophageal speech training. Specifically, rapid production sequences, particularly in the isolated sound stage (e.g., /p/) may provide an opportunity for small amounts of air to inadvertently transgress the PE segment. If this occurs in a continuous manner, insufflation will continue in an additive manner.

Thus, insufflation of vast volumes of air is not the goal of esophageal voice training protocols[4]; rather, insufflation, regardless of the amount of air, is the key element constituting success. Given the capacity of the esophageal reservoir, which has been estimated at approximately 80 cubic centimeters (cc) of air (van den Berg & Moolenaar-Bijl, 1959), this offers an additional advantage to the patient. That is, while small amounts of air insufflation may indeed be insufficient for the purposes of speech sound production, recurrent injections of the same amount of air will eventually meet a level from which the patient can fully experience and appreciate the egressive, esophageal voicing mechanism. The esophageal reservoir, therefore, need not be charged to maximal capacity in order to function as an alaryngeal (accessory) power source. In fact, several studies have indicated that insufflation to maximum capacity may not be necessary for acceptable levels of speech production (Snidecor, 1978a; Snidecor & Isshiki, 1965).

The egressive flow of air through the PE segment has the most dramatic effects on PE segment function. This suggestion is consistent with a conceptual desire to have the patient inject air into the esophagus in both a direct and indirect manner. Specifically, although initial insufflation may be accomplished using direct, volitionally controlled tongue maneuvers, additional insufflation may also occur indirectly during the process of speech production (i.e., via consonantal injection). This has rather considerable effects on the overall pause time that may exist before recharging the system.

Once previously discussed skills (CV and CVC stimuli) are established, the program presented by Gardner (1971) is then shifted from the plosive-based construction to a stimulus expansion that involves addition of the alveolar sibilant /s/. This involves first asking the patient to produce the isolated /s/ and then placing it in the final consonantal position (e.g., "kiss"). If sibilant production is difficult for the patient, Gardner (1971) suggests that the speech-language pathologist can request production of /s/ by compressing air while the tongue is in contact with the alveolar ridge. This consequently will result in a production of /ts/. Once this is achieved, the patient may then add this construction to the end of a plosive-vowel pair (e.g., "cuts," "cats," etc.). The final stage of this transition in the training program involves pairing /s/ with /p/, /t/, and /k/; thus, the patient is presented with tasks which facilitate injection of air from an /s/-blend context.

The final level of Gardner's (1971) program attempts to train the patient to successfully insufflate the esophagus using additional sounds. Most often, the best success may be found when /s/, /ʃ/, or the unvoiced affricate /tʃ/ are used. Similar to other stages in the esophageal voice training program, the clinician should attempt having the patient produce training stimuli (consonants) in both initial and final phonetic contexts. Training materials have been provided by Gardner (1971), Lauder (1989) and others. However, the speech-language pathologist may wish to develop his or her own lists of stimuli as he or she becomes

---

[3]Examples of word stimuli have been presented by Gardner (1971), Lauder (1989), and others.
[4]Over-insufflation of air into the esophagus may result in air-induced hypertonicity (Henderson, 1983).

more comfortable and experienced in training the laryngectomized patient to insufflate the esophagus for alaryngeal speech acquisition and development.

Pacing Associated with Voice Training

Controlling the speed of stimuli production, or pacing, may offer advantages to some patients. An advantage of clinical pacing that is on the brisk side rests in the fact that patients may not have time in between trials to "posture" their oropharyngeal system in a manner not conducive to insufflation. That is, rapidly sequenced trials may avoid unnecessary generation of PE segment tension. Such increases in tension can prove detrimental to esophageal sound production (Gardner, 1971; Shanks, 1986a).

Pacing also may involve moving rapidly across different stimuli. This may facilitate improved production in patients who demonstrate "generalization." For patients who meet with inconsistent success, rapid pacing may limit the sense of "failure" for more problematic targets. What is important to note is that if one particular sequence cannot be achieved, the speech-language pathologist should move on to the next step *and then return* to the previous step once success has been obtained (Gardner, 1971).

Similarly, use of voiced stop-plosives may in some cases prove to be successful stimuli in that the entire esophageal system may be more relaxed due to lower intraoral pressure levels. Although limited data exist in the literature, many clinicians have reported that use of affricatives provide a very valuable context from which insufflation may occur. Perhaps affricatives provide an advantage in that the pressure build-up is less rapid when compared to stop-plosives and muscular tension may be decreased. Affricates also have the advantage of exhibiting pressure increases over a longer period of time. This may be beneficial to the patient.

The Glossal and Glossopharyngeal Methods of Air Insufflation

Although the *glossal* and *glossopharyngeal press* methods of insufflation are considered distinct maneuvers to facilitate esophageal air insufflation (Weinberg & Bosma, 1970; Diedrich & Youngstrom, 1966), and appear in some reports to differ from the classic description of "plosive-injection" (Moolenaar-Bilj, 1953), clinicians should realize that some patients ultimately develop what might be best described as hybrid methods of injection.

In fact, several authors have provided information that would support use of multiple methods of injection by excellent esophageal speakers (Diedrich & Youngstrom, 1966; Snidecor, 1978a; Snidecor & Isshiki, 1965). A distinction between methods may further emanate from the fact that in the consonant injection technique, a specific speech sound serves to initiate the injection movement. In contrast, other pressure/compression maneuvers which require tongue movement may instruct a specific pattern of movement that has no direct representation to that of speech. Nevertheless, it is important to outline specific details associated with the glossopharyngeal method of injection in hope of understanding basic physiologic processes that occur in the oral cavity prior to esophageal insufflation.

Diedrich and Youngstrom (1966) have noted that two methods of air injection were discerned from cinefluorograms of their experimental speakers. They termed the two methods the *glossal* and the *glossopharyngeal press*. According to Diedrich and Youngstrom (1966), the glossal press involves the following sequence of events:

> The tip of the tongue was in contact with the alveolar ridge and frequently the middle of the tongue contacted the hard and soft palate. The posterior portion of the tongue made a dorsad (backward) movement, but did not touch the posterior pharyngeal wall. Velopharyngeal clo-

sure was always present. The lips may or may not be open. (p. 37)

In contrast, Diedrich and Youngstrom (1966) described the glossopharyngeal press to occur following a different sequence:

> Both the tip and middle portions of the tongue were in contact with the alveolus, hard palate, and soft palate. The posterior portion of the tongue made a dorsad movement contacting the posterior pharyngeal wall. Sometimes the posterior wall made a ventrad movement during this phase. The hypopharyngeal cavity was frequently obliterated by the backward movement of the tongue. The velopharyngeal port was always closed. The lips may or may not be open. (p. 37)

Based on these descriptions, one can appreciate that unique (although one may argue slight) physiologic patterns differentiate the two methods. Both methods, however, represent techniques that require movement of the tongue in order to compress air within the (oral)pharyngeal chamber.

Diedrich and Youngstrom (1966) note, however, that these generalized patterns of movement were subject to individual speaker variability. This was particularly evident in association with speakers who used the glossopharyngeal press method of injection. This may account in part for Snidecor's (1978a) clustering of the glossopharyngeal press and the plosive-injection methods as a unitary phenomenon. Further, Diedrich and Youngstrom did not find either of these two methods (or that of inhalation) to result in better speech skills. Therefore, either method may be used by an esophageal speaker without adversely affecting their speech capabilities.

Which Method Is Best?

What is important for the speech-language pathologist to understand about the glossal and glossopharyngeal methods is that they require the patient to learn patterned movement of the tongue in the oral cavity. Thus, Snidecor's (1978a) statement that injection by the tongue and related structures, and that related to the glossopharyngeal press or plosive method "are rather closely related" (p. 165) may be quite true. It is obvious that oral compression must be achieved in order for injection to take place; the focus of this goal should not, therefore, be placed on how it occurs clinically, but rather *whether it results in esophageal insufflation*. Esophageal voicing cannot occur without insufflation.

When one considers this issue, there appears to be a clear rationale for use of a plosive-injection method. This recommendation is based on the fact that it requires patients to perform an act they have performed millions of time—produce a phoneme! While the clinician carefully instructs the patient on "getting a feel" for where his or her tongue is located in the oral cavity, and on how to move the tongue in an upward and/or backward direction, the essence of the consonant-injection task is familiar to the patient. Many patients will also no doubt make their own idiosyncratic adjustments that may facilitate injection. Yet the issue of "self-generated" methods of insufflation may also exist in an overlapped fashion on those more commonplace insufflation methods.

For example, Gately (1976) recommended an injection technique seldom referenced in the literature. This technique involves the following sequence of events. First, the patient is asked to inflate the cheeks by sealing his lips and then pushing the tongue against the palate. Next, the patient is asked to relax his velopharyngeal seal, thus, allowing oral air to escape through the nose. In the final step of this injection process, the patient is asked to perform the first two steps; however, this time he closes his nose manually. Gately (1977) states that this maneuver will result in esophageal insufflation if the patient's lips are not blown apart. While it should be clear that this technique has functional limitations in regard to verbal communication, it does permit another method for achieving insufflation. Often, the simple experience of successful insufflation is enough to trigger some degree of awareness regarding *what structures are involved* and *what sequence of events* can be expected.

Few would disagree with the suggestion that attempts to teach a patient novel behaviors (e.g., glossopharyngeal press) in lieu of a previously well-learned behavior (e.g., consonant production) would run contrary to good clinical practice. If the clinician must teach through example, the use of phoneme-based tasks achieves a level of salience to the patient that vague descriptions of lingual "stroking" cannot; the use of imagery can only go so far (Lauder, 1971). Again, however, clinicians *should not* exclude consideration of positive pressure injection methods other than plosive injection. It does imply that capitalizing on facile acts of behavior is both quite practical and clinically expedient.

The "Modified Swallow" Technique of Esophageal Insufflation

Another method of air injection that may be used has been referred to in the literature as a "modified swallow," or "half-swallow" method (Diedrich & Youngstrom, 1966; Salmon, 1986d). Martin (1963) has referred to this method as the "swallow-belch." Although a clear-cut definition of what constitutes this method cannot be easily teased from the literature, some themes are recurrent.

In large part, the modified swallow technique may share considerable similarities to other "tongue and related structures" injection methods noted in the literature (see Snidecor, 1978, pp. 161–163). As noted by Gardner (1971, p. 43), any injection method that involves the term "swallow" may be interpreted to be the "equivalent to a command to perform the act of deglutition." It is indeed true that the motor act that constitutes a "modified

swallow" may in many cases have no clear resemblance to the true act of swallowing. Perhaps some inferences to "swallowing" have evolved due to suggestions that "soda drinks" be used in conjunction with esophageal voice training (Snidecor, 1978, p. 162). Swallowing air is, nevertheless, an insufficient means of esophageal air insufflation from both temporal and mechanical standpoints.

Salmon (1979) has stressed the need for clinicians to avoid using the term "swallowing" and, in fact, has noted that she instructs the patient *not to swallow*. Snidecor (1978a) cautioned against use of the term in all instances. This concern is based on the simple fact that the mechanism of swallowing does not permit adequate volitional control for the duration of the air injection. Successful air injection must be accomplished in all cases (except when using the inhalation method) by having the patient actively manipulate oral and pharyngeal structures. If such control is not exhibited, the patient's ability to initiate and maintain "rapid, fluent, and normal appearing" esophageal speech will be minimized (Duguay, 1977, p. 358). Shipp (1970) has shown that esophageal insufflation is essentially invariant provided that a "swallowing pattern" is not used. Use of the term "modified swallow" (Diedrich & Youngstrom, 1966) may, therefore, be the by-product of observations that a combination of injection maneuvers are used by a given speaker (Duguay, 1977).

Esophageal Insufflation Using the Inhalation Method

The second general method of esophageal air insufflation is the "inhalation" method (Diedrich & Youngstrom, 1966; Lauder, 1989; Salmon, 1986d). The inhalation method of insufflation operates on an entirely different principle from that of positive pressure maneuvers (Diedrich, 1968; Diedrich & Youngstrom, 1966; Gardner, 1971; Snidecor, 1978a). While this method requires that a pressure differential between oropharyngeal (atmospheric) and esophageal air be created, this differential is achieved in an indirect manner.

The generalized physiologic requirements that differentiate positive pressure methods of injection and that of inhalation rests in the fact that the former demands a "tight oral-pharyngeal chamber," whereas the latter requires quite the opposite (Gardner, 1971). Successful insufflation of air using the inhalation method requires that the oral-pharyngeal compartment is open and relaxed. Diedrich and Youngstrom (1966) have observed that the two basic methods of air insufflation (i.e., injection and inhalation) can be distinguished based on lingual contributions. Positive pressure approaches require substantial activity of the tongue, whereas inhalation requires nonmovement of the tongue.

Using the inhalation approach, the patient is required to inhale air through the tracheostoma. It is essential that inhalation is quite rapid. This is easily perceived by the patient and observed by the clinician. Rapid inhalation results in the creation of a negative thoracic pressure.

Recalling that the structure of the trachea is characterized by a series of horseshoe-shaped cartilages with the "open" portion of the horseshoe directed posteriorly, a soft tissue separation exists between the posterior trachea and the esophagus which is situated directly behind it. Due to this anatomical orientation, creation of a negative thoracic pressure in response to rapid inhalation of air creates an increase in a preexisting negative pressure within the esophagus[5] (Atkinson, Kramer, Wyman, & Ingelfinger, 1957).

While a negative pressure *is always present* in the esophagus, it is decreased substantially during inhalation. This results in a greater negative pressure in the

esophagus (Diedrich, 1968; Duguay, 1977). Once the negative pressure is sufficient to meet minimum requirements of the system for "equalization" of pressures to occur, insufflation follows. Thus, the active event of inhalation permits a passive increase in negative pressure within the esophageal lumen. As such, the "normal" atmospheric pressure that characterizes the oral-pharyngeal cavity becomes positive relative to that of the esophagus. This event thereby initiates the transgression of air across the PE segment into the esophageal reservoir.

Cinefluorographic data presented by Diedrich and Youngstrom (1966) has provided the following description of oral structures during inhalation insufflation:

> The tongue never occluded the oral cavity and little or no dorsad movement of the posterior tongue was visible. The lips were open and the velopharyngeal port was usually closed. A completely patent airway was maintained between the lips and the pharyngo-esophageal junction. (p. 37)

This method clearly differs from other methods of insufflation in that the oral cavity *must remain open and relaxed*. Inhalation, therefore, requires the primary muscular activity associated with achieving insufflation to occur with the diaphragm. The muscular initiation must, however, be rapid for esophageal insufflation of air to occur. By doing so, a more rapid pressure differential may be generated, and hence, insufflation may then be facilitated.

Training the Inhalation Technique

Several methods have been suggested in regard to teaching the inhalation method. The most common involves asking the patient to "take a quick breath" (Duguay,

---

[5]The typical resting pressure within the esophagus for both normal and esophageal speakers has been reported by Salmon (1979) to be in the range of –4 to –7 mm Hg below that of atmospheric. Upon inspiration, the negative pressure may decrease to –15 mm Hg (Salmon, 1979, p. 7).

1977; Gardner, 1971; Diedrich, 1968; Snidecor, 1978). Interestingly, this method may be used with both an open-mouth, as well as a closed-mouth approach. The open-mouth approach relies on cues to the patient such as "breathe through your mouth" (Salmon, 1986d). Although the patient is in actuality unable to breathe through their mouth, such instructions may permit an open and, hopefully, relatively relaxed oropharyngeal system (Diedrich & Youngstrom, 1966).

In contrast, the closed-mouth approach centers on having the patient breath through their nose, or to "sniff" (Diedrich & Youngstrom, 1966) in a somewhat aggressive fashion. Both the open-mouth and closed-mouth approaches should be performed following a request to fill the lungs about one-half to three-quarters of maximum capacity. Again, while sniffing is not possible due to laryngectomy, it may facilitate an easy yet rapid inhalation.

If injection via inhalation is successful, the patient is then encouraged to immediately produce esophageal sound in the form of an esophageal vowel. Vocalic productions can then be paired with consonants (Diedrich & Youngstrom, 1966). In this circumstance, it may be best to move from isolated vowels to CV syllables utilizing stop-plosives, affricatives, and sibilants. VC pairings may also be appropriate in some circumstances (Duguay, 1977; Gardner, 1971). Similar to other methods of air insufflation, use of unvoiced phonemes may facilitate concomitant recharging of the esophageal reservoir during syllabic production.

Duguay (1991), has recommended two additional techniques for inhalation insufflation which differ somewhat from the more traditional descriptions in the literature. In the first of these, Duguay states that the patient is requested to "relax and to yawn as deeply, easily, and realistically as possible" (p. 66). This technique does not rely on an atypical behavior and, hence, may be very useful. It would also appear to have the advantage of creating a rather open and unrestricted pharyngeal region. Because of this relaxation, oropharyngeal air is unrestricted at the time the PE segment opens. The second method presented by Duguay (1991) involves asking the patient to digitally close his or her airway (tracheostoma) following several sequences of inhalation and exhalation. Upon the final exhalation and airway closure, the patient opens his or her mouth and "injection" (via inhalation) may occur. If this method is used to train inhalation insufflation, the clinician should carefully assure the patient that he or she cannot suffocate in the period of time that the airway is occluded.

What the clinician needs to keep in mind with such instructions is that the patient has had many years of practice breathing through the mouth and nose. Consequently, a request for the production of these behaviors is not new to the patient. As noted, tasks such as those outlined must be performed in the presence of an open and relaxed airway. Should any tension in the oropharyngeal musculature exist during the inhalation, the creation of sufficient pressure differentials may be more difficult. The speech-language pathologist should then ensure that the patient is comfortably seated and relaxed.

It must be noted, however, that during the inhalation task(s) in the laryngectomized individual, there is essentially no resistance offered by the airway to inhalatory flow. So, the patient's ability to perform this task should be relatively easy. The speech-language pathologist must carefully monitor the patient's breathing patterns to eliminate overly aggressive and deep inhalations. If this occurs, hyperventilation is a real possibility, and while this poses no great risk to the patient, it can be quite disconcerting.

Developing a Protocol for Speech Reacquisition

Numerous reports in the literature have suggested a variety of modifications to organizational protocols in teaching esophageal sound production. Generally, however, the clinician should not feel that unique protocols exist for individual methods of injection. That is, in most cases the sequence of training speech will not differ dramatically regardless of whether the patient uses injection or inhalation, or both methods. Protocols may also be scaled down (as far as the level of demand placed on the patient) dependent on how long the patient is seen postsurgery.

Duguay (1977) stated that the sequence of speech reacquisition should be guided by two goals, one for the patient and one for the clinician. According to Duguay (1977), the first requirement centers on reducing the chance that "tension and anxiety" will be created in the patient, which may be detrimental to the process. Second, the clinician strongly desires to have the patient produce at least his first esophageal sound during that session. Duguay states that while this places pressure on the clinician, this pressure is unknown to the patient.

Finally, Duguay (1977) has provided an overview of several general "approaches" that may be used by the speech-language pathologist to undertake alaryngeal voice therapy. Duguay has described these strategies as the *indirect, semidirect,* and *direct approaches.* Although all have clinical merit, the approach undertaken with most patients will be based on the clinician's own philosophy of therapeutic intervention. The essential components which underlie Duguay's approaches may be simply characterized as differences in the manner in which the clinician will *observe, identify,* and *reinforce* behaviors and the method(s) used to *model, modify,* and *instruct* the patient. Different patients require different approaches, and, hopefully, the clinician exhibits the capacity to adapt in the clinical situation. A summary of tasks and objectives to be undertaken in the beginning stages of esophageal speech training are provide in Table 10–2.

Esophageal Speech Training: Fundamental Objectives

According to Berlin (1963) and Weinberg (1983a, 1983b) the initial emphasis of any alaryngeal voice re-acquisition program should involve the following goals: (1) the production of alaryngeal voice both quickly and reliably, (2) the ability to sustain the duration of alaryngeal voicing so that short phrases can be produced, and

---

TABLE 10–2.
Tasks and Objectives Associated with Initial Stage of Esophageal Speech Training

---

Task 1: Train air insufflation: injection or inhalation
Objective: Successful "loading" or "charging" of esophageal reservoir.

Task 2: Voice production on demand following insufflation.
Objective: To achieve a level of reliability equal to 100%

Task 3: Repeated productions of voice following insufflation
Objective: Habituation of behavior

Task 4: Monitor development of detrimental behaviors during insufflation and/or sound production.
Objective: Eliminate disruptive associated behaviors (grimacing, stoma blast, etc.).

Task 5: Reduce the degree of articulatory contact associated with insufflation and voice production.
Objective: Facilitation of voicing control, refinement of speech production.

Source: Adapted from Berlin (1963) and Weinberg (1983a).

(3) the ability to sustain voicing for production of all voiced phonemes (vowels and voiced consonants). These three goals have clear implications for the development of alaryngeal speech that can fully support functional communication.

In regard to the acquisition of esophageal voicing, these goals require that the patient is able to exert some degree of control over both ingressive and egressive aspects of esophageal speech. That is, the patients must demonstrate the capacity to "load" the esophagus with air in order to supply the power source for oscillation of the PE segment. As noted by Snidecor (1978a) an essential goal of any esophageal voice and speech treatment program is to "get air in" and then to "get air out." If insufflation of the esophageal reservoir cannot be done in an expeditious manner, the individual is unlikely to be able to meet the general goal pertaining to rapid production of esophageal voice.

All remaining aspects of Weinberg's (1983a) goals center around the efficient generation and maintenance of esophageal voicing at a variety of levels (single sound through short phrases). Therefore, the ultimate success of alaryngeal speech acquisition in general, and of esophageal speech in particular rests with the patient's ability to carefully manipulate the system in order to facilitate insufflation of the esophageal reservoir, followed by controlled, egressive flow for alaryngeal speech purposes.

Beyond the First Esophageal Sound

Once the patient is able to successfully insufflate air into the esophageal reservoir and, hence, provide the basis of a power supply to the PE segment, the elements of air expulsion do not need to be adjusted in accordance with the preferred method of insufflation. Generally, a simple sequence should move from vowel production, to that of CV syllables, and then to CVC syllables. It is important that vowel

production be achieved at high levels of performance, namely, production must move toward a goal of 100% production on demand (Berlin, 1963; Weinberg, 1983a). Inconsistent production of isolated vowels will require continued work at this level prior to proceeding to later stages of the program (Gardner, 1971).

It may not be unusual to observe that transitions across stimulus subtypes, for example, moving from isolated vowels to CV syllables, may create difficulty for some patients. In such instances, the speech-language pathologist needs to carefully assess why this is occurring. Has the patient lost or shifted concentration? Is the patient posturing oral structures in a different manner? Are extraneous behaviors becoming overlaid on the old behavior? These, and many more questions will be raised in circumstances where a patient is unable to successfully shift from what the clinician believes is one simple task to another. But it must be remembered that training, particularly for esophageal speech, is frequently initiated fairly early postoperatively. There are always changes in postoperative anatomy that still are resolving (e.g., tenderness, edema, etc.). Although this is a natural phenomenon associated with the healing process, slight adjustments in oropharyngeal anatomy may be substantially more problematic for some patients. The speech-language pathologist must be sensitive to the potential contribution and influence of these types of changes and modify programs accordingly. Although it may be safe to say that the overall format followed in attempts to teach not only the first esophageal sound but later refinements is *relatively* consistent from patient to patient, adjustments based on the needs of individual patients will always be necessary.

Although the speech-language pathologist ultimately desires the patient to speak as quickly as possible, care must be taken to ensure that the patient is successfully acquiring the base skills that will serve his or her speech later on (Duguay,

1977; Gardner, 1971; Weinberg, 1983a, 1983b). Thus, erring on the side of too much "drill work" early on in treatment is likely preferable to moving ahead following insufficient work. Even though "clinical intuition" may suggest that the program should advance, the speech-language pathologist will find it necessary to review data obtained and make the appropriate decision for modifications or advancement based on these data.

In many instances early in therapy, the clinician may be working at quite an artificial level (e.g., sustained vowels, nonsense syllables, etc.). Unfortunately, these levels are necessary early in the treatment process and will provide a method for the clinician to systematically assess strengths and weakness for given injection methods, classes of stimulus sounds, and so forth. The clinician should, however, aggressively work toward the transition to "real words" and meaningful speech as soon as possible. This has significant functional (communicative) and motivation value to the patient.

Advanced Levels of Esophageal Voice and Speech Training

The ability of patients to refine esophageal voice and further develop their esophageal speech proficiency is a long-term process. Continued use of esophageal speech will in many cases serve to improve the individual's ability to make such changes. The primary influence upon one's ability to acquire advanced skill, however, centers on what has occurred early on in the rehabilitative process. Inappropriate behaviors or those that interfere with communication (e.g., stoma noise, facial grimaces, etc.) must be identified and reduced or eliminated before they become habitual (Shanks, 1986a; Weinberg, 1983a). Thus, the speech-language pathologist must be vigilant in identifying and modifying such negative behaviors. Identification of problem areas

serve to direct the clinician towards establishing more advanced methods of training to remediate the perceived deficit.

Numerous approaches to the development of advanced esophageal speech skills have been provided previously in the literature (Amster, 1987; Gardner, 1971; Lauder, 1979; Martin, 1986; Snidecor, 1978a; and others). Recommendations differ somewhat in the general composition of tasks; however, they do share one specific component. Regardless of the materials or tasks employed, all programs follow an organized, systematic approach to training. Treatment is structured so that patients can acquire skills that are progressively more challenging (Berlin, 1963; Weinberg, 1983a).

The skills to be developed in the intermediate or advanced stages of esophageal speech training are seen to cross many discrete areas of performance. Yet overall assessment of how proficient the speaker has become must also be evaluated in a combined manner. Specific dimensions of speech performance and proficiency may be objectively assessed to determine changes that occur over time. For example, acoustic and temporal attributes, intelligibility, and so forth can be monitored on a regular basis. This focus on discrete elements of esophageal speech should not replace global judgments of performance (overall communicative success) as this is what the nonprofessional listener will encounter. A summary of advanced objectives associated with esophageal speech training is provided in Table 10–3.

The generic therapy program outlined by Weinberg (1983a) also addressed several additional areas that are essential components of proficient esophageal communication (see Table 10–3). This includes the development and refinement of skills in the areas of: (1) speech rate and temporal patterning, (2) articulatory function and associated speech intelligibility, (3) the overall reduction of extraneous behaviors that may coexist with voice and speech

TABLE 10–3.
Advanced Objectives Associated with Reacquisition
and Refinement of Alaryngeal Speech Production.

Goal 1: Seek to maintain voicing throughout progressively more lengthy utterances.
Goal 2: Maintain levels of high intelligibility.
Goal 3: Work to minimize the presence of any associated noises or behaviors that may interfere with communication.
Goal 4: Seek to maintain an adequate rate of speech during productions of increasing length.
Goal 5: Seek to acquire ability to signal linguistic contrasts and prosodic features of speech (e.g., lexical stress, intonation, juncture, etc.).

Source: Adapted from Weinberg (1983a).

output, and (4) the speaker's ability to realize and successfully produce prosodic and linguistic contrasts.

In regard to speech rate and the temporal patterning of speech, Weinberg (1983a) has suggested that the patient seek to increase the number of words (or syllables) produced, while at the same time maintaining a constant level of intelligibility. This goal is typically met under the clinician's direction by having the patient become aware of his or her own productive limitations based on levels of air support. This also involves rather careful attention to pause behavior.

Treatment Monitoring and Evaluation of Progress

The early stages of speech and voice rehabilitation must be structured in a manner that has the potential to offer both the clinician and the patient direct feedback on their performance. This feedback serves two distinct purposes. First, if a system of quantifying the patient's ability to acquire particular "base" skills for esophageal speech (or any other method of alaryngeal communication) is utilized by the clinician, progress also can be noted by the patient. The patient's ability to appreciate the fact that he or she is acquiring early skills which form the basis of later steps in the treatment program can be encouraging and motivating.

The second purpose serves both the patient and the clinician. Specifically, careful monitoring of progress can indicate whether a given patient is acquiring essential behaviors that form the foundation of further voice and speech development and refinement. If progress is not being made, the clinician can observe this directly, and modify the program accordingly. The treatment program, thus, can be modified in two ways dependent on the quantitative data obtained.

In the case where progress is slow, or more importantly when the acquisition of basic skills is not occurring, the clinician is posed with two options. The logical first step is for the clinician to assess whether or not a modification in the program (e.g., changing the air insufflation technique, etc.) will result in some positive changes.

Obviously, each program seeks to train the same basic introductory skills in the training of esophageal speech; however, the approach(s) used may vary from patient-to-patient. Thus, it is incumbent on the clinician to assess whether a minor adjustment will facilitate the patient's ability to learn a particular skill, or whether large scale changes in the program must be undertaken.

The other potential scenario that may emerge and with which the clinician must deal pertains to the patient who cannot acquire basic skills, even once modifications are undertaken and exhausted. Although this scenario is not pleasant to acknowledge, the clinician should never have this occur unknowingly. That is, if simple, yet careful quantitative data are collected on a session-by-session basis, the clinician should always be able to assess how the patient is performing over the course of initial treatment. If progress is not being made, this lack of progress will be noted early on in the program and, therefore, the clinician is provided with two specific alternatives: (1) modify the existing program based on clinical observations, or (2) prepare treatment sessions to include ongoing counseling which may *redirect the patient* to use an artificial laryngeal device (although ideally the patient *should* be using an artificial device concurrently during esophageal speech training).

Related Problems Observed During the Acquisition of Esophageal Phonation

It can be seen that the instruction of esophageal speech requires that primary concerns are placed on the insufflation of air into the esophagus. Once this goal has been mastered by the patient, tasks which center on ensuring reliable and consistent egressive flow of that air through the PE segment for voicing purposes take precedent (Berlin, 1963; Weinberg, 1983a). However, other behaviors may come into play at this time and must be assessed and, if necessary, modified in a timely and effective manner. Related behaviors that may be noted by the speech-language pathologist may be associated with the injection phase or simultaneously with the production of esophageal voice (Diedrich & Youngstrom, 1966).

The two most common behaviors that require modification by the speech-language pathologist are (1) "klunking" which occurs with injection of air into the esophageal reservoir; and (2) "stoma noise," which is a result of exhalatory airway turbulence that exists simultaneously with esophageal voice production. While other behaviors have been noted to develop in some individuals who are attempting to acquire esophageal speech (e.g., lip smacking, facial grimacing, etc.), klunking and stoma noise appear to be most prevalent.

Air Injection Noise

The term "klunking"[6] has been used to refer to the sound made when air moves through the tonically closed PE segment in an effort to insufflate the esophagus. Edels (1983) has referred to this sound as "thumping." Thus, an audible sound is frequently associated with insufflation. This sound does appear to be more commonly associated with positive pressure methods of air injection (Diedrich, 1968; Diedrich & Youngstrom, 1966; Kallen, 1934; Snidecor, 1978a).

Injection-related noise may also be uncommon with consonant injection methods although the sound may be masked to some degree by the explosive release of the target phoneme. Diedrich and Youngstrom (1966) noted that klunking was not observed when inhalation methods of esophageal insufflation were used. Similarly, Gardner (1971) has suggested that when excessive levels of klunking are noted, teaching the patient to inhale in synchrony with an injection maneuver may decrease this behavior substantially. This does not,

---

[6]The term "klunking" has been noted by Diedrich and Youngstrom (1966, p. 102) to be synonymous with the term "gulping" used by others authors. However, Diedrich and Youngstrom are opposed to the term gulping to describe the phenomenon of noise in association with esophageal insufflation. Their rationale stems from a belief that "gulping" has a strong association to the act of swallowing, which is believed to be an ineffective manner of esophageal air insufflation.

however, imply that injection via the use of inhalation is a silent process; yet it may be less audible (Diedrich & Youngstrom, 1966). When insufflation noise in response to inhalation occurs it has been identified as a "click" (Logemann, 1983).

Although several differences of opinion as to what constitutes this injection-related noise have been offered, it is safe to say that this noise is a consequence of air violating the closed sphincter. Edels (1983, p. 137) has stated that klunking informs the clinician that insufflation is occurring with "too much air, too quickly, and with too great a force." This may indeed be true, but other physical factors can also influence this response.

For example, the creation of pressure differentials between the hypopharynx and the esophageal reservoir must overcome PE segment resistance. Hence, a springlike response of the sphincter must occur in order for air to move into the reservoir. Although no data exist in regard to the possible relationship between resting pressures of the PE segment and the audibility (amplitude) of klunking during injection, the severity of this klunking sound appears to correspond to the "ease" with which egressive airflow occurs. Despite one's ability to create sufficient pressure differentials that will eventually violate the closed PE segment, a tighter sphincter may result in a relatively more audible klunk. In some cases this does not involve use of too much air in too quick a manner, but rather it results because very high pressures must be created to overcome the resistance of the muscular junction between the hypopharynx and esophagus. Thus, "force" issues may carry the best explanation of excessively loud injection noise.

Within the literature on esophageal speech training, there is substantial agreement that substantial amounts of injection-related noise is a negative feature. When this noise is significant, it may serve as a distraction to the overall communication process. Thus, the speech-language pathologist must attempt to decrease the level of klunking noise; such modification must occur relatively early in the treatment sequence.

In the initial stages of esophageal speech training, however, klunking serves a valuable function to the patient and clinician. When Snidecor's (1978a) recommendation that the essential goal of esophageal speech training is to get air into the esophageal reservoir then expel it volitionally is considered, klunking offers direct feedback to both patient and clinician. This is particularly true in patients who experience egressive flow difficulties in the early period of training. These patients may be successful getting air in, but they are still unable to manipulate its output. The clinician must reinforce the fact that the patient has met the first requirement of esophageal voicing—that is, to charge the system. It also signals that insufflation has occurred. This may be of benefit to patients who are inconsistent in their ability to insufflate the esophagus. As the patient develops more control over the ability to produce voice, the resistance of the sphincter may become reduced (Shanks, 1986a), and this may result in a corresponding reduction in injection noise. Nevertheless, reinforcement should always be tempered by informing the patient that injection noise will need to be decreased later in the acquisition process because it serves as a communicative distraction.

Modifying Excessive Levels of Insufflation Noise

In patients who continue to demonstrate unacceptable levels of injection noise, several therapeutic tactics may be employed. The general focus of these goals centers on having the patient monitor his or her own productions in an attempt to reduce klunking noise. In many cases, however, the clinician must attempt to provide salient feedback to the patient. This is particularly true in those who exhibit substantial degrees of hearing loss.

One of the easiest methods is to use a stethoscope (Gardner, 1971). The patient is instructed to listen to the sound associated with insufflation while the clinician places the diaphragm of the stethoscope on the neck at a level consistent with likely location of the PE segment (C5–C7). This provides direct "amplified" feedback to the patient, and this may be used in a manner where noise can be reduced. It is best for the clinician to view the level of reduction as a *relative shift* in its presence. That is, some noise will always exist although it may be quite minimal; therefore, any reduction should be acknowledged as a positive change.

The second method that can be used to reduce injection noise uses somewhat indirect instruction on the reduction of effort involved in insufflation. This is best approached by having the speech-language pathologist instruct the patient to "slow" the process that *precedes* injection. If the presence of injection noise is primarily a consequence of an extremely hypertonic PE segment, the patient cannot really decrease effort in relation to building the necessary pressure to overcome sphincter resistance. However, by modifying the temporal sequence of events, opening of the sphincter may be less abrupt. Using this method may permit the patient to insufflate the esophagus by "sneaking" air through the PE segment rather than having it "rush" through.

If the spring analogy holds true for the PE segment, creation of sufficient pressure over an extended period (albeit very brief and on the order of milliseconds) will be less likely to generate a rapid and perhaps extremely audible closure response (Shipp, 1970). The clinician should also continually provide an excellent model of easy and relaxed speech (Gardner, 1971). It should be remembered that patients need not only meet pressure requirements for injection of air, but they also need to try and reduce the tension of the sphincter (Diedrich & Youngstrom, 1966; Gardner, 1971; Shanks, 1986a; Weinberg, 1983a). In doing so,

insufflation is not only facilitated, but it is facilitated with greater ease.

Reduction in effort appears to have a considerable impact on how the PE sphincter responds to increasing levels of pressure in the hypopharynx. Once again, the overall effort level may be observed to decrease over the early acquisition period as the patient develops both greater control over their new alaryngeal voice production system, as well as increasing his or her awareness of the need to coordinate and control a variety of related systems (e.g., oral mechanism, respiratory system, etc.).

The Presence and Reduction of Respiratory Noise During Production of Esophageal Voice

Like the problem of injection-related noise, the problem of excessive respiratory noise during esophageal speech production has long been noted. The presence of respiratory noise, or *stoma noise*, is best viewed as competition to that of the speech signal. Levels of noise associated with respiratory flow can in some cases be substantial, and consequently, detract considerably from speech (Clark & Stemple, 1982). The absence or presence of stoma noise can also be viewed as a powerful perceptual feature associated with listener judgments of alaryngeal speech proficiency (Shipp, 1967).

Addressing the problem of stoma noise necessitates a basic understanding of why it occurs. Unlike that of other extraneous behaviors that may be observed in association with esophageal speech production (e.g., facial grimacing, lip smacking, etc.), stoma noise may be viewed as a natural phenomenon. Prior to laryngectomy, patients had habituated on the fact that in order to produce speech they needed to exhale. The postsurgical disconnection of the oropharyngeal pathway and that of the airway postlaryngectomy eliminates that requirement; however, the habit remains. Although the patient does not need to exhale to produce esophageal speech, the sequential "set" associated with speech production on exhalation remains. The presence of stoma noise is, therefore, a consequence of a normal lifelong process and its modification involves either reducing the explicit presence of this behavior or teaching an entirely new set of behaviors. It can be generally stated that the former approach may be best for improving overall esophageal speech proficiency.

Substantial attention has been directed toward understanding relationships between respiratory patterns and that of esophageal speech production (Diedrich & Youngstrom, 1966; Isshiki, 1978; Isshiki & Snidecor, 1965; Robe et al., 1956; Snidecor & Isshiki, 1965). Isshiki (1978), Isshiki and Snidecor (1965), and Snidecor and Isshiki (1965) evaluated the relationship between respiratory movement, direction of airflow (in or out), and whether voicing was present. They found that eight distinct patterns of performance or phase relationships existed. A summary of these phasic relationships as outlined by Isshiki (1978) is provided in Table 10–4.

Although these eight patterns were observed to occur in the majority of esoph-ageal speakers ($n = 6$) studied by Isshiki (1978), he did state that regardless of whether insufflation was accomplished using injection or inhalation, that "Most speakers employ both synchronic and asynchronic intake or air in various degrees" (p. 142). Isshiki (1978) went on to state that in the majority of speakers studied more air charging was achieved in a synchronous manner. That is, synchrony implies that the insufflation of air occurred with inspiration and expulsion of esophageal air occurred with exhalation, behaviors consistent with the normal speech process.

Based on Isshiki's (1978) data, the esophageal speaker appears to exhibit a predilection toward maintaining the respiratory-phonatory relationship that was used prelaryngectomy. These speakers typically follow the "normal" pattern of events in which inspiration precedes expiration and speech production. Thus, therapeutic attempts to modify behaviors (i.e., reducing the degree of expiratory effort), as opposed to eliminating them through training of "new" behaviors (i.e., control of expiratory flow), has an increased likelihood of culminating in success.

Given that stoma noise is a result of rapid and relatively unimpeded airflow

TABLE 10–4.
Categories of Phase Relationships Among Oral Airflow, Tracheal (Respiratory) Airflow, and the Presence of Voicing During Esophageal Speech Production.

	Direction of Airflow and Presence of Voicing		
	Oronasal	Tracheal	Voicing
1.	In	Out	No
2.	In	Out	Yes
3.	In	In	No
4.	In	In	Yes
5.	Out	Out	No
6.	Out	Out	Yes
7.	Out	In	No
8.	Out	In	Yes

Source: From Isshiki, N. (1978). Airflow in esophageal speech. In J.C. Snidecor (Ed.), *Speech rehabilitation of the laryngectomized,* 2nd, (pp. 137–150), Springfield, IL, Charles C. Thomas, reprinted with permission.

through the tracheostoma, a rather simple clinical approach to reduce its presence can be undertaken. This task involves having the patient produce esophageal voice with less expiratory effort. Decreasing the level of effort to produce speech will often reduce the rate of expiratory air flow, and noise will be minimized.

Diedrich and Youngstrom (1966) provided methods that involve having patients directly control their expiration. Contrary to the notion that the patient should be taught to hold their breath and "fix" their chest while speaking, Diedrich and Youngstrom (1966) suggest the patient simply be instructed to exhale in a slower manner. Diedrich and Youngstrom (1966) believed that the use of breath holding may be detrimental to the treatment process. Specifically, requiring the patient to stop a normal physiologic pattern (exhalation) may result in more aggressive levels of output after speech production. If this occurs, it serves only to provide an additional obstacle to communicative effectiveness.

In contrast, Weinberg (1983a) has suggested a technique that relies on the use of tidal breathing as a point of reference. The technique initially involves having the patient sit quietly and breath normally. If no stoma noise is present, Weinberg suggests that vowels and monosyllabic stimuli be produced *without* stoma noise. Patients are encouraged to use "as little force of the chest wall as possible" (Weinberg, 1983a, p. 117). This suggestion is of value because it does not request the patient to stop thoracic movement, but only limit movement to some extent. The patient is modifying rather than eliminating a normal pattern of respiratory movement. Weinberg (1983a) carefully acknowledges that if stoma noise is observed during the quite tidal breathing task, speech production is unlikely to be performed without such competing noise.

Two additional methods may be used clinically to reduce stoma noise. The first involves use of a stethoscope similar to that noted for the reduction of klunking associated with injection. For stoma noise, how-

ever, the diaphragm is placed over but not covering the tracheostoma. This permits auditory feedback to the patient. A second method also involves the auditory monitoring of flow through the stoma. Gardner (1971) has recommended that a rubber tube be positioned with one end near the stoma and the other near the speaker's face, ear, or eye. Excessive expiration associated with stoma noise will be noted by the patient quite effectively using this technique. This technique may be upgraded with simple modification of a housing from a tracheostoma breathing valve (Blom, Singer, & Hamaker, 1982) and some surgical tubing.

It should be noted that some patients respond very well to tactile cues associated with expiration. Therefore, placing one's hand several inches away from the stoma during quite breathing and then during different speech production tasks (vowels, monosyllables, etc.) may provide excellent feedback to the patient (Diedrich & Youngstrom, 1966; Weinberg, 1983a).

Feedback can also be provided through implementation of a microphone set within a tracheostoma adaptor and a playback system that uses headphones. Using such a device, Till, England, and Law-Till (1987) have shown that auditory feedback may permit reductions in stoma noise up to levels of 5–10 dB. Interestingly, Till et al. (1987) reported that stoma noise was observed to be significantly greater for voiceless consonants when compared to voiced phonemes. Thus, early training of esophageal speech that out of necessity may rely on use of voiceless phonemes due to intrinsic pressure characteristics, may also serve as the impetus for the development of excessive stoma noise. These data suggest that more systematic approaches to remediating stoma noise, particularly in the early phase of esophageal speech training may be of substantial benefit to the patient's long-term rehabilitation success.

The final method that can be used involves providing direct visual feedback to the patient. Weinberg (1983a) has noted that airflow from the stoma can be directed to a pnuemotachograph; the output can then be input to an oscilloscope or other visual device (Weinberg, 1983a). The patient can then be trained to modify levels of output in a systematic fashion in hope of reducing stoma noise. While single forms of feedback such as auditory, visual, or tactile may be of value to the patient, combined forms should also be entertained in the clinical reduction of stoma noise.

Summary

This chapter has addressed a broad range of issues related to esophageal speech. Both structural considerations, as well as in-depth issues related to clinical management, have been addressed. This has included discussion of factors specific to the PE segment and the potential effects of esophageal speech acquisition. A detailed presentation of methods of esophageal insufflation and associated treatment techniques has been provided. Additionally, aspects related to stimulus consideration, program structure, and monitoring of treatment have been pursued. Finally, considerations related to the clinical modification of extraneous behaviors frequently observed as a consequence of esophageal speech training have been highlighted.

Artificial Laryngeal Speech

CHAPTER

The clinical application of extrinsic methods of alaryngeal speech through use of a variety of electronic artificial laryngeal devices has been acknowledged by many as an extremely viable voice and speech rehabilitation option following laryngectomy. Yet provision of an artificial laryngeal device does not ensure that adequate verbal communication will occur. As stated so succinctly by Snidecor (1978b), "The acquisition of an artificial larynx gives little promise that clear and intelligible speech will automatically result" (p. 208). The speech-language pathologist will, therefore, play a major role in facilitating and training the best speech possible using the artificial larynx. Thus, the purpose of this chapter is to present information related to the general function and use of the electronic artificial larynx. Based on the belief that bias should never be introduced into the presentation of any postlaryngectomy communication option, advantages and disadvantages of the artificial larynx will

be outlined. Controversies surrounding use of the artificial larynx will also be addressed. Finally, specific issues underlying clinical treatment will be presented.

An Overview of Artificial Laryngeal Communication

The concept underlying the artificial larynx has a lengthy history associated with its development and refinement. Keith and Shanks (1986) have provided a comprehensive review of this history since the mid-1800s and the evolution of the artificial larynx as a broad group of alaryngeal speech devices. An excellent discussion of a variety of topics related to contemporary artificial laryngeal devices also has been presented in the book *The Artificial Larynx Handbook* (Salmon & Goldstein, 1978).

Although early development of pneumatic (air driven) devices which utilized vibratory systems similar to that of a reed have received considerable attention, this type of artificial larynx is best viewed from a historical perspective (Lebrun, 1973). That is, despite the fact the some of these pneumatic devices provided an adequate alaryngeal sound source, they were subject to considerable problems. Many of the problems were directly associated with connections of this type of prosthetic device to the patient's tracheostoma. This frequently created tissue irritation, increased the potential for respiratory problems, as well as a host of other difficulties such as fear that the airway would be impeded (Duguay, 1983).

Solutions to these problems were sought; however, the problems continued to occur even during the modern era of their development (Taub & Bergner, 1973; Taub & Spiro, 1972). Perhaps the only device that gained any serious, although somewhat limited, clinical attention was the simple pneumatic reed device termed the *Tokyo* artificial larynx. The Tokyo device was shown to result in intelligibility levels that were similar to those of normal and excellent esophageal speakers under "optimal signal-to-noise" conditions (Weinberg & Riekena, 1973). Additionally, Bennett and Weinberg (1973) reported that speech produced with a Tokyo device was judged by listeners to be more acceptable when compared to other artificial laryngeal methods.

The primary artificial laryngeal devices that are currently used in a majority of clinical settings are electronic artificial laryngeal devices (Salmon & Goldstein, 1978). In many clinics the most common devices found are typically the Cooper-Rand (intraoral) device and the Western Electric, Servox, Neovox, or Aurex (transcervical) devices. Regardless of the type of device or who manufactures it, substantial similarities exist across artificial larynges as a group of electronic alaryngeal speech devices.

Artificial Laryngeal Communication

Features of the Ideal Artificial Larynx

Barney (1958) provided a set of "design objectives" which addressed the essential requirements of what features characterize the "ideal" artificial laryngeal device. The objectives outlined by Barney (1958) were based on the opinions of individuals who had undergone total laryngectomy and physicians. These design objectives are presented in their entirety in Table 11–1. With these objectives outlined Barney and

---

TABLE 11–1.
Design Objectives and Essential Features That Characterize the "Ideal" Electronic Artificial Laryngeal Device.

---

1. Produces speech (vocal) intensity that is equal to that of a normal laryngeal speaker.
2. Provides speech quality and pitch inflection that is similar to that of a normal speaker.
3. Is small and unobtrusive, without wires, tubes, and so forth.
4. Provides reliable, trouble-free operation.
5. Is hygienically acceptable to the user.[a]
6. Is inexpensive to purchase and operate

Source: Adapted from Barney, H.A. (1958). A discussion of some technical aspects of speech aids for postlaryngectomized patients. *Annals of Otology, Rhinology, and Laryngology, 67,* 558–570. Reprinted with permission.
[a]This is perhaps the most prominent negative feature associated with use of pneumatic or reed-fistula type artificial laryngeal devices.

his colleagues (Barney, Haworth, & Dunn, 1959) provided the first contemporary prototype for an electronic artificial larynx (Western Electric #5) of which refined versions are still being used today.

Although these objectives were provided by Barney (1958) 36 years ago, the ultimate artificial larynx is still characterized by these six basic requirements. While many devices have unique features that expand their functional capabilities, such as intensity and frequency control, rechargeable batteries, and so forth, artificial laryngeal devices have essentially remained the same in principle and function, but have been "fine-tuned" over the years (Salmon & Goldstein, 1978).

Interestingly, Barney (1958) was careful to point out that one additional feature also needed consideration. Specifically, he noted that the artificial larynx should be "simple to operate so that a minimum of training is required" (p. 558). Therein lies the primary advantage of the artificial larynx once Barney's (1958) first six design objectives are met. The most significant strength associated with the artificial larynx is that for most patients speech can be learned (at least in basic form) in a relatively short period of time.

Snidecor (1978b) stated that therapeutic intervention that targets optimizing the patient's use of the artificial larynx is "much less arduous" than that associated with esophageal voice and speech training. In this respect it may also be less problematic when compared to tracheoesophageal speech. This is due primarily to the care and maintenance associated with use of a tracheoesophageal (TE) puncture and TE puncture voice prosthesis (Singer & Blom, 1980; 1981). Snide-cor (1978b) also implies that one should not assume that the treatment process undertaken with the artificial larynx is conducted with any less physical vigor or clinical rigor than that associated with other alaryngeal speech options.

Acquiring essential skills that form the basis of excellent artificial laryngeal speech requires a concerted clinical effort between the patient and the speech-language pathologist. If provided with clear and concise direction, a majority of patients can learn to use the artificial larynx quite successfully in a variety of communicative settings following a relatively brief period of training. The postoperative application of the artificial larynx should always be considered as a potential speech rehabilitation option in those who undergo total laryngectomy. It is hoped that the relative strengths and weaknesses of each alaryngeal method can be presented to the patient in a fair and unbiased manner so that each can be evaluated carefully.

Primary Methods of Artificial Laryngeal Speech

While the general principle that underlies the basic function of any electronic artificial laryngeal device is the same, its use manifests in two specific forms: (1) *oral* devices and (2) *neck-type* (or transcervical) artificial larynges. Thus, the artificial larynx provides the voicing source for speech production via its application directly into the oral cavity (oral-type), or through external application to tissues of the anterior or lateral neck (neck-type).

Oral artificial laryngeal devices involve the presentation of an electronic voice source into the oral cavity by transmission through a tube. Once the source is introduced into the oral cavity articulation takes place. In contrast, when a neck-type device is used it is placed in firm contact with neck tissues and then activated. This external voice source is transmitted through soft tissues of the neck into the vocal tract where it can then be articulated into the sounds of speech.

For both the oral and neck-type artificial larynx an extrinsic, electronic device provides the power supply and vibratory element (i.e., vocal source) for alaryngeal communication. However, introduction of the electronic voice source into the vocal tract involves two different routes. Neither the oral or neck-type artificial laryngeal device relies on any intrinsic structures for the purposes of providing a *voice source* in the patient who has undergone total laryngectomy. Although a wide variety of artificial laryngeal devices are available commercially, some of which can be adapted to provide either an oral or transcervical source (Blom, 1978; Zwitman & Disinger, 1975; Zwitman, Knorr, & Sonderman, 1978), they all function on the same general principles.

Controversies Surrounding the Use of the Artificial Larynx

Historically, the artificial larynx has received considerable attention in the clinical literature with numerous types of devices introduced over many years (see Keith & Shanks, 1986). Whereas significant advances in the general design and output characteristics of artificial laryngeal devices have not taken place over the past two decades[1] (Weinberg, 1985), the artificial larynx still offers an important option to the individual who undergoes total laryngectomy. Despite the functional utility of the artificial larynx, it has been viewed as a less favorable option relative to esophageal speech and more recently tracheoesophageal (TE) speech (Gates, Ryan, & Lauder, 1982; Luboinski et al., 1989; Salmon & Goldstein, 1978).

Use of the artificial larynx (regardless of type) most notably has carried with it its own particular stigma. Diedrich and Youngstrom (1966) have acknowledged that issues related to the "relative merits" of the artificial larynx as a method of

postlaryngectomy voice and speech have provided one of the common areas of dispute over the years. However, Diedrich and Youngstrom (1966) strongly urged those involved with individuals who undergo laryngectomy to forsake this "dichotomy" between methods (i.e., esophageal speech vs. artificial laryngeal speech). This advice clearly focused on having clinicians dissolve any bias they may have had toward the artificial larynx (Duguay, 1978, 1983; Salmon & Goldstein, 1978). Diedrich and Youngstrom (1966) were among the first to actively support a more open consideration of the artificial larynx as a potential voice and speech rehabilitation option.

The Advantages and Disadvantages of the Artificial Larynx

Rothman (1982) has provided a comprehensive summary of literature related to the reasons for and against the use of the artificial larynx. A synopsis of both viewpoints is provided in Tables 11–2 and 11–3, respectively. From a practical communicative perspective it appears obvious that the reasons for use of an artificial larynx sufficiently outweigh those against its use.

When one carefully inspects the collection of reasons for and against the use of the artificial larynx (Rothman, 1982), a clear distinction in the evolution of "pro and con" arguments becomes apparent. Specifically, many of the reasons against recommending or supporting use of the artificial larynx have no sound rationale based on experimental data provided in either the applied or basic scientific literature. In fact, many reasons provided in Table 11–2 are steeped in the rather

---

[1]The Aurex Corporation has recently provided information on two new *Neovox* artificial laryngeal devices. The first has been designed to provide a more "natural" electronic voicing source and quieter operation. The second is designed for use by women and is reported to have a "slightly higher" pitch level and is less powerful than other models, which results in "softer-voiced" speech production.

TABLE 11–2.
Justification Provided in the Literature Against the Use of an Artificial Laryngeal Device.

1. The device serves as an unnecessary crutch to the patient.
2. It interferes with the acquisition of esophageal voice and speech.
3. May cause speech to be unintelligible and/or noisy.
4. Requires use of one hand.
5. Requires use of an instrument.
6. The artificial larynx calls attention to an infirmity.
7. Artificial laryngeal devices require expensive maintenance.
8. If device fails to operate, the individual is left speechless.

Source: From Rothman, H.B. (1982). Acoustic analysis of artificial laryngeal speech. In A. Sekey (Ed.), *Electroacoustic analysis of alaryngeal speech* (pp. 95–118). Springfield, IL: Charles C. Thomas. Reprinted with permission.

TABLE 11–3.
Justification Provided in the Literature for Recommending and Supporting the Use of an Artificial Laryngeal Device.

1. The artificial larynx is a psychological and economic necessity for individuals who have been recently laryngectomized.
2. If esophageal speech cannot be acquired in the immediate postoperative period due to surgical trauma, the artificial larynx provides a simple method of verbal communication.
3. Artificial laryngeal speech is often more intelligible than esophageal speech in a variety of communicative situations.
4. Artificial laryngeal speech is easily understood over the telephone.
5. It may allow the speaker to communicate more effectively in situations involving stress.
6. Provides greater speech intensity.
7. Allows prompt and immediate speech.
8. Use of an artificial larynx is easily learned for most patients.
9. The artificial larynx can be used by older individuals and those in poor health.
10. The artificial larynx can be used by those who fail to acquire esophageal speech.
11. There is no difficulty in using esophageal and artificial laryngeal speech in an alternating fashion.

Source: From Rothman, H.B. (1982). Acoustic analysis of artificial laryngeal speech. In A. Sekey (Ed.), Electroacoustic analysis of alaryngeal speech (pp. 95–118). Springfield, IL: Charles C. Thomas. Reprinted with permission.

narrow perception of those other than the patient. For example, reasons such as "calls attention to an infirmity" in reality may not be a significant issue for many patients.

The loss of one's ability to verbally communicate in any manner may call much more "attention" to one's "infirmity" than using the artificial larynx. Further, many attributes that have been considered by clinicians to be negative features inherent to use of an artificial larynx may now, at least in some cases, be rendered less important based on contemporary attitudes toward disability (Gorenflo & Gorenflo, 1991). A majority of patients have the simple desire to *verbally communicate* postsurgically regardless of method. Clinicians must strive to meet this basic rehabilitative goal.

The Artificial Larynx: A Primary or Secondary Method of Alaryngeal Speech?

Some authors have implicity identified that the artificial larynx should be considered as a secondary method of alaryngeal communication when attempts at acquiring intrinsic methods (i.e., esophageal speech) prove unsuccessful (Duguay, 1978). This suggestion is at times quite subtle, but, nevertheless, it portrays the artificial larynx as being a method of last resort for postlaryngectomy communication (Luboinski et al., 1989). Rather than focusing on a single method, it may be best for clinicians to be more open in their approach to therapy; a sole method need not be offered to the patient.

There is nothing wrong with concurrently teaching two methods of alaryngeal speech. Duguay (1978) has strongly supported the concept of a "dual track" (p. 6) approach to postlaryngectomy speech rehabilitation and has acknowledged that this may indeed be a common clinical occurrence (Duguay, 1983). Despite the apparent openmindedness of such treatment, some clinicians may still introduce concurrent methods of alaryngeal speech training in a manner that presents one method as superior to others. In instances where multiple methods of alaryngeal speech rehabilitation are instructed concurrently, the clinician is advised to present both methods as reasonable and viable options.

Duguay (1978) has stated that the ultimate goal of clinicians who work with laryngectomized individuals should be to develop each method to its fullest level. This advice serves both the patient and clinician well. If successful, this very practical approach to alaryngeal speech rehabilitation affords the patient an additional opportunity to assess each option in a realistic manner. This may permit the patient an opportunity to acknowledge that he or she is capable of efficiently utilizing more than a single method of alaryngeal speech. The patient might then be less likely to choose only one method which may be limiting in some circumstances (Duguay, 1978, 1983).

In contrast, other authors have been quite explicit in their disdain for the use of the artificial larynx in any form, citing that its use is unacceptable in all cases (see Gates, Ryan, & Lauder, 1982). This opinion exists regardless of data which indicate that use of an artificial larynx does offer the speaker "highly intelligible and functionally similar" voice and speech (Weinberg, 1985, p. 113). The view that an artificial larynx is totally unacceptable is simply intolerant and has sufficient potential to decrease the patient's ability to acquire a truly functional method of verbal communication postlaryngectomy. If a functional method of alaryngeal speech *is not* acquired by the patient, rehabilitation has failed. Thus, all methods of alaryngeal speech must be considered as potentially viable options.

Changing Attitudes Toward Use of the Artificial Larynx

The past 10 years have seen a dramatic change in the role and scope of those professionals who deal with individuals with communicative impairments. Important advances in the area of computerized technology has certainly permitted more widespread applications for those individuals traditionally labeled as nonspeaking. The specialized area of augmentative and alternative communication has perhaps had an indirect influence on those who undergo total laryngectomy for laryngeal carcinoma. The use of a variety of voice synthesis devices for the nonspeaking population has likely resulted in greater acceptance of the communicatively impaired into society at large. At least some of those factors cited by Rothman (1982) as justification for *not* recommending the use of an artificial larynx may now be somewhat outdated. Thus, social influences and changing attitudes may render invalid some of the reasons offered.

Of those few items listed in Table 11–2 that are indeed factual (i.e., "requires the use of one hand," "requires use of an instrument," and "may leave the individual speechless if mechanical breakdown occurs"), only the concern of mechanical breakdown carries any real merit. The others are simply factual items that have no real bearing on the *communicative effectiveness* of the individual who uses an artificial larynx. Again, the individual's ability to speak may be viewed as a substantial counterbalance to many of the reasons outlined. The combined group of concerns that have been presented historically may in large part be non-issues in contemporary society. Although this belief in no way assumes that disability is not perceived in a unique fashion by some, it does suggest that many may be more tolerant today compared to 10 years ago or longer.

Whether the negative bias that has been directed toward artificial laryngeal devices is presented implicitly or explicitly, there has been a rather distinct disregard for the patient's ultimate communication needs. Issues pertaining to the method of alaryngeal communication have been the primary focus of these discussions, rather than the ability of the artificial larynx to provide the patient with functional communication. Consequently, clear and accurate information on the relative advantages and disadvantages of the artificial larynx should be provided to the patient along with discussion of any specific concerns the patient may have about this alaryngeal option.

Treatment Issues

Essential Components of Artificial Laryngeal Speech

The electronic artificial larynx is in principle a rather simple device for postlaryngectomy alaryngeal communication. Substantial changes in the basic design and functional flexibility of electronic artificial laryngeal devices have occurred since their initial introduction in the early 1940s (Keith & Shanks, 1986). Diedrich and Youngstrom (1966) have subdivided the use of an artificial larynx into three specific compo-

nents: (1) sound generation, (2) sound transmission, and (3) articulation.

Types of Artificial Laryngeal Devices

Perhaps the most widely used intraoral artificial laryngeal device is the *Cooper-Rand* device. Although transcervical type artificial larynges can be adapted for use as an intraoral devices (see Blom, 1978; Zwitman & Disinger, 1975), the commercial availability of the Cooper-Rand in both the United States and Canada makes such modifications infrequent events except in unique patient situations. This device is shown in Figure 11–1.

Several neck-type artificial larynges are also encountered clinically. The best known devices are those manufactured by Western Electric and AT&T in the United States. These devices are quite similar in design and construction. While the AT&T device is currently the most frequently found, the Western Electric device continues to be used in some centers. Examples of the Western-Electric and AT&T neck-type devices are shown in Figures 11–2 and 11–3, respectively. The primary difference between these devices is that the Western Electric device uses a variable pressure activation switch while the AT&T device uses a simple binary on-off button-type switch.

Although many other artificial laryngeal devices are used worldwide, one of the most frequently used is the Servox artificial larynx which is manufactured in Germany. An example of this durable device is shown in Figure 11–4. This device has the advantage of being entirely rechargeable. An example of the Servox artificial larynx along with its portable battery charger is shown in Figure 11–5.

Approaches to Treatment

Numerous approaches are indeed available for the clinician to employ in various

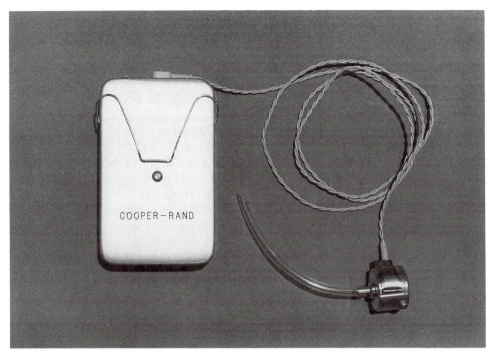

Figure 11–1. The Cooper-Rand intraoral artificial larynx. Device is comprised of electronic source, connecting wire, and intraoral tube assembly with on-off switch.

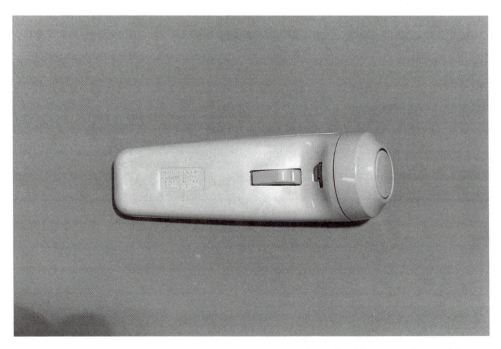

Figure 11–2. The Western Electric neck-type (transcervical) artificial larynx with variable pressure on-off and pitch control switch.

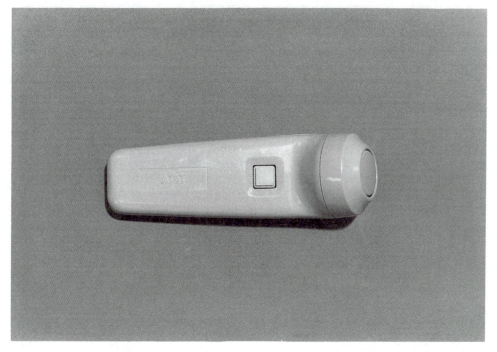

Figure 11–3. The AT&T neck type artificial larynx with single-pole button activation switch.

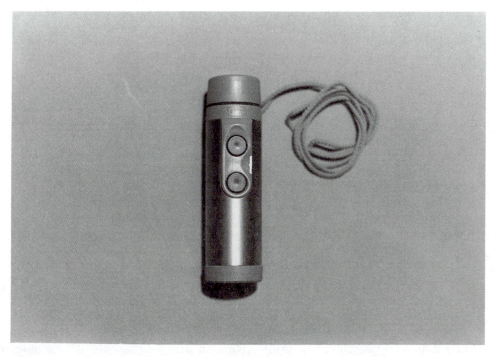

Figure 11–4. The Servox transcervical artificial larynx.

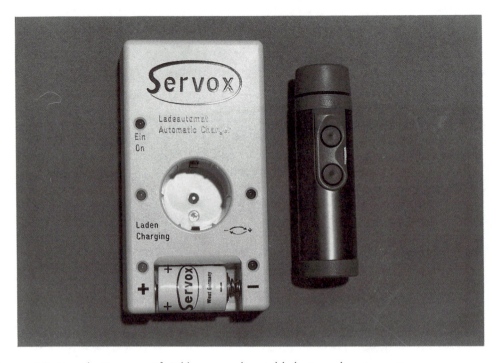

Figure 11–5. The Servox artificial larynx and portable battery charging unit.

phases of training use of the artificial larynx. Yet it does not really matter what stimulus items are used by the clinician provided that problem areas of production are targeted in therapy. Regardless of stimuli, care must be taken to identify problem sounds so that they can be targeted in treatment. Attention should always be paid to variations in phonetic position when drill work is undertaken. What is important though is *how* the program is implemented and monitored. Careful monitoring by the clinician will permit effective identification of problem areas so that goals for modification can be implemented in treatment.

Although the "behavioral" treatment paradigm in its strict form is a historical relic, some of the basic stimulus-response premises can be used effectively in alaryngeal speech training. The acquisition of alaryngeal speech in general, and of artificial laryngeal speech in particular, will necessitate that multiple trials and multiple sets of particular target behaviors are performed in treatment. Thus, the clinician needs to establish base units that must be achieved in order for the patient to move to the next step of treatment (e.g., 90% correct over 10 consecutive sets of 10 trials each). Establishing the number of trials and the number of sets from which success for any given task will be derived is clearly arbitrary. For alaryngeal speech, however, one should probably seek high levels of performance, for example, levels of 90 to 100% accuracy (Weinberg, 1983a, 1983b).

Drill work is essential during the early phase of alaryngeal speech rehabilitation. It is also important for the patient to realize the benefits of such a repetitive treatment protocol; this is best accomplished by setting up several simple but more natural communicative tasks (e.g., going to the hospital cafeteria for coffee, etc.). This type of task permits the patient an opportunity to see that he or she is able to communicate in a basic manner; however, it also frequently brings to the patient's attention the need for further refinement of skills. Many requirements identified for determining successful acquisition of early esophageal speech skills have demanded high levels of performance (Berlin, 1963). The clinician should always set goals that are high for the patient who is attempting to learn proficient use of the artificial larynx. However, the clinician should not be inflexible and delay opportunities for a patient who is experiencing difficulty meeting a particular percentage goal. If this occurs, the criterion for success needs re-evaluation and possible modification. This is where the clinician needs to carefully and comprehensively assess the patient's performance along a number of speech and nonspeech behaviors (Weinberg, 1983a, 1983b). The goal of therapy is always directed at providing the best possible alaryngeal speech for any given patient.

Fortunately, in many patients progress is relatively rapid, and a transition to less artificial and more meaningful speech tasks can be accomplished after a fairly short period of therapy. Some patients will be slower at acquiring skills, and use of more structured stimulus-response paradigms may offer a consistent method of determining change in performance. This can be done quite simply using daily (session) calculations of percent correct across a variety of target behaviors (e.g, isolated consonants, monosyllabic words, etc). In this case, even if progress is slower than that typically noted for the majority of patients, progress *can be monitored and evaluated*. Identification of progress can then serve both the patient and the clinician by demonstrating that a positive change is occurring (although it may not be at an ideal or desired pace).

Defining Successful Communication for Artificial Laryngeal Speech

Although the term "functional communication" may be subject to many different definitions, it is best to view this terminology with respect to whether the artificial larynx permits the individual to communicate basic wants, desires, and needs. The speech-language pathologist and other members of the rehabilitation team should employ this simple communication metric as the minimum basis of successful alaryngeal communication. Too often in the rehabilitative process the patient may become a secondary player rather than the primary one. It should be the patient who ultimately decides what will best serve his or her specific communication needs.

With direct input from the patient the rehabilitative emphasis is placed on *the patient's ability to be a successful communicator* as opposed to the desires of others. This allows the clinician to focus on meeting the patient's primary communicative needs, which will then define the success of preliminary speech rehabilitation. That is, a continuum of "success" should be avoided (particularly in the initial stages of treatment), and a binary decision-making process should be instituted. The binary decision is contingent upon whether the artificial larynx (or other method of alaryngeal communication) can serve to facilitate *at least* the basic communication needs of the patient. Once established, a more continuum-oriented approach can be employed to determine communicative effectiveness and proficiency.

Training Use of the Artificial Larynx: Primary Goals of Treatment

The focus of rehabilitation efforts using the electronic artificial larynx should primarily be directed at three specific clinical goals. These goals require the patient to successfully acquire the following skills in a consistent manner: (1) *proper placement* of the artificial larynx (whether intraoral or transcervical) to ensure maximum generation, transmission, and resonance of the acoustic signal in the vocal tract; (2) use of a *slowed rate of speech* and "over-articulation" to ensure correct coding of phonemic units (particularly with intraoral devices); and (3) synchrony in the patient's ability to manipulate *on-off control*. Within these three specific goals, other behaviors such as creating optimal vocal loudness and maintaining normal phrasing (Snidecor, 1978b; Weinberg, 1983a) may be acquired by the patient in an indirect fashion or they can be directly targeted in treatment. Although other goals will be pursued during the rehabilitative process (see Duguay, 1983), the consistency with which these three goals are acquired and used will form the foundation for the successful use of the artificial larynx regardless of the device employed.

Proper Placement and Contact Pressure and the Use of the Artificial Larynx

In regard to the first goal, two particular problems may be encountered with patients. First, the clinician must work with the patient to determine *where*, either on the external aspect of the neck (transcervical) or within the oral cavity (intraoral), the electronic artificial larynx provides its most complete transmission of the electronic voicing source. With transcervical devices care must be taken to locate a region of the neck that does not physically impede transmission of this external source (e.g., scar tissue or fibrosis). Diedrich and Youngstrom (1966) have noted that proper placement of the artificial larynx is perhaps the most common obstacle encountered with an transcervical electronic artificial laryngeal device.

Identification of the best location for transmission of the artificial sound source is also influenced by how much pressure is applied. For transcervical artificial larynges transmission of sound is conducted via the contact of an oscillating diaphragm

assembly with the tissue of the neck (Diedrich & Youngstrom, 1966; Duguay, 1983; Salmon & Goldstein, 1978, Snidecor, 1978b). In addition to ensuring that the *best location* is found, attention also must be paid to two specific aspects of diaphragm-skin coupling.

The first of these centers on *contact* or *coupling pressure.* The clinician and patient must ensure that diaphragm-neck coupling pressure is not achieved with either too little or too much pressure. In cases where too little pressure is applied, signal transmission will be degraded because of insufficient contact. In contrast, if too much pressure is applied, movement of the oscillator will be impeded, and sound transmission will not occur. Examples of this can easily be demonstrated for the patient by providing too little or too much coupling pressure either on the palm of the patient's hand or through variations in pressure directly on tissues of the neck. However, the clinician may wish to demonstrate on the patient's hand first, given that sensitivity in many cases may be better on the hand than on the postsurgical tissues of the neck.

In the early stages of training in the use of an artificial larynx, the patient's neck may still be tender as a result of surgery; thus, use of moderate-to-extreme pressures may cause some level of discomfort to the patient. Use of a transcervical type of artificial larynx in the early postoperative period may also pose one additional problem. Tissues of the neck often may be rather edematous postoperatively and as a result, signal transmission through such tissue may be impeded to a greater extent. Should this occur, the effectiveness of signal transmission is reduced as is that of the speech produced. It should also be noted that such contact difficulty may also be observed in patients who receive radiation treatment.

The second area related to correct placement of the artificial larynx which needs to be addressed clinically involves ensuring that the face plate of the oscillating diaphragm is in complete contact with neck tissue. The entire diaphragm head and tissues of the neck must be in *parallel contact* with one another. Incomplete contact of the oscillating diaphragm and neck tissue will result in inadequate transmission of the source into the vocal tract and the simultaneous generation of extraneous noise. Such inadequate contact between the vibratory head of the device and the skin will result in production of sufficient extraneous noise from the oscillator of the electronic artificial larynx. This "noise" will override that of the signal which is successfully transmitted into the vocal tract for speech purposes and be disruptive to verbal communication.

Therefore, ensuring that the patient understands the importance of correct placement of the artificial larynx will eliminate several potential problems that are likely to influence the effectiveness of this form of alaryngeal communication. If these skills can be established early in treatment the patient's overall success using the artificial larynx will be enhanced.

Effects of Medical Treatment on the Effectiveness of Sound Transmission

A second area of concern related to successful use of the artificial larynx is influenced by the postsurgical and postradiation status of the patient's neck. That is, anatomical changes in the structure and compliance of neck tissues can disrupt the transmission of the electronic sound source for speech production purposes. In those who have received radiotherapy as part of their treatment regimen the clinician needs to adequately access whether any radiation-induced tissue *fibrosis* is present. Fibrotic changes in neck tissue will reduce its supple nature and, thus, reduce the ability of this tissue to adequately transmit the external source through into the vocal tract. Although the extent of tissue fibrosis is variable from individual to indi-

vidual, it must always be considered as a potential limitation for patient's who desire to use a neck type artificial larynx.

The effects of radiation may be compounded by two specific anatomical changes as a result of the laryngectomy procedure. First, development of scar tissue in and around the surgical incision line(s) subsequent to laryngectomy and any related neck dissection may limit the efficient transmission of the electronic alaryngeal sound source (Diedrich & Youngstrom, 1966). Like that of radiation-induced tissue fibrosis this change will be permanent and, therefore, must be carefully evaluated in the early stages of alaryngeal voice and speech rehabilitation.

The second anatomical change that may influence the successful transmission of the electronic sound source relates to postoperative tissue edema. This change may pose a significant problem for some patients in the early postoperative period; however, these effects are typically transient in nature. The extent of tissue edema may be exacerbated in some patients who receive postsurgical radiation as an adjunctive therapy.

Correct Placement Using an Intraoral Artificial Larynx

In the case of intraoral artificial laryngeal devices such as the Cooper-Rand, placement concerns must address an additional variable that is not encountered with neck type devices. The very nature of the intraoral artificial larynx necessitates that the transmission tube is placed within some portion of the oral cavity. Because of this requirement the possibility exists that tongue excursion will be restricted and, hence, articulatory precision will be disrupted. This might then decrease the patient's speech intelligibility.

The typical recommendation of speech-language pathologists when working with the patient using an intraoral device is to try to locate a suitable location for tube placement. This is often in a lateral region of the posterior oral cavity. In most patients the tube should not be inserted greater than 1–2 inches into the oral cavity. One area of concern related to placement of the tube may offer an additional area of controversy.

Good clinical commonsense suggests that lateral placement of the tube will serve to reduce any potential disruption of lingual movement for articulatory purposes. The consideration of using a "midline" placement has, therefore, been strongly discouraged by many clinicians. Duguay (1983) and others have suggested that use of a midline oral placement has the likelihood of disrupting production of anterior phonemes due to the oral tube limiting tongue excursion and articulatory contact. For some patients, however, the clinician may wish to pursue such anterior midline placement. One need only see a patient using such a tube placement effectively to appreciate this placement option. Although the long-held recommendation for lateral placement of the intraoral tube is recommended, the clinician should not exclude "variations on a theme" including consideration of midline placement in selected patients. If midline placement is unsuccessful this may be presented to the patient as a further indication for consistent lateral placement. Thus, experimentation with different oral positions may at worst be considered "negative practice" (Van Riper, 1978).

Directional orientation (upward or downward) of the intraoral tube is unlikely to create difficulty as the patient begins to acquire basic skills in the operation and use of an intraoral artificial larynx. However, one specific problem may be encountered in the early phase of treatment. If the distal end of the tube is positioned in a downward fashion between the teeth and tongue, there is sufficient opportunity for the tube to become clogged by saliva. This not only disrupts transmission of the electronic sound source into the oral cavity where it can be resonated and articulated

into speech, but may result in a variety of concerns for the patient (e.g., hygienic concerns, efficient function of device, etc.).

Eliminating Difficulties Associated with Saliva Blockage

The problem of saliva blockage may be solved by using a "saliva tip" affixed to the oral end of the tube (Duguay, 1983). The less penetrable characteristics of the saliva tip relative to that of the oral tube provide some restriction to the entrance of saliva into the end of the tube. Another option is to cut the distal end of the tube on an oblique (45 degree) angle (Duguay, 1983). This simple clinical modification is frequently successful in eliminating the rapid clogging of the tube by saliva because it has increased the "open" area of the tube commensurately. Saliva blockage may persist, although it will not occur as frequently as that noted with the unmodified tube. If this modification is utilized, one further recommendation is offered.

Following cutting of the intraoral tube by the clinician, an emery board or piece of emery cloth should be used to smooth the freshly cut edges of the tube. This simple addition eliminates the possibility that the occasionally sharp edge of the tube will irritate the patient's oral cavity. This may be a particular problem in individuals who have reduced intraoral sensation due to surgery or other factors. The final issue to be addressed requires that the patient is aware of basic hygiene issues related to the oral tube.

Patients should be instructed to clean the tube regularly. This is easily done on a daily basis with soap and water. Salmon (1989) has suggested that tubes be soaked overnight in water with a few drops of bleach added to help reduce unpleasant odors related to saliva entering the tube. Another option is to soak tubes in a solution of water and hydrogen peroxide. Regular tube replacement also can be facilitated in a rather easy manner without purchasing new tubes directly from the manufacturer. Patients should be instructed that they can purchase bulk tubing of a similar diameter through a local pet or aquarium supply store. This tubing is typically used for air line hook-ups and is quite inexpensive. New tubes can be cut quite easily directly from longer lengths using either a sharp knife or scissors. This recommendation may help to reduce hygienic problems that occur with intraoral tubing, as well as reducing unnecessary ordering from the supplier.

Development of Clinical Tasks: Articulatory Proficiency

Numerous suggestions on clinical tasks, goals, and protocols may be employed during training in the use of the artificial larynx (Diedrich & Youngstrom, 1966; Duguay, 1983; Salmon & Goldstein, 1978; Snidecor, 1978b). As Snidecor (1978b) has pointed out, many drills and exercises that exist for esophageal speech training (particularly those drills that highlight production of vowels, diphthongs, and consonants) may have similar application in the training of artificial laryngeal speech. This relates to the fact that esophageal sound production is also "all voiced" as is that of the artificial larynx. It is then recommended that similar to esophageal speech training, teaching the use of an artificial larynx should also involve highly systematic programs.

Many clinicians have developed their own protocols and "target word lists" given the commercial availability of many word (stimuli) books which are segmented by phonetic context (Griffith & Miner, 1979; Keith & Thomas, 1989; and others). Others have developed a hybrid from information and suggestions of other clinicians. Again, however, the three primary goals associated with training in the use of the artificial larynx (i.e., proper placement,

slowed rate of articulation, and manipulation of on-off control) are essential skills that must always precede articulatory refinement of artificial laryngeal speech.

The Voiced-Voiceless Distinction

Perhaps the most obvious areas of refinement addressed clinically pertain to phrasing and articulatory precision (Duguay, 1983; Gardner, 1971; Diedrich & Youngstrom, 1966; Salmon & Goldstein, 1978; Snidecor, 1978b). One particular area where clinical efforts must be directed has been noted in relation to the production of voiceless consonants. Because the electrolarynx is an "all voiced" system of sound production, voiced-for-voiceless perceptual errors for consonant cognate pairs has been frequently documented in the literature (Weiss & Basili, 1985).

To successfully code voiceless consonants, it is generally believed that the speaker must be trained to utilize intraoral-pharyngeal air (Duguay, 1983; Diedrich & Youngstrom, 1966) in order to create the necessary turbulence. Salmon (1979) has suggested a very simple task which initially targets production of voiceless plosives (/p, t, k/), fricatives (/f, s, ʃ/) and the voiceless affricate (/tʃ/)in isolation without access to an artificial larynx. The next upgraded task requires the patient to produce these voiceless sounds in words (e.g., path, chalk, fish, etc.) in combination with use of the electrolarynx (Salmon, 1979). This is particularly important for patients learning to use the intraoral artificial larynx. This is due to placement of an intraoral tube; adequate closure of the lips may not always occur and, therefore, pressure consonants may be more difficult to produce.

A related goal that is addressed during this type of consonant-vowel-consonant (CVC) task centers on having the patient continue to produce intraoral and pharyngeal air pressure while at the same time avoiding creation of a "stoma blast."

Although these tasks may apply equally to those who use a transcervical or intraoral type of artificial laryngeal device, some increased difficulty may be encountered using an intraoral device. This is due to possible disruption of articulatory movements resulting from tube placement within the oral cavity. Voiceless consonant production may be improved in those using an intraoral device if careful and consistent feedback is provided to the patient. Again, pressure build-up in the oral cavity may be a problem in those who use an intraoral device.

Duguay (1983) has stressed the importance of working at the isolated sound level similar to that recommended by Salmon (1979). Duguay (1983) also suggests that tasks such as blowing strips of paper, or blowing out matches may facilitate the development and use of intraoral air. The essence of Duguay's (1983) training protocol is clearly directed at having the patient produce "loud and strong" targets. If this goal is accomplished, sound created via intraoral air compression and turbulence may precede or override that provided by the artificial larynx.

Secondary Goals

In addition to primary goals that must be achieved consistently by the patient when using an intraoral electronic artificial laryngeal device, Duguay (1983) has identified several other areas that should be addressed by the speech-language pathologist. These issues pertain to *pitch and volume control* and the patient's *hand preference.* Many artificial laryngeal devices permit the user to adjust pitch and loudness levels. The clinician and patient should work together to identify a pitch level that is best suited to the patient. The goal is to find the best match between source frequency and vocal tract transmission. When this is determined the clinician may wish to mark this setting on the device for the patient. This is easily accomplished with fingernail polish. While one

always desires that the pitch level used will be consistent with the patient's gender, this is not possible in many cases with female patients. Consequently, a setting that permits the best possible voice quality is recommended if more flexible devices are not available to the patient.

In regard to loudness, patients should be instructed to set the loudness level to meet general communicative needs. Louder output will be required in situations where background noise is present. If greater loudness is required several new and rather convenient pocket amplification systems may be obtained through many electronic shops. However, patients must also be informed that loudness levels be carefully monitored in dyads. That is, loudness levels should be maintained at a level which permits some degree of privacy when the patient speaks in public places. This is frequently best learned by trail and error, but sufficient guidance can be provided by the speech-language pathologist.

Patients must also become more sensitive to hearing loss by some family members and peers (Clark, 1985). This will require that adjustments of vocal output be adapted to specific situations in a variety of settings. The speech-language pathologist should identify the advantages of direct facial contact with those who have reductions in hearing sensitivity in order to optimize their communication interactions.

In regard to hand preference, there is no consensus of which hand (dominant or nondominant) is best. Use of the dominant hand will often be somewhat easier for the patient, particularly in early therapy. However, the patient may wish to learn use of both hands in order to meet unique situational needs (e.g., needing to write while speaking on the telephone). Discussion with the patient will often identify which hand is preferred, and this should be honored in most cases unless a compelling reason exists (e.g., limited mobility of an upper extremity due to surgery, etc.).

Patients should also have at least a basic understanding of the general function of the artificial larynx they will use. The patient must also be informed of, as well as trained in, simple issues of device maintenance should breakdown occur (Duguay, 1983). This includes how to clean the device, replace or recharge batteries, and in the case of intraoral artificial laryngeal devices, how to clean and replace tubes and connecting wires. Instructing the patient in these areas will provide a greater sense of independence and in most cases will eliminate unnecessary visits to the speech-language clinic for simple problems.

Observing and Assisting the Patient

Similar to many other behaviors which the speech-langauge pathologist seeks to teach and establish in any patient's repertoire, good skills must also be modeled for the laryngectomized speaker. This is particularly true in the case of those who are attempting to learn proper use of an artificial larynx. The three basic goals of good placement, a reduced rate of speech to facilitate articulatory precision, and careful synchrony associated with on-off control of the artificial larynx must be firmly established as *automatic behaviors* if the best possible speech is to be achieved. These skills may, however, be strongly influenced by a variety of other factors. Thus, it is incumbent on the speech-language pathologist to teach by example.

Not only is demonstration of a given device advantageous for the patient, but the clinician should accept the primary role for identifying all target behaviors in the early stages of treatment. The clinician should manipulate the artificial larynx for the patient until the patient fully understands the demands required. By having the clinician place the device and ensure that a proper seal is achieved, as well as initiating and terminating sound production, the patient is better able to "get a feel" for what is occurring through use of this new voicing device.

Adjusting Treatment Demands

Clinicians must remember that this is a time in the recovery period when considerable demands are placed on the patient. Foremost among such demands, the patient will need to absorb and at least partially understand substantial amounts of new and often complex information. If the patient is able to focus attention on monitoring (auditory, visual, tactile) the ideals that he or she will soon be evaluated on, it is not unreasonable to assume that the acquisition of artificial laryngeal speech will be expedited. This does not imply that the patient should be discouraged from accepting increasing levels of responsibility if progress occurs quickly. However, placing too many demands on the patient too early in the rehabilitation process may create frustration; this in turn may retard early progress in treatment. As for any other patient with a communicative disorder, the clinician needs to be a careful observer of behavior in those who are laryngectomized. Subjective judgments of the patient's daily status in regard to pain and discomfort, fatigue, and depression should certainly factor into a clinician's judgment of what tasks will be undertaken on any given day. A good rule-of-thumb is to always begin and end a treatment session on a positive note (i.e., a successful outcome).

Additional Considerations

During the initial stages of teaching the use of an artificial larynx, Duguay (1983) has identified several factors that may play a significant role in the patient's chance of successfully using the device. Although the factors presented by Duguay (1983) are in no way exhaustive or mutually exclusive they may be categorized into motor capabilities (e.g., manual dexterity, tremor of the hand), intellectual and psychological abilities (e.g., alcoholism, dementia, acceptance of responsibility), and the presence of concomitant communicative limitations (e.g., illiteracy, aphasia, hearing loss). Clearly, numerous other factors may play a key role in a given patient's rehabilitation progress (Diedrich & Youngstrom, 1966; Gardner, 1971; Snidecor, 1978). These concerns must also be identified and addressed. If necessary, treatment protocols should be adapted or modified based on the patient's limitation(s).

Ideally, the introduction of an artificial larynx will not be new to the patient. If the program of rehabilitation has transpired in its best form, the patient may have had some exposure to the device during the preoperative period. In many instances the patient may have the term "artificial larynx" introduced in a preoperative counseling session; but the patient will not likely have significant exposure to one until the postoperative period.

Summary

The artificial larynx should hold a significant role in the rehabilitation of individuals who undergo total laryngectomy. While considerable bias against the use of the electronic artificial larynx (whether a transcervical or intraoral device) has been observed, this bias is wholly unwarranted. The ultimate goal of postsurgical rehabilitation for those who lose their larynx is perhaps complex in nature, but simple in its focus. That is, postsurgical rehabilitation should focus on having the patient achieve the capacity for functional communication. *The method with which functional verbal communication is achieved is irrelevant.* The artificial larynx certainly appears to offer such an opportunity to the patient, particularly in the early postoperative period of rehabilitation. It is essential to acknowledge, however, that use of the artificial larynx in no way limits either the patient's consideration or use of other methods of alaryngeal communication. The artificial larynx does provide a viable option for postsurgical verbal communication and, therefore, should be given fair consideration as a method of postsurgical alaryngeal speech for all who undergo total laryngectomy.

Tracheoesophageal Speech

CHAPTER

Until the 1980s laryngectomized patients were provided with two primary alaryngeal speech options, esophageal speech and the artificial larynx. Development of the tracheoesophageal (TE) puncture technique (Singer & Blom, 1980) and TE puncture voice prosthesis has offered an additional alternative for the laryngectomized patient over the past decade. TE speech has the benefit of being supported by pulmonary air, thereby distinguishing it from traditional esophageal speech. This difference has been shown to favorably affect the overall acoustic aspects of TE speech (Robbins, 1984; Robbins et al., 1984) as well as intelligibility and acceptability (Doyle, Danhauer, & Reed, 1988; Tardy-Mitzell, Andrews, & Bowman, 1985; Williams & Watson, 1985).

TE speech also requires a rather unique approach to clinical treatment. Specifically, the majority of clinical interactions will focus on the function, use, and insertion of the voice prosthesis. The patient must also understand aspects of problem solving

once he or she leaves the clinic. Thus, in contrast to other alaryngeal methods, intervention involves a variety of issues specific to the prosthesis as opposed to direct speech modification tasks. The purpose of this chapter is to review information regarding the TE puncture technique, design and function of the TE voice prosthesis, and its use. Further, information on variations in the surgical technique (secondary versus primary) and use of cricopharyngeal myotomy are presented. Procedures for clinical training of patients who receive TE puncture are also outlined. Finally, several areas of voice modification and refinement are addressed.

The Method of Tracheoesophageal Speech

During traditional esophageal speech, intraoral air is typically trapped in the oral cavity and then forced down the pharynx and into the esophageal reservoir. This air is then forced back up through the pharyngoesophageal (PE) segment which creates vibration of these muscular tissues for voice production. The voiced esophageal sound source then moves through the vocal tract where it is articulated into speech. In TE speech a fistula is surgically created between the trachea (primary airway) and the esophagus (vicarious voicing source). Thus, pulmonary air serves as the power or "driving source" for TE speech production. Not only is the amount of air available substantially different between esophageal and TE speech, but the pulmonary air source is under greater voluntary control. This difference contributes substantially to the acoustic composition of TE speech production.

The Tracheoesophageal Puncture Technique

The voice restoration procedure developed by Singer and Blom (1980) created new hope in the area of postlaryngectomy speech rehabilitation. The surgical procedures employed are vastly different from those associated with air-bypass mechanisms (Shedd, Schaaf, & Weinberg, 1976; Weinberg, Shedd, & Horii, 1978) or the VoiceBak device (Taub & Bergner, 1973; Taub & Spiro, 1972). The surgical procedure itself evolved from the pioneering work of Conley, DiAmesti, and Pierce (1958) and Conley (1959) using venous grafts. Although numerous prior attempts at postlaryngectomy voice restoration using other similar techniques have been reported (Amatsu, 1978; Griffiths & Love, 1978; Komorn, 1974; Sisson, McConnell, Logemann, & Yeh, 1975; and others), success was limited.

The surgical technique for TE puncture is performed using an endoscopic technique (Singer, 1983; Singer & Blom, 1980; Singer, Blom, & Hamaker, 1983, 1984). This technique was originally conducted under general anesthesia as a one-step

secondary procedure after completion of laryngectomy. The goal of the procedure was to create a "controlled midline tracheoesophageal puncture" (Singer & Blom, 1980). The puncture is created between the common posterior wall of the trachea and the anterior wall of the esophagus. Several modifications of the original procedure for creating the TE fistula have been reported (Spofford, Jafek, & Barcz, 1984; Stewart & Sherwen, 1987). Further Hamaker, Singer, Blom, and Daniels (1985) have presented the puncture technique as a *primary procedure* performed at the time of laryngectomy. Following TE puncture, the TE "port" is stented with a catheter prior to insertion and fitting of the voice prosthesis.

Once stenting of the fistula is discontinued post-TE puncture, the prosthesis is inserted into the TE puncture. The TE voice prosthesis acts as a one-way valve capable of shunting pulmonary air from the trachea into the esophagus. Several varieties of prosthesis are available commercially. The prosthesis is made of silicone and varies in length (ranging from 1.8 cm to 3.6 cm) to accommodate various depths of the puncture site. An example of a duckbill and low-pressure prosthesis along with their insertion devices are shown in Figure 12–1. Once inserted, the prosthesis is taped to the superior portion of the patient's tracheostoma. Upon insertion, the prosthesis passes through the TE puncture with the posterior (valve) end of the device located just below the pharyngoesophageal (PE) segment. The one-way valve construction of the TE voice prosthesis allows pulmonary air to be diverted into the esophagus, while eliminating aspiration resulting from reflux of esophageal contents into the tracheal airway.

Following insertion of a prosthesis, the patient is instructed to digitally close the tracheal stoma, thus diverting pulmonary air into the esophagus via the prosthesis. Closure can also be achieved using a tracheostoma valve which eliminates the need for digital closure for voice production (Blom, Singer, & Hamaker,

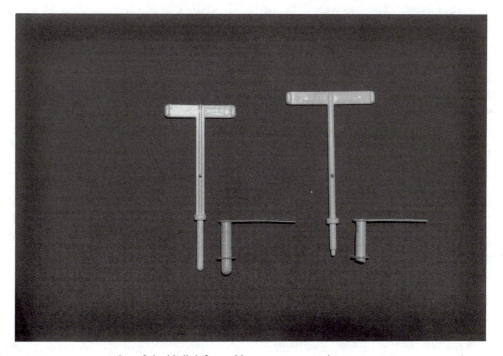

Figure 12–1. Examples of duckbill (left) and low-pressure (right) TE puncture voice prostheses and respective insertion devices.

1982). Esophageal air insufflation is then obtained almost instantaneously on exhalation (Singer & Blom, 1980). Once fitting is completed the speech-language pathologist instructs the patient in correct breath control, articulation, and, if needed, muscle relaxation. Finally, although the prosthesis remains in place continuously, the patient must be instructed in hygiene and re-insertion, as well as use of the prosthesis. If the prosthesis is removed from the fistula and the TE puncture is left open, the puncture will spontaneously close.

Surgical-Prosthetic Speech Restoration: Early Clinical Findings

In the initial report of findings using the TE puncture technique and voice prosthesis, Singer and Blom (1980) presented results from 60 patients, 43 of whom had undergone radical neck dissection. Only 4 patients had achieved some functional esophageal speech prior to TE puncture. TE punctures were performed on patients who had been laryngectomized from 4 weeks to 19 years. Fifty-four in this initial series of patients achieved "successful" speech. Singer and Blom (1980) defined successful speech as being "intelligible and fluent" to listeners. This introduction of the procedure signalled a hallmark in contemporary alaryngeal speech rehabilitation.

In a follow-up to their initial report, Singer, Blom, and Hamaker (1981) presented findings based on 40 months of experience conducting the procedure. Singer et al. (1981) evaluated results of 129 patients and found that 113 (88%) patients acquired voice successfully (success was again based on intelligibility and fluency). Nine patients, although successful in voice production, were unable to maintain the prosthesis and discontinued its use. Fourteen of the patients who were not successful in voice acquisition agreed to undergo further evaluation and revision myotomy of pharyngeal constrictor musculature. When 8 of these patients were assessed using a transtracheal insufflation test and simultaneous videofluroscopy, all revealed pharyngeal masses consistent with pharyngeal constrictor spasm. A selective parapharyngeal nerve block was used with all 14 patients prior to myotomy and revealed that all were capable of producing fluent speech. Ten patients underwent selective myotomy which resulted in successful speech. Based on these findings and those of Singer and Blom (1980), the problem of pharyngeal spasm which may limit postoperative speech production appeared to be alleviated in a high percentage of patients who had previously been unsuccessful in voice acquisition.

Additional findings on the restoration of voice following the TE puncture technique and use of the Blom-Singer voice prosthesis were presented by Johns and Cantrell (1981) for 26 patients. Twenty-four of these patients acquired "good to excellent" speech. The definition of success appears consistent with that of Singer and Blom (1980), with Johns and Cantrell specifying that the two unsuccessful patients exhibited intelligible yet nonfluent speech. Further, they stated that the quality of speech was noted to improve with time and practice. The longest that a prosthesis had been used in this series was 7 months. However, as in prior reports, no objective data on parameters of speech production were compiled. Such data might possibly have indicated the expected progression and proficiency of a patient's newly acquired TE voice.

Wetmore, Krueger, and Wesson (1981) reported findings on 18 patients who underwent TE puncture. Punctures were conducted from 5 weeks to 6 years postlaryngectomy. Speech proficiency prior to TE puncture (esophageal speech) was rated from poor (7 patients) to excellent (3 patients). Thirteen of the patients were reported to be using the prosthesis as their primary means of communication. Ratings of speech proficiency by the investigators reportedly ranged from poor to excellent, with an average rating of fair. Overall, these patients were reported to have increased their preoperative speech intelligibility following the TE puncture.

In the area of TE puncture and use of the Singer-Blom voice prosthesis, Wetmore, Krueger, and Wesson (1981) were the first to report some objective measures of speech production. They collected measures from talkers while counting on a single breath, prolonging production of the vowel /a/, and producing the maximum number of syllables per breath (SPB) within conversational speech. Results revealed a range of counting from 10 to 70, with the mean count being 30 on a single breath; a mean duration of 14 seconds (range 3 to 30 seconds) for vowel prolongation was also noted. The mean number of SPB was revealed to be 14 (range 4 to 28). However, note that 59 syllables would be needed for counting to 30, and this may be a misleading mean value in that the measured range of SPB peaked at 25. The discrepancy noted with the measure of counting on a single breath may be accounted for by second and third breaths unnoticed by the investigators. This problem has been noted previously with esophageal talkers (Isshiki, 1978; Isshiki & Snidecor, 1965; Snidecor & Isshiki, 1965), and is, no doubt, an important variable to control. Although these data were limited, they provided the first basis for comparison to esophageal talkers.

Wetmore, Johns, and Baker (1981) presented a second report on 63 patients who underwent TE puncture. Patients were followed-up from 1 to 12 months postpuncture. Fifty-six (89%) were reported to have acquired fluent speech. Whereas Wetmore, Krueger, and Wesson (1981) gathered some objective data, no qualitative or quantitative data were reported by Wetmore, Johns, and Baker (1981). Although the overall success rate reported was good, only 45 patients (71%) were using the Blom-Singer prosthesis as their primary mode of alaryngeal communication. Subjectively, all TE talkers in this report were judged to be better than traditional esophageal talkers.

In another investigation of the TE puncture technique, 23 patients were studied (Donegan, Gluckman, & Singh, 1981). All patients receiving TE puncture for voice restoration had been unsuccessful in acquiring esophageal speech following 6 months of therapy. Preoperatively, all patients were given a transnasal insufflation test in an attempt to predict postpuncture success, but Donegan et al. (1981) reported the insufflation procedure to be of limited predictive value for either success or failure.

Donegan et al. (1981) used the previously established criteria (Singer & Blom, 1980; Singer et al., 1981) for determining speech success (fluency and intelligibility), as well as the patients' ability and willingness to maintain the prosthesis hygienically. Of the 23 patients, 13 were classified as successful. Of 10 failures reported, 7 resulted from the patients' inability to maintain and care for the prosthesis outside the hospital, despite having acquired *fluent* speech. The primary maintenance problem pertained to difficulty in manipulation and positioning of the prosthesis. Additionally, several patients inadvertently left the prosthesis out, thus allowing the TE puncture to close spontaneously. Three patients reportedly suffered from pharyngeal spasm which rendered the production of voice impossible.

Wood, Rusnov, Tucker, and Levine (1981) presented results from 32 patients who underwent TE puncture. These investigators presented selection criteria for patients to receive the puncture. Identified in their criteria were motivation, learning, and patient expectation factors; the need for adequate manual dexterity and vision; features related to the anatomy, size, and maturity of the stoma; general physical health; and results of insufflation testing. Results of the Wood et al. (1981) study indicated that 28 patients were classified as

successful speakers following surgery. Of two failures, one eventually acquired speech after undergoing myotomy. Overall, TE speech proficiency for all patients was subjectively judged by a speech pathologist to be better than that demonstrated by esophageal speakers for parameters of fluency, pitch volume, phrasing, and extraneous noise factors (stoma noise).

Based on early data, viability of the TE puncture technique for voice restoration was supported. Although additional reports have appeared in the literature over the past decade, similar trends in success have been noted. However, after the initial series of clinical reports many modifications in the device and pre-selection of patients came to the clinical forefront. As such, several different types of devices have been used and clinical reports cannot be generalized across prosthesis type and patient populations. The TE puncture technique has gained widespread application worldwide and has been shown to be a highly effective method of voice restoration. Effectiveness is enhanced when careful preoperative evaluation is employed (Andrews, Mickel, Monahan, Hanson, & Ward, 1987; Singer, 1983, 1988; Singer & Blom, 1980; Singer et al., 1981, 1983).

Assessing Candidacy

Since introduction of the Singer-Blom method of TE puncture and use of the valved voice prosthesis (Singer & Blom, 1980), considerable information has been collated regarding candidacy for this procedure. This has resulted in the identification of numerous factors that may be used to assess an individual's chance of successfully using the TE voice prosthesis. This information has been provided to reduce the chance that unsuitable individuals will undergo the surgical procedure. Few patients meet all necessary requirements.

Although many factors have the potential to be contraindications for successful use, the identification of one or more factors is not exclusionary in all cases. Factors that have been identified serve as a *guideline for candidacy* rather than a checklist of inclusionary or exclusionary criteria. It is the clinician's responsibility to fully understand the reason that particular factors may influence a patient's chance at achieving success following TE puncture. The experienced clinician will be able to discern which factors are substantive and which may be remedied or overcome with advance training of the patient. A summary of these criteria are provided in Table 12–1.

Esophageal Insufflation Testing

One of the most widely reported methods for assessing candidacy for TE puncture is termed the *esophageal insufflation test*. This method was first reported by van den Berg and Moolenaar-Bilj (1959); procedural details in the contemporary literature were best presented by Taub (1980) who identified the method as the "air-blowing test." Taub's use of the air-blowing test as a *preoperative method* of determining a patient's candidacy for such a procedure appears to provide a valuable tool for assessment and evaluation of esophageal function (Taub & Bergner, 1973; Taub & Spiro, 1972).

Goals of Esophageal Insufflation Testing

The impetus for use of the air-blowing test was twofold. The first goal was simply to identify the anatomical location of the esophageal inlet and reservoir; the second goal sought to determine whether the esophagus in a given individual could serve as an alaryngeal voicing source (Taub, 1980; Taub & Bergner, 1973; Taub & Spiro, 1972). By insufflating the esophageal reservoir with a continuous supply of air, the capacity of the PE segment to serve as an alaryngeal voicing source is permitted. Blom, Singer, and Hamaker (1985) recommended that insufflation testing be performed "to identify patients at risk for voice failure." Yet several issues regarding the use of the esophageal insufflation test as a predictor of esophageal function have been raised. Further, alterations in the method of assessment may influence results obtained and, therefore, must be considered carefully when interpreting data on esophageal insufflation.

TABLE 12–1.
Criteria for Candidacy to Receive the TE Puncture Procedure.

1. Patient must be motivated.
2. Patient must have adequate understanding of postsurgical anatomy.
3. Patient must have basic understanding of function of the TE puncture voice prosthesis.
4. Patient must demonstrate adequate manual dexterity to manage prosthesis.
5. Visual acuity must be sufficient for purposes of managing tracheostoma and prosthesis.
6. Patient must exhibit ability to care for prosthesis.
7. Patient should not have significant hypopharyngeal stenosis.
8. Patient should demonstrate positive results following esophageal air insufflation test.
9. Patient must have adequate pulmonary support for prosthesis use.
10. Patient should have stoma of adequate depth and diameter for prosthesis to avoid airway occlusion.
11. Patient should be mentally stable.

Source: From Andrews et al. (1987), Major complications following tracheoesophageal puncture for voice rehabilitation, *Laryngoscope, 97,* 562–567, The Laryngoscope, St. Louis, MO; reprinted with permission.

Method of Esophageal Insufflation Testing

Early reports on esophageal insufflation testing (Taub, 1980) involved a relatively simple protocol for assessment. The initial step in this process involves transnasal insertion of a catheter into the region of the upper esophagus below the PE segment. This procedure is typically performed by the otolaryngologist, although a speech-language pathologist may perform this task under supervision of a physician in some multidisciplinary clinics. Catheter insertion permits introduction of air into the esophageal reservoir in order to ascertain the functional capacity of the PE segment as a possible alaryngeal voicing source.

Careful assessment of the literature on esophageal insufflation testing indicates some degree of inconsistency on the type of catheter that best serves this purpose. Although many reports indicate use of a Foley-type urinary catheter, the diameter of the catheter used is not consistent (e.g., No. 12 to a No. 18 French). Others have suggested use of more rigid catheters such as the Levin-type stomach tube (Reed, 1983a). Regardless of the catheter used, the final placement of the distal end of the catheter rests in the esophageal lumen. If insertion extends too far below the esophageal reservoir, air will be directed toward the stomach; if it is positioned too high, a weak, turbulent sound will be produced by structures of the pharyngeal tissues (see Finkbeiner, 1978). Changes in positioning of the catheter usually result in clear, perceptually distinct voice qualities.

The introduction of air into the esophageal lumen via the catheter has been done using several methods. Until the mid-1980s, air was usually introduced by having the examiner expire into the end of the catheter. This method has several advantages; however, the disadvantages were significant. Although air insufflation by the examiner permitted at least a subjective evaluation of the pressure required to initiate oscillation of PE segment tissues, the potential for over-insufflation did exist.

Over-insufflation was not uncommon during insufflation tests performed by introducing air provided via a small compressor; the esophagus has been shown to be sensitive to air distention (Henderson, 1983). Hence, the possibility of inducing reflexive contraction of the muscle fibers comprising the upper esophageal sphincter clearly existed. If such reflexive contraction occurred because either too great a volume of air or insufflation at too rapid a rate was introduced into the esophageal reservoir, some form of PE spasm may have been noted.

This response ostensibly limited the vibratory capacity of the PE segment because of the reflexive muscular contraction of the sphincter. Consequently, this reflex limited the potential for voicing and a "failed" esophageal insufflation test was proclaimed. Although multiple trials of the test were typically reported, it was not unusual to observe a consistent pattern of failure with the ultimate result being labeled "cricopharyngeal spasm" (Singer & Blom, 1981) Thus, direct insufflation by the examiner may have introduced a methodological variable which modified the individual's ultimate outcome. Although it is important to note that some cases of true cricopharyngeal spasm may have existed with many individuals who failed an insufflation test, numerous clinicians who have performed the insufflation test by this method have anecdotally noted that different outcomes were at times observed based on the amount of effort used to insufflate the esophagus.

Another factor associated with this potential confound in the observed response of a given individual to esophageal insufflation rests with the difference in catheter size noted above. From a strictly physical standpoint, smaller diameter catheters require the examiner to provide higher exhalatory pressures to "charge" the esophageal reservoir. In instances where insufflation was provided via compressed air, fine adjustment in the volume of air introduced is not always possible, and insufflation may occur too quickly, thus triggering reflexive contraction. The diameter of the catheter also has the potential to alter the rate at which air moves into the esophagus during the insufflation procedure. Modifications in the esophageal insufflation procedure may have eliminated potential confounds in preoperative assessments of esophageal function for alaryngeal voice purposes (Blom et al., 1985).

Perhaps the most obvious disadvantage of the above discussed insufflation method rests with simple concerns regarding general hygiene and issues of infection control that are now so important in all health care settings (ASHA, 1989, 1990). Direct insufflation by the examiner poses a clear risk to both individuals undergoing and performing the insufflation. Thus, the esophageal insufflation test *should never*

be performed using direct insufflation. Currently, it is recommended that all esophageal insufflation testing be conducted using the procedures developed and outlined by Blom et al. (1985).

The procedure recommended by Blom et al. (1985) was developed to address three critical issues pertaining to esophageal insufflation testing: (1) use of a measured catheter would permit correct placement of the catheter in the esophageal lumen, (2) the method would use self-insufflation by permitting individuals to insufflate their own esophageal reservoir with their own pulmonary air, and (3) the method would provide a replicable, standard protocol for esophageal insufflation testing. This procedure involves use of a disposable (i.e., single-use) insufflation system which includes a 50 cm rubber catheter (No. 14 French), a tracheostoma housing assembly, and related adhesives. This system is shown in Figure 12–2. The catheter

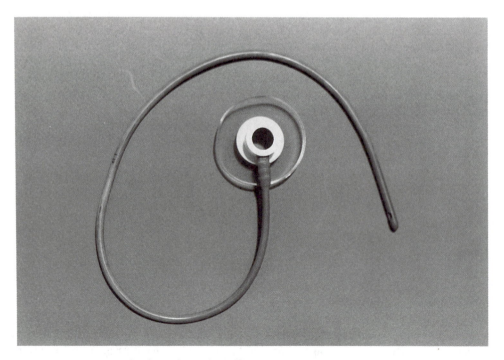

Figure 12–2. Transtracheal esophageal insufflation system. System is comprised of catheter, adapter, and tracheostoma housing.

is marked at a distance 25 cm from the tip. It is recommended that the catheter be inserted transnasally until the 25 cm mark is at the nostril, thus permitting insertion which ensures that the tip is located in the upper thoracic esophagus (Blom et al., 1985). Due to the flexible nature of the catheter, Blom et al. (1985) note that the examiner must carefully insert the catheter and confirm that the distal end has entered the esophagus rather than coiling in the pharynx.

The next step in the process requires that a liquid adhesive, as well as a stick-on adhesive disk be applied to the peristomal region and back of a flexible, open housing, respectively. Next, the housing is carefully placed over the tracheostoma. The tracheostoma housing does not interfere with the individual's breathing at any point during the preparation for or performance of the esophageal insufflation test. A plastic interfacing adapter which comes attached to the catheter is then inserted into the housing (see Figure 12–2). The adapter, similar to a ring, is also open and, therefore, does not restrict respiration. Once this three-step procedure is completed, the individual is instructed about the tasks he or she will perform.

Instructions to the Patient

Patients should be instructed that they will be required to follow a simple, three-step procedure for insufflation testing: (1) patients are asked to take a normal breath, (2) they are then asked to manually occlude the open portion of the adapter which is now inserted into the tracheostoma housing, and (3) they are then asked to exhale with their mouth open and attempt to produce the vowel /ɑ/. It is important, however, to ensure that the patient (1) is not inspiring too deeply (i.e., well beyond levels typically observed for normal speech breathing), (2) is fully occluding the open portion of the adapter, (3) is not pressing excessively on the adapter and tracheostoma housing, and (4) has opened his or her mouth for sound production. It is also helpful to ask the patient to avoid trying to say anything specific and to "just let the sound come out." Blom et al. (1985) also suggest a brief practice period. Once the clinician is comfortable that the patient understands the tasks to be performed, the clinician should request that a vowel be sustained for as long as possible on a single breath. Thus, the esophageal insufflation test mimics the basic method used for evaluation of maximum phonation time (MPT).

Once the patient is comfortable with requirements of the task, the assessment can begin. Blom et al. (1985) recommend that *at least five trials* of vowel prolongation be performed; additionally, the patient is requested to count from 1 to 15 in several trials. During counting, the clinician must encourage the patient to do so on a single inspiration. Following completion of these tasks a clinical interpretation of results can be achieved.

What Defines a Successful Outcome?

According to Blom et al. (1985), a successful insufflation will culminate in the patient being able to sustain a vowel "without interruption" for at least 10 seconds. In their training tape on TE puncture and use of the voice prothesis, Blom, Singer, and Hamaker (1989) have revised this guideline to a minimum of 8 seconds. Performance on the counting task should be consistent with that for the sustained phonation task. Blom et al. (1985) note that a "successful response to transnasal esophageal insufflation" is characterized by voice production that is "essentially devoid of any strained quality." It is, however, prudent to weigh this factor carefully.

The primary purpose of esophageal insufflation testing is by definition an attempt to determine the utility and, perhaps, the efficiency with which the PE segment may function as a vicarious voicing source. Although the competent clinician certainly needs to observe more global aspects of the patient's alaryngeal voice, the main objective centers on whether the individual is capable of producing (tracheo)esophageal voice for *a minimum period of time without interruption*. It is unreasonable to assume that a patient would be classified as exhibiting an unsuccessful response to insufflation based on judgments of voice quality or other parameters that are independent of those related to temporal components of sustained alaryngeal phonation.

From a practical clinical standpoint, esophageal insufflation testing is best viewed as a binary event; either the assessment has been successful (sustained esophageal voicing for ≥ 8 seconds) or it is unsuccessful (< 8 seconds). Although this binary judgment is indeed arbitrary, it does appear to have merit in regard to minimum expectations for "continuous" voicing that may be required for functional speech purposes. The overall continuity of voicing is what will ultimately distinguish TE speech from traditional esophageal speech and, therefore, must be addressed within that context. Yet Blom et al. (1985) are clear to point out that "airflow-induced pharyngeal constrictor spasm" may be observed in a variety of forms unique to each individual. Some individuals may exhibit such severe spasm that they are unable to initiate even a brief burst of voicing, whereas others may exhibit more intermittent forms of spasm.

The intermittency observed when airflow-induced spasm occurs is typically characterized by short-to-moderate periods of esophageal voicing followed by complete cessation of voicing. This type of pattern may also be observed to ebb and flow in that voicing may be initiated, then cease abruptly, only to have voicing return and cease again in a repetitive pattern. It should be clear then that *cricopharygeal or pharyngeal constrictor spasm is not a unitary phenomenon* although its occurrence is globally interpreted as being discontinuous voicing.

Specifically, continuity of alaryngeal voicing likely has its greatest impact on overall communicative effectiveness. If a given speaker (regardless of whether he or she uses esophageal or TE speech) is unable to produce voicing of adequate duration, the listener may judge the effectiveness of the communication negatively (Bennett & Weinberg; 1973; Hoops & Noll, 1969; Shipp, 1967). The duration of continuity has a primary effect on the patient's rate of speech; shorter durations of voicing require the speaker to pause more frequently (even if the pause is itself short in duration) which alters the naturalness of the speech produced. The underlying goal of esophageal insufflation testing clearly centers around determining who is "at risk" for (tracheo)esophageal voice acquisition failure (Blom et al., 1985).

Pharyngoesophageal Spasm

Over 20 years ago Gardner (1971) directly addressed problems associated with the inability of the patient to open what he termed an "overly tense" PE segment. If this tonic contraction does not permit insufflation, then no power source exists for the production of esophageal voice. These concerns re-emerged in relation to observations made in some patients who were unable to generate "esophageal" voicing following TE puncture.

Identification of suspected "pharyngoesophageal spasm" was reported by Singer and Blom (1980) in their first report of patients who underwent TE puncture for voice restoration. In that report, Singer and Blom (1980) stated that five or six patients ($N = 60$) experienced difficulty with voice production and this was believed to be the result of spasm. Considerable interest in this phenomenon was generated, and a rather substantial controversy emerged as to whether the observed spasm was a normal or abnormal response (Doyle, 1985; McGarvey & Weinberg, 1984). Singer and Blom (1980) believed that if the spasm could be eliminated, fluent TE speech would then be possible. This concern also resulted in a general reassessment of PE segment function (Zwitman, 1986) and, once again, the acknowledgment that the extent of surgery and subsequent reconstruction could influence (tracheo)esophageal voice production (Callaway, Truelson, Wolf, Thomas-Kincaid, and Cannon, 1991; Lewin, Baugh, & Baker, 1987).

The Clinical Value of Esophageal Insufflation Testing

The potential value of esophageal insufflation testing in assessing the functional integrity of the PE segment appears, at least at face value, to have clinical merit. The value of such an assessment can be viewed to occur at two basic levels of clinical inquiry, one that centers its attention on the use of this procedure to determine potential candidacy for those who wish to acquire TE speech and one that centers on broader issues of esophageal function. Although use of esophageal insufflation testing may indeed provide a presurgical indication of the potential for postsurgical (i.e., TE puncture) success in the acquisition of TE voice and speech, false positive and negative results may occur. This issue creates a variety of clinical dilemmas.

At the second level of clinical inquiry noted, esophageal insufflation testing would appear to offer extremely valuable information about the function of the postlaryngectomy (reconstructed) PE segment. Although false positive and false negative results appear to be just as likely, the use of this technique would seem to hold great promise in identifying patterns of PE segment behavior in response to insufflation at various time intervals postlaryngectomy (Welch, Gates, Luckmann et al., 1979; Welch, Luckmann, Ricks et al., 1979). This issue is raised because of the very nature of total laryngectomy and subsequent surgical resection performed. Because of the type and

extent of surgery performed for laryngeal cancer which necessitates total laryngectomy, several concepts of postlaryngectomy function must be addressed.

Function of the pharynx and the esophagus in the normal human system is complex (Henderson, 1983). When the structural components that comprise these two distinct anatomical regions are altered due to laryngectomy, several considerations must take place (Singer, 1988). The essence of such considerations rests with the fact that the overall structure of the PE segment proper is significantly influenced by (1) the extent of surgical reconstruction which is guided by tumor extension and disease-free surgical margins and (2) the individual's postoperative course.

It is without question that total laryngectomy influences the amount of tissue that forms the postlaryngectomy PE segment, the overall relationship of muscular tissue to that of nonmuscular (connective) tissue that exists in continuity with the newly reconstructed upper digestive tract and lower vocal tract, the composition of the muscular fibers which comprise the PE segment, as well as both static and dynamic function of the PE segment postlaryngectomy (Damste, 1986; Gates, Ryan, Cantu, & Hearne, 1982; Singer, 1988; Zwitman, 1986). Therefore, postlaryngectomy PE segment function is altered and influenced by anatomic, physiologic, and neurologic variables that are likely to be highly individualized (Doyle, 1985).

When these variables are viewed collectively, it should become obvious that the essential behavior that the speech-language pathologist is interested in determining through the use of esophageal insufflation testing is multifaceted. Due to system interactions (anatomical, physiological, and neurological) in the postlaryngectomy PE segment, there exists great potential that this mechanism will exhibit substantial alteration in its responsivity to air insufflation (Doyle, 1985). Although it has been suggested that use of an esophageal insufflation test preoperatively may identify those individuals who will exhibit spasm (Lewin, Baugh, & Baker, 1987; Blom et al., 1985; Singer & Blom, 1980), both false positive and false negative responses may occur (Singer & Blom, 1980).

Only two studies in the literature have attempted to provide a replicable method of esophageal insufflation testing. Lewin et al. (1987) evaluated the effectiveness of esophageal insufflation testing as a pre-operative assessment of individuals who were to undergo TE puncture. Lewin et al. (1987) developed and employed an objective procedure for determining intraesophageal pressures in 27 laryngectomized patients. The goal of this investigation sought to identify the predictive value of esophageal insufflation testing. Data obtained indicated that intraesophageal pressures appeared to correspond to postoperative speech abilities. Specifically, lower pressures were related to "fluent" speech production; in contrast, higher pressures appeared to correspond to "nonfluent" speakers or those who were "nonspeakers." Combined data were interpreted to be indicative of the value of esophageal insufflation testing.

In a recent report, Callaway et al. (1992) sought data on the potential predictive value of esophageal insufflation testing. Callaway et al. (1992) evaluated the performance of 14 individuals who had undergone total laryngectomy. Prior to TE

puncture, esophageal insufflation testing was performed on all 14 subjects following the objective method presented by Lewin et al. (1987) using compressed air presented at a rate of 3 to 4 liters per minute (LPM). Thus, direct objective measures of "resistive esophageal pressures" (in mm Hg) could be gathered for comparative purposes. Measures were acquired while subjects sustained the vowel /a/ and during counting. Although all subjects were assessed preoperatively (TE puncture), only 7 subjects underwent a second, post-TE puncture insufflation test. These pre- and postoperative pressures ranged from a low value of 15 to a high of 70 mm Hg. Subjective perceptual evaluation of each patient's speech was also performed using an ascending 5-point scale for parameters of loudness, quality, and fluency. The aggregate sum of the ratings for these three parameters were then used to determine "success" of TE speech.

Although an intelligibility rating was obtained for each subject, specific details were not reported. Callaway et al. (1992) arbitrarily defined successful TE speech for those individuals who exhibited combined perceptual ratings of ≥ 10, or a fluency rating that *met or exceeded 4*. A summary of the comparative esophageal pressure measures obtained for the 7 subjects who underwent both pre- and postoperative insufflation is provided in Table 12–2.

TABLE 12–2.
Esophageal Insufflation Pressures (in mm Hg) Obtained from 7 Subjects Prior to TE Puncture and at > 6 Months Following TE Puncture.

Subject	Pre-TE Puncture	> 6 Months Post-TE Puncture
1	40	25
2	45	55
3	40	40
4	40	20
5	40	25
6	16	22
7	15	20

Source: Adapted from Callaway et al. (1992).

Based on the combined data collected by Callaway et al. (1992), significant improvements were noted over time for fluency and the combined rating scores. The mean combined rating score increased from 7.7 pre-TE puncture to 12.2 postoperatively (i.e., > 6 months). Speech intelligibility ratings were also found to be associated with the combined ratings at 6 months. The resistive pressure measures obtained during esophageal insufflation testing were not, however, successful in predicting acquisition of TE speech.

Although Callaway et al. (1992) hypothesized that pressures below 20 mm Hg would increase the likelihood that TE speech would be acquired and, conversely, that pressures exceeding 20 mm Hg would result in failure, statistical evaluation did not support this assumption. Thus, pre-TE puncture pressure values *did not appear to be indicative of eventual long-term speech outcomes* in the 7 subjects who were evaluated at both points in time. Interestingly, of 11 subjects who exhibited successful TE speech 6 months or later post-TE puncture, 7 demonstrated "speech failure" during the initial fitting of the TE puncture voice prosthesis. Further, evaluation of the raw data they presented indicated that the patient who exhibited the lowest pressure (15 mm Hg) in the pre-TE puncture assessment and the subject who exhibited the highest value (70 mm Hg) both exhibited combined ratings scores of 14 for speech performance at 6 months post-TE puncture or longer.

In summary, data presented by Callaway et al. (1992) indicate that (1) TE voice and speech improved with time (i.e., from pre-TE puncture assessment to ≥ 6 months post-TE puncture) and (2) that objective evaluation of esophageal insufflation testing does not appear to be a good predictor of successful TE speech acquisition. However, Callaway et al. (1992) noted that patient performance at the time of prosthesis fitting may provide an index of later patient performance. This suggestion indicates that the puncture procedure itself may introduce additional variables that

should be considered in assessments of the long-term success in postoperative speech acquisition (Singer, 1988). Given these data, careful consideration regarding information provided to a patient who demonstrates "success" during a preoperative esophageal insufflation test is warranted. Although an individual may exhibit a favorable response during insufflation, the puncture procedure itself, as well as the introduction of a valved voice prosthesis, may alter esophageal performance.

Surgical Methods, Modifications, and Refinements

Over the past 14 years since the TE puncture technique and TE puncture voice prosthesis were initially introduced (Singer & Blom, 1980), numerous modification and refinements in the surgical method(s) have been observed (Hurbis, Tesenga, Goodman, & Wenig, 1991; Maniglia, 1982; and others). While the original technique presented by Singer and Blom (1980) is still used as a secondary method of TE puncture, experience has dictated that modifications are necessary with particular subgroups of patients. As use of the TE puncture technique and TE puncture voice prosthesis moves into its second decade of usage in the 1990s further use (Heatley & Anderson, 1992), as well as modifications and refinements, will likely continue.

Primary Versus Secondary Surgical Procedures

It was originally suggested that TE puncture for voice restoration be performed as a secondary procedure (Singer & Blom, 1980). The term *secondary* indicated that the TE puncture was performed at some point following total laryngectomy. This involved at least a 6 month waiting period postlaryngectomy. The use of TE puncture as a secondary procedure for voice restoration resulted in good success rates (Singer & Blom, 1981; Yoshida, Singer, Hamaker, Blom, & Charles, 1989). Thus, a majority of reports represented data from use of TE puncture as a secondary procedure, and the procedure was supported by a majority of head and neck surgeons (Lopez, Kraybill, McElroy, & Guerra, 1987).

It was believed that secondary application of the TE puncture technique was appropriate because the initial problems associated with total laryngectomy, those relating to changes in anatomy and physiology, could be dealt with directly and remedied before introducing a new set of demands on the individual. Secondary TE puncture offered distinct advantages in regard to tissue healing, radiation induced tissue changes, and so forth. Thus, TE puncture as a secondary procedure found its foundation in potentially reducing the overall chance of a variety of complications that may have occurred if the technique was employed at the time of laryngectomy (Andrews et al., 1987).

One of the most significant changes in TE puncture emerged in 1985 (Hamaker et al., 1985) when it was suggested that the procedure could be performed at the time of laryngectomy. Hamaker et al. (1985) believed that several advantages for use of a *primary* procedure existed when compared to *secondary* procedures; the most compelling reason for performing TE puncture as a primary procedure involved the fact that "improved exposure" of the surgical field was provided. Controversy continues as to which method is best, although success appears to range from approximately 65% to 100% (Hamaker et al., 1985; Maves & Lingeman, 1982; Morrison & Ogrady, 1986; Stiernberg, Bailey, Calhoun, & Perez, 1987; Yoshida, Hamaker, Singer, Blom, & Charles, 1989). Use of primary TE puncture does not appear to sacrifice aspects of safety that are related to surgical management of the malignancy (Trudeau, Hirsch, & Schuller, 1986). How-

ever, it is clear that more careful consideration of individual patient factors influencing success with either method needs to be addressed in a comprehensive manner. To date, a clear indication of who is likely to be the best candidate for primary TE puncture is largely unidentified.

Complications associated with primary TE puncture are quite varied and range from serious to minor problems. This includes fistula formation, infection, closure of the puncture site, development of granulation tissue, and salivary leakage (Ho, Wei, Lau, & Lam, 1991; Maniglia, Lundy, Casiano, & Swim, 1989; Singer et al., 1989; Wenig, Mullooly, Levy, & Abramson, 1989; Yoshida et al., 1989). Yet similar complications are not uncommon in those who undergo secondary procedures (McConnel & Duck, 1986; Silver, Gluckman, & Donegan, 1985; Singer & Blom, 1981). Despite findings by Wenig et al. (1989) that complication rates for primary TE puncture may be "slightly higher" when compared to patients who undergo secondary procedures, they suggest that both methods are "equally effective in permitting the development of tracheoesophageal speech." Although problems associated with long-term use, management, and success of the prosthesis have been reported in patients receiving primary TE puncture (Trudeau, Hirsch, & Schuller, 1986), they do not appear more prevalent compared to patients undergoing secondary TE puncture.

Trudeau et al. (1986) attempted to determine if differences in recovery patterns for patients who had received secondary and primary TE punctures could be identified. They evaluated 36 patients, 21 who had undergone primary voice restoration and 15 who had received secondary procedures. Trudeau et al. (1986) reported that patients who received primary TE puncture were "no more prone to serious complications" than those who had TE puncture performed as a secondary procedure. These authors did note, however, that patients who had undergone primary

TE puncture were more likely to acquire another method of alaryngeal communication if TE puncture failed.

Approaches to Management of Pharyngoesophageal Spasm: Myotomy and Neurectomy

Two general approaches to the elimination of PE segment spasm have been offered in the literature: *selective myotomy* (Chodosh et al., 1984; Henley & Souliere, 1986; Mahieu, Annyas, Schutte, & van der Jagt, 1987; Singer & Blom, 1981;) and *pharyngeal plexus neurectomy* (Singer et al., 1986). Although the underlying neurophysiologic mechanism that influences spasm is somewhat controversial, it is generally agreed that pharyngoesophageal spasm is a direct response of the segment to air distention in the esophageal reservoir. Myotomy seeks to diminish muscular contraction by dissecting muscle fibers[1] that form the sphincter. The muscles involved in myotomy are typically the cricopharyngeus, as well as the inferior pharyngeal constrictor and the middle pharyngeal constrictor (Singer, 1988). It is also important to note that the myotomy is done *unilaterally*. In contrast, neurectomy involves dissection of the nerve trunks that form the pharyngeal plexus (components include fibers from cranial nerves IX, X, and XI). This dissection of neural innervation serves to diminish the tonicity of the PE segment without incising muscles which form the sphincter. Thus, medical approaches to management have sought to disrupt the degree of contraction by dissecting muscular components of the sphincter (myotomy) or by disrupting the neural control to the sphincter (neurectomy).

Myotomy and neurectomy form the two most commonly used approaches to

reduce pharyngoesophageal spasm in response to airflow. Generally, the results of these two methods have been favorable in reducing tonicity of the sphincter (Singer, 1988; Singer & Blom, 1981; Singer et al., 1986). It has also been suggested that management of PE segment tonicity be undertaken as a primary procedure in an attempt to avoid difficulties with TE (or esophageal) voice acquisition in the postlaryngectomy period (Hamaker et al., 1985). The rationale underlying application of myotomy or neurectomy at the time of laryngectomy is based on a desire to eliminate the need for a secondary procedure should spasm be observed. This does not entirely reduce the possibility that spasm will occur postoperatively (Hamaker et al., 1985; Singer & Blom, 1981; Singer et al., 1981).

The use of myotomy or neurectomy has potential applications in voice and speech restoration following laryngectomy. Nevertheless, both procedures carry some degree of risk. The most common complications associated with selective myotomy appear to be related to post-myotomy fistula formation and infection (Hamaker et al., 1985; Singer & Blom, 1981; Singer et al., 1986). Complications of this type may be increased in patients who have received previous radiation therapy (Lewin et al., 1987; Singer, 1988; Singer et al., 1986). Although these complications appear in less than 10% of patients (Singer, 1988) they are serious and must not be disregarded. Fistula formation or tissue breakdown are unlikely in cases of neurectomy. If such complications occur, speech treatment must be delayed and the delay is often substantial. Therefore, the introduction of an artificial larynx is essential in order to provide the patient with an alternative method of communication should problems arise. The use of an intraoral artificial laryngeal device is recommended in these cases in that difficulty associated with placement (skin-device

---

[1]It should be noted that this dissection is incomplete both in regard to the depth and length of the muscular incision.

coupling) may be encountered with neck type devices.

Evolution of the Voice Prosthesis

Since introduction of the TE puncture voice prosthesis, considerable modifications in its design have been undertaken. Modifications such as the addition of a retention collar, implementation of a single neck strap, and the refinement of insertion devices which decrease rotation of the prosthesis on the inserter have reduced many clinical problems. An example of single and double-strap duckbill prostheses are shown in Figure 12–3. The design of voice prostheses that exhibit lower resistance to

airflow also appear to offer considerable advantages to the patient. Consequently, a variety of voice prostheses are now commercially available to patients who choose to undergo TE puncture for voice restoration. A variety of specialty prostheses have also been developed (Shapiro & Ramanathan, 1982). For example, several varieties of combined TE puncture voice prostheses and tracheostoma vent devices are available. Two examples of these devices are shown in Figure 12–4. Finally, in-dwelling devices will soon be available in North America.[2]

Considerable disagreement between clinicians has been apparent in regard to which prosthesis is "best." Suffice it to say, no one device is perfect. What is more important than questions about the prosthesis itself, however, is what prosthesis is best with any given patient. Prostheses

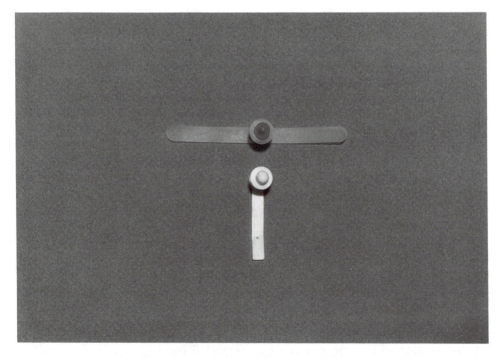

Figure 12–3. Examples of single strap and double-strapped TE puncture voice prostheses.

---

[2]Personal communication, E.D. Blom (1993).

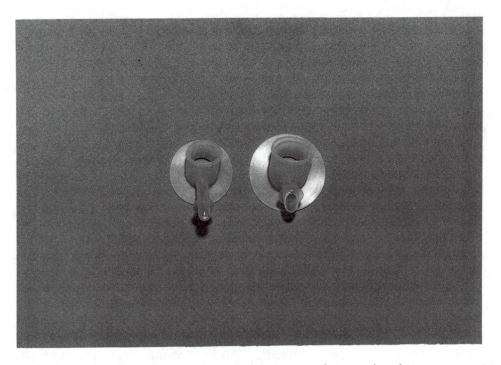

Figure 12–4. Examples of combined TE puncture voice prostheses and tracheostoma vents. Note duckbill-type prosthesis unit (left) and low-pressure prosthesis unit (right).

that offer less resistance to airflow appear to have distinct advantages from those that exhibit higher resistances. Yet some low resistance devices might exhibit other attributes that may prove to be problematic for a given patient.

One of the most obvious factors in this consideration pertains to the diameter of the prosthesis. For example, a larger diameter prosthesis may have lower overall resistance but it also results in more circumferential area around the prosthesis for potential leakage. Larger diameter prostheses also may be unsuitable for patients with smaller tracheostomas because they occlude too much of the airway. The clinician must, therefore, consider multiple factors in assessing which prosthesis will best serve the patient. Most clinicians admit that they might prefer one particular type of prosthesis from another. It would be unfortunate, however, if a clinician failed to consider the relative merits of another prosthesis if it appeared to offer some advantage to the patient. If possible, clinicians should avoid unnecessary bias in their consideration and recommendation of TE puncture voice prostheses.

Management Issues Associated with Surgical-Prosthetic Methods of Voice Restoration

The role of the speech-language pathologist in voice and speech rehabilitation following TE puncture is quite multifaceted. Ideally, the speech-language pathologist will have preliminary information on the patient's ability to generate "esophageal" voice via preoperative esophageal insufflation testing. Although a positive insufflation test in no manner guarantees that voice will be achieved postoperatively, it may provide the clinician with what should be expected once the puncture is completed. The ideal clinical situation would also rely on the combined expertise of the speech-language pathologist and surgeon in addressing all aspects of TE puncture and prosthesis concerns.

Initial Considerations

As with all other methods of postlaryngectomy voice and speech rehabilitation, numerous additional concerns specific to TE puncture frequently must be addressed by the speech-language pathologist. Much of this additional information pertains to the TE puncture and the puncture prosthesis. Similar to other alaryngeal options, considerable instruction is always required to ensure that the patient understands the basics of "what" the prosthesis does and "how" it works. Use of diagrams and/or teaching aids may be beneficial for this purpose (Smith, Reisberg, Hill, & Maddox, 1985). Regardless of whether the TE puncture is done as a primary or secondary procedure, the clinician is now faced with the additional responsibilities that emerge from use of an "internal" prosthetic device not found with traditional esophageal speech, or the use of an electrolarynx. Therefore, before formal voice and speech treatment is begun, several important steps must be undertaken.

Prior to initiation of direct voice and speech treatment following TE puncture, several preliminary steps are typically required. The areas which need to be addressed may be segmented into several discrete areas. The primary goal centers around the general evaluation of the puncture site itself. This involves assessing the TE puncture and then sizing and fitting the patient with the TE puncture voice prosthesis. This goal is also extended to include the evaluation of in vivo performance of the TE puncture prosthesis; that is, the

speech-language pathologist must assess patient performance with the prosthesis in place.

The next area of clinical concern relates to "trouble-shooting" problems that may arise (Bosone, 1986). In cases where problems arise early in the management process, the speech-language pathologist must identify the cause and then attempt to correct the problem (Bosone, 1986). Should a patient experience difficulty initiating voice following TE puncture or insertion of a TE puncture voice prosthesis, the underlying cause must first be identified. The clinician will work with the patient at this time to determine whether the problem is a result of (1) anatomical-physiological problems, (2) prosthesis difficulties, or (3) a combination of both factors. Thus, many preliminary steps which are not related directly to speech production precede formal treatment in those who undergo TE puncture for voice restoration.

Initial Assessment of the TE Puncture Site: Preparing for Prosthesis Insertion

The initial step in training patients who undergo TE puncture for voice restoration involves providing information on the puncture itself. Patients must understand that the puncture site provides a direct link between their airway and the pharynx/esophagus. Due to this, the puncture site must be stented to avoid salivary leakage and possible aspiration. Further, stenting eliminates spontaneous closure (which may be quite rapid) of the fistula. Stenting can be done using either a prosthesis or a catheter. The patient must also understand that should partial or complete closure occur, secondary surgery to correct the problem may be required. Accordingly, the patient's first responsibility in the training process is to learn how to remove and insert a catheter or similar stent. The clinician must ensure that each patient fully understands these tasks as it will often save both the patient and clinician from encountering future problems.

The best method for training should be done in a well-lighted room in front of a mirror. The clinician should then ask the patient to take one or two dry swallows to clear the pharynx of secretions. Once this is completed, the patient should be asked to avoid swallowing for several minutes. At this point the clinician should begin removing the catheter from the TE puncture site while explaining that he or she is gently extracting it. On removal, the clinician should immediately point out the puncture site to the patient and then reinsert the catheter into the fistula. When the tip of the catheter is through the port, the patient may be asked to swallow as this will help to direct the catheter in a downward direction.

Catheter insertion should be demonstrated using a consistent and easy pace, possibly facilitated by gentle rolling of the catheter between the fingers. The patient is then asked to remove and reinsert the catheter while the clinician provides direct feedback. Patients who exhibit reduced visual abilities or manual dexterity problems may need additional instruction to ensure that they are able to successfully replace the catheter. The number of trials required is rather arbitrary; however, the speech-language pathologist should continue trials until it is evident the patient would be able to successfully insert the catheter should a problem arise outside of the clinic. Following this important preliminary step in the training process, the clinician and patient should advance to assessment of the puncture site and prosthesis sizing and initial fitting.

Assessing the TE Puncture

The first step of speech rehabilitation following TE puncture involves the clinician's assessment of the TE puncture site and the patient's ability to use the puncture as an air shunt. There are considerable differences

of opinion related to when this initial session should be conducted. Initial reports suggested that prosthesis "fitting" could be conducted on the second day post-TE puncture (Singer & Blom, 1980). Since that time, however, TE puncture has evolved from one which was only performed as a secondary procedure to one which may now also be performed at the time of laryngectomy (Hamaker et al., 1985). As a result, more lengthy waiting periods may be required. Patients who have undergone selective myotomy or neurectomy (Singer et al., 1981; Singer et al., 1986) for cricopharyngeal spasm which was identified presurgically may need to wait for longer periods postoperatively prior to initial prosthesis fitting. Adjustments will also need to be considered in patients who develop postsurgical complications (e.g., infection). Finally, this initial session may vary dependent on whether the patient is seen as an inpatient or outpatient. In considering these factors, as well as the variability associated with each patient, it is probably best for the speech-language pathologist to ask the surgeon when fitting can occur. This again points out an advantage of having cooperative efforts from both speech-language pathology and medical specialists. Initial evaluation and fitting sessions might occur from 2 to 14 days post-TE puncture depending on the patient and whether it was done as a primary or secondary procedure.

During the initial postoperative session, the speech-language pathologist will remove the catheter from the TE puncture site. As with any clinical task, the clinician should always explain to the patient what he or she will be doing in each progressive step of this process. Prior to removal of the catheter, the patient should be asked to swallow several times. This will help to decrease pooled secretions that remain in the pharynx. In doing so, the chance that salivary drainage will occur through the open port into the airway will be lessened. However, once the catheter is removed, the patient should be asked to avoid swallowing. If the patient feels the need to swallow, he or she should indicate this to the clinician. At that time, the catheter can be replaced for a brief period to accommodate the patient's needs.

In the process of removing the catheter from the TE puncture for the first time, the clinician may find that it has become "stuck" in the puncture site. This is quite common due to the normal response of the puncture site to "heal" postoperatively. Remember that the catheter has been inserted into the TE puncture in order to resist the normal healing process and, therefore, maintain patency of the puncture site. Removal of the catheter should be done by applying gentle pressure on the catheter during its withdrawal from the puncture. Catheter removal may also be aided by gently rolling the catheter between the thumb and index finger during withdrawal. It is essential to note that once removed the TE puncture should not be left "unstented" for an extended period of time. Once removed, the catheter, dilation stent, or prosthesis should be replaced in no more than several minutes. This is particularly important during periods when the clinician and patient are discussing aspects of the prothesis and its use, which is common during this session.

Initial Generation of Tracheoesophageal Voice

The most important step in this initial process involves the speech-language pathologist's assessment of the patient's ability to successfully generate TE voice production. This task is initially performed with an open port; that is, with the catheter removed the patient should be able to shunt tracheal air through the puncture site into the esophageal lumen. By performing this maneuver without a voice prosthesis in place, the patient avoids the need for overcoming prosthesis resistance.

Once the catheter is fully removed from the TE puncture, the patient should

be informed that he or she will need to inspire and that the clinician will manually close the patient's stoma. It is important to notify the patient that the airway will be closed for a brief period. If not informed, some patients become uncomfortable with such closure. Once notified, the patient is requested to take a normal breath and to exhale in a normal manner with the mouth open. The patient should also be instructed to "just let the sound come out" in the form of a sustained vowel.

The clinician should pay particular attention to the depth of the patient's inspiration. Full inspirations should be avoided. During expiration, the clinician should observe the smooth, fluent production of TE voicing. While initial attempts in voice production should be short in duration so as not to require excessive effort by the patient, each progressive production should be extended. In most patients, a normal inhalation should provide sufficient pulmonary air to vibrate the PE segment for a minimum of 6–8 seconds. An extended fluent duration of 8 seconds should rule out the presence of cricopharyngeal spasm (Blom & Singer, 1983; Singer & Blom, 1981; Singer, Blom, & Hamaker, 1989). If voice production is successful, the catheter should be replaced for a brief period while prosthesis sizing, insertion, and use is discussed. If the patient experiences difficulty with voice production, the cause must be identified (Bosone, 1986). Causes may range from those that are simple to those that are more complex.

Difficulty in Generating Sound Through an Open TE Puncture

If TE voice production is unsuccessful through an open TE puncture, the nature of the problem needs to be determined immediately. Identifying the problem will often be facilitated by what was observed by the clinician. Two primary determinants always emerge: (1) was voice production intermittent or effortful? and (2) was voicing unable to be generated? In the case of either intermittent or effortful voice production, the clinician should always consider the potential for cricopharyngeal spasm (Bosone, 1986; Singer & Blom, 1981). However, several additional options also exist. Because of the relative ease with which these potential problems can be assessed the clinician is encouraged to evaluate their possible contribution first.

When TE voice production is intermittent, the speech-language pathologist should evaluate two aspects of the TE voicing procedure. First, he or she should attempt to determine if the patient attempted to produce voicing with an adequate amount of air (Blom & Singer, 1983). Some patients may take rather shallow breaths prior to their attempts to produce TE voicing. Because the resistance of the PE segment to airflow is generally believed to be substantial (Weinberg et al., 1982), a reduced volume of respiratory air may be insufficient to excite the esophageal voicing source. The catheter should again be removed, and the patient should be encouraged to inhale again, perhaps by taking a bit deeper breath. The clinician might instruct the patient by asking him or her to fill the lungs to "about half way" or "about three-quarters" of their maximum capacity. The speech-language pathologist should carefully monitor the patient to ensure that full capacity breaths are not taken. On reinstruction, voicing is again attempted while the clinician digitally occludes the stoma. If voicing is achieved successfully, the process can continue with formal prosthesis sizing and fitting. If voicing difficulties persist, spasm must still be considered.

The second method to assess the patient's difficulty with TE voice production involves varying the closure pressure during phonatory attempts. That is, if too much digital pressure is applied to the tracheostoma for airway closure, the esophageal lumen may be compressed.

This may then in turn result in "distortion of the airflow tract" (Blom & Singer, 1983) which limits the smooth flow of air through the PE segment. The clinician must have the patient attempt additional productions while decreasing levels of closure pressure. Hopefully, this will result in successful TE voicing.

If voicing is still not achieved, the final consideration by the speech-language pathologist prior to assessing the integrity of the esophageal lumen and PE segment via esophageal insufflation testing involves ensuring that the suprapseudo-glottal region is unconstricted. Clinicians may at times be quite focused on digital closure and breathing issues during initial voicing attempts. Although instructions have been provided to the patient, the patient may often forget to open the mouth for sound production. Thus, the clinician needs to ensure that adequate oral posturing to facilitate the transfer of the alaryngeal sound into the vocal tract occurs.

Further, some patients may be observed to lock their tongue against the hard palate during attempts at voicing. This behavior has been noted in several patients who have been unsuccessful in the acquisition of traditional esophageal speech. Thus, they may have some carryover of injection maneuvers which may be detrimental to the successful acquisition of TE voicing. If this occurs, airflow may initially move past the PE segment and create voicing; however, voicing ceases when air fills the cavity between the sphincter and the tongue-palate closure. Patients should then be observed carefully and, if this is suspected, they should be asked to simply relax and open their mouths during exhalation. This more relaxed posturing will often result in a successful attempt at voicing.

One other voicing outcome may also be observed in a small number of patients. Specifically, with the port open, the patient will be observed to work quite hard with limited voice output. The patient does not exhibit intermittent voicing but, rather, a somewhat low intensity and effortful voice. In those few patients in which this pattern of initial voicing has been noted, it appears that they experience rather substantial edema in the region of the PE segment post-TE puncture. Following discussion with the surgeon, information may be provided which indicates that difficulty was encountered during insertion of the esophagoscope. The patient's esophageal tissue may have been manipulated in a more aggressive manner with subsequent development of edema in the post-TE puncture period. In these patients, a decision to wait an additional 72 hours prior to initial fitting may be best. However, the puncture must be patent. Following this waiting period, patient's achieve voicing with minimal effort and without suggestion of cricopharyngeal spasm. Thus, if the speech-language pathologist can be assured that the TE puncture site is open, a decision to wait several days longer is recommended. It is important for the clinician to explain to the patient why a delay is advised in order to help alleviate any anxiety the patient might have during the additional waiting period.

Evaluating TE Puncture Integrity Using Esophageal Insufflation Testing

If the previously discussed tasks do not result in successful trials of fluent TE voice production, the functional integrity of the TE voicing system must be evaluated further. This evaluation is required in order to rule out or confirm the presence of cricopharyngeal spasm (Blom et al., 1985). In doing so, the clinician will be required to perform an esophageal insufflation test. Blom and Singer (1983) have suggested that this type of post-TE puncture evaluation can be performed by placing a clean catheter through the puncture site and into the esophagus and then having the clinician blow through the catheter. Although this method will provide needed informa-

tion to the speech-language pathologist and the surgeon, it is not recommended due to hygienic and infection control concerns (ASHA, 1989, 1990). This testing can be performed by having the patient insufflate his or her own esophageal reservoir using the system that is now widely used for preoperative esophageal insufflation assessments (Blom et al., 1985).

In instances where the patient is unable to generate any voicing through an "open" TE puncture site, several concerns must always be entertained by the speech-language pathologist. First, spasm is typically an intermittent phenomenon. That is, voice production may begin, but then will terminate rather rapidly. Should even a very brief burst of phonation be noted, spasm is quite likely. The nongeneration of voice suggests that the puncture is not open.

If partial closure is suspected, the clinician should carefully inspect the puncture site visually to determine if any blockage is present. Bosone (1986) has provided a series of guidelines which suggest closure of the puncture site. One method for determining whether at least some degree of closure exists can be done by asking the patient to swallow with the catheter removed. If the puncture is open, some saliva will be observed to pass through the surgically created fistula. Bosone (1986) has pointed out that if no leakage is observed "it is a reasonable assumption that at least the esophageal end of the track has closed" (p. 197). Bosone (1986) also notes that it is quite "rare" to observe no leakage of saliva during swallowing if the puncture site is open. If voice production is nonexistent, the clinician should immediately consult with the surgeon.

If the closure is in the initial stages, the surgeon may be able to dilate the puncture without a second surgery. If closure is incomplete, the speech-language pathologist may be able to systematically dilate the puncture via insertion of progressively larger catheters into the puncture site (Bosone, 1986). This process should be done sequentially, with an adequate waiting period once a catheter is inserted. Thus, this process may permit expansion of the shrinking puncture site. Should complete closure occur or be suspected, it is always the responsibility of the surgeon to manage this problem. The speech-language pathologist *should never* attempt to open a TE puncture site that is suspected of closure.

Esophageal Insufflation Testing Following TE Puncture: Determining the Cause of the Intermittent or Nongeneration of Voicing

In patients suspected of cricopharyngeal spasm or those unable to generate any TE voicing, the clinician can perform esophageal insufflation testing to assess the status of the sphincter. This can be done using the esophageal insufflation kit that is commercially available (Blom et al., 1985). This evaluation should be done with the cooperation of the physician. Recall that this device has a housing that can be affixed directly to the patient's tracheostoma, as well as a housing "insert" in which a rubber catheter is attached. However, the procedure to be conducted for testing requires a simple modification due to the presence of a puncture. Briefly, the tracheostoma housing should be positioned over the patient's stoma and then affixed in the usual manner using double-faced tape and liquid adhesive. During this placement, it is best to leave the original catheter in place within the TE puncture site and slip the housing over the externalized portion of the catheter. By leaving the catheter in place, the chance of puncture site shrinkage will be eliminated.

Once several minutes have elapsed, the catheter assembly can be positioned in the housing. Now, rather than inserting the catheter transnasally, the catheter tip should be brought to the front of the housing insert and then inserted into the TE puncture through the stoma. The clinician will need to ensure that (1) the catheter *is not* being pushed down into the trachea,

and (2) once inserted into the puncture site, that the catheter is directed inferiorly. If the catheter enters the airway, the patient will respond accordingly by attempting to cough it out. It is important that the speech-language pathologist avoid this problem by carefully attending to the task. Good lighting is essential. Once positioning of the catheter is completed, esophageal insufflation testing can proceed.

Evaluation will follow standard procedures for testing with one exception. Although the clinician will provide digital closure of the housing insert in order to permit air to move through the catheter into the esophageal lumen, several adjustments are required. Because the catheter is now "wrapped around" the front of the catheter-insert assembly, care must be taken to ensure that an adequate digital seal is achieved *without* crimping the catheter. That is, closure needs to be complete but the clinician will need to avoid compressing the catheter tube against the edge of the insert. In many cases use of the thumb may provide an adequate degree of "fleshiness" that will conform to the diameter of the insert opening without compromising the catheter. Some clinicians may find this to be problematic. Should this occur, a seal may be achieved using a piece of rubber dental dam that has been folded over into multiple layers. This may then permit an adequate seal when placed between the housing insert and the finger or thumb. The clinician *should not use small pieces of dental dam* to avoid any threat to the airway. The evaluation can then be conducted using the typical procedure outlined with standard esophageal insufflation testing. If spasm is confirmed, the patient will need to be followed by the surgeon to determine if the problem can be remedied through selective myotomy or neurectomy.

Prosthesis Fitting: Initial Sizing

On confirmation that the TE puncture is open and that voicing can be achieved with the catheter removed, the next step in the treatment process involves prosthesis fitting. Once the clinician confirms that the puncture site is open, and that TE voicing can be produced without difficulty, prosthesis sizing and the initial fitting can commence. Several methods for fitting have been provided in the literature (Blom & Singer, 1983, Reed, 1983a; Singer & Blom, 1980). Some have suggested that prosthesis sizing be done using a formal sizing device which is shown in Figure 12–5, while others have recommended that a more informal approach be undertaken (use of a swab to measure depth under direct vision). The clinician might also fit the prosthesis by beginning with a longer prosthesis and then moving to relatively shorter prostheses until an optimal fit is obtained. Regardless of which sizing method is used, the primary goal of initial fitting is to obtain the best possible fit *without underfitting*. That is, the clinician should always err on the side of "over-

fitting" the patient with a prosthesis that is too long, as opposed to the alternative.

The essence of proper initial prosthesis fitting involves identifying a TE puncture voice prosthesis that is sufficient in length to penetrate the entire thickness of the tracheoesophageal wall (in which the puncture is located) while at the same time avoiding excessive extension of the prosthesis into the tracheostoma. If the prosthesis is too long it may be pushed into the puncture upon digital closure of the tracheostoma. Should this occur, the esophageal end of the TE puncture voice prosthesis will push against the posterior esophageal tissue and may impede airflow into the lumen. The speech-language pathologist must also take into account the general structural configuration of the trachea and the location of the puncture site itself. That is, steeply sloping tracheas may require shorter length prostheses, whereas more angular tracheas may require a longer

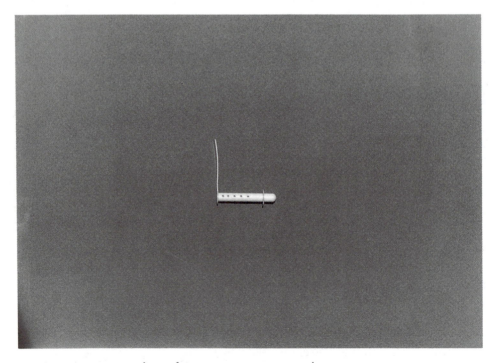

Figure 12–5. Measuring device for TE puncture voice prosthesis.

prosthesis. It is critical to stress once again that the clinician should always opt for a prosthesis that is slightly longer. Should underfitting occur, the retention collar of the prosthesis will not open on the anterior esophageal wall. This will result in closure of the puncture in the posterior aspect of the fistula (Bosone, 1986). Ideally, all speech-language pathologists should learn prosthesis fitting from clinicians who have substantial experience in this area, first through direct observation and then through direct hands on experience.

Prosthesis Downsizing

Another major issue that deserves mention in regard to initial sizing of the TE puncture voice prosthesis relates to *downsizing* at a later date. Downsizing involves refitting the patient with a shorter prosthesis (usually one size shorter) at some point 3–6 weeks post-TE puncture. This downsizing is believed to reflect changes in general tissue thickness that may have been altered as a result of the surgical procedure (e.g., edema). Thus, while patients may initially utilize one length prosthesis, it is not uncommon to have them convert to a slightly shorter prosthesis at some point in the postoperative period. This may be particularly true in cases of primary TE puncture where sufficient tissue changes are evidenced in the postoperative period.

Prosthesis Insertion

Initial insertions of the TE puncture voice prosthesis are always undertaken by the speech-language pathologist or surgeon. Once initial sizing is determined, the prosthesis and its inserter are prepared. The catheter is then removed from the puncture, and the clinician inserts the prosthesis into the port. Generally, the same process is used whether a duckbill, or low-pressure, voice prosthesis is used. Insertion must be done under direct vision to ensure that the

attitude of insertion is consistent with that of the puncture. The patient should be informed that he or she will feel some pressure during insertion.

To aid insertion, slight dilation using progressive, increasing diameter catheters has been recommended (Blom & Singer, 1983). Additionally, dilation may be achieved using a commercially available dilation stent (Figure 12–6). Insertion has also been aided with the recent introduction of TE voice prosthesis "gel cap." This gelatin shell is placed on the tip of the prosthesis prior to its insertion. Once inserted, the gelatin safely dissolves within the esophageal lumen. An example of a low-pressure voice prosthesis with and without a gel cap is shown in Figure 12–7.

Prior to insertion of the prosthesis the clinician should always inspect the prosthesis to guarantee that the valve (duckbill or hinged-flap) is functional. Occasionally, the valve may be stuck during fabrication, and this will eliminate its ability to serve as an air shunt. If this is identified, it can often be resolved quickly. For duckbill prostheses the clinician can use a razor to separate the valve at the point of adhesion; for internal hinge-type valves the stick end of a swab can be inserted through the prosthesis, and the valve can be dislodged via gentle pressure. The clinician should be careful not to "spring" hinge-type valves during an attempt to release it. If the problem persists, the clinician should obtain another prosthesis and return the original to the manufacturer.

Insertion begins by inserting the prosthesis into the puncture and then gently pushing it into the tract. Often, this may be facilitated by rotating the inserting tool between the thumb and index finger (similar to that of catheter insertion). An example of both duckbill and low-pressure voice prostheses on their respective inserters is shown in Figure 12–8. Insertion should continue until the retention collar enters the esophageal lumen and again springs back to its original configuration. During insertion the collar will collapse as it passes

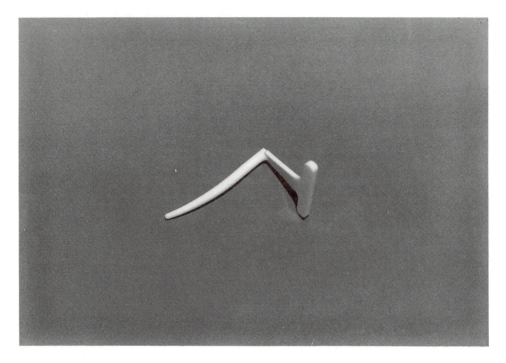

Figure 12–6. Dilation stent (In-Health Technologies, Santa Barbara, CA).

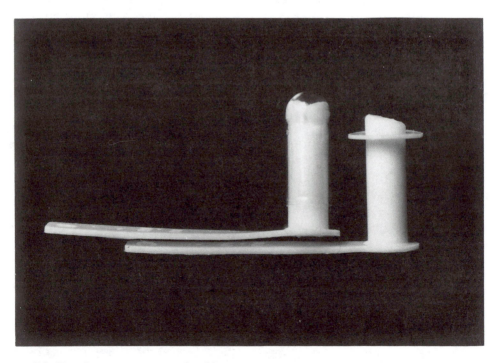

Figure 12–7. Comparative example of low-pressure type TE puncture voice prosthesis with (left) and without (right) gel-cap. (Compliments of Eric D. Blom, Ph.D.)

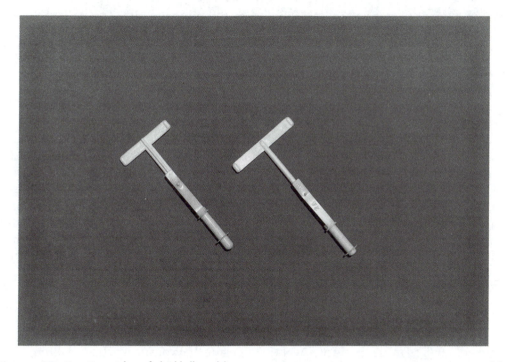

Figure 12–8. Examples of duckbill and low-pressure TE puncture voice prostheses prepared for insertion.

through the puncture. Clinicians and patients have often reported that when the retention collar enters the lumen an audible "pop" can be heard.

Correct insertion of the prosthesis can be confirmed by removing the insertion tool from the prosthesis and then pulling on the strap of the prosthesis. If the collar is fully expanded in the esophagus, the prosthesis will be retained even with rather aggressive tugging on the neck strap. If the prosthesis is easily removed during this procedure, the clinician has not correctly inserted the prosthesis, and the insertion process should be repeated. If difficulty with expansion of the retention collar is noted, the clinician should carefully reassess the prosthesis to ensure that it is of sufficient length to pass through the entire length of the puncture. In cases where several attempts at insertion are attempted, the catheter should be replaced regularly to eliminate any shrinkage of the puncture site, which will reduce ease of insertion.

The speech-language pathologist needs to understand that repeated attempts at insertion, whether in the process of determining sizing or in assuring that a complete insertion has occurred, may create a tissue response that may make the process more difficult. Specifically, during initial fittings the puncture site is essentially unhealed and, thus, will respond to irritation associated with insertion. This may in turn result in some minor tissue swelling which might further reduce insertion effectiveness. Some minor bleeding may also be noted. However, once fitting is completed and the puncture has the opportunity to re-epithelialize during the healing process, bleeding and irritation will be decreased substantially, if not entirely eliminated. Finally, it is recommended that the initial fitting be performed in the morning if possible so that follow-up can occur in the afternoon. This will permit the clinician to identify any immediate problems that have occurred. The most important problem to identify is that of underfitting, should it occur.

Initial TE Voice Production with the Puncture Prosthesis Inserted

Once the prosthesis is inserted, the next step is to request sound production. In preparing the patient, the clinician should again indicate that following a normal breath the clinician will manually seal off the airway. Similar to that performed with the open puncture, the patient will be asked to inhale and then exhale with the mouth open. This should result in production of an extended vowel. If problems with voice production are encountered, the clinician needs to determine the reason.

It is common to observe some minor degree of change in the patient's overall voice quality when the prosthesis is in place. Voice production should not, however, be strained or highly effortful for the patient. If the patient is unable to generate voice with the prosthesis in place, the clinician will need to assess several potential causes for this problem. Provided the clinician has checked the prosthesis before insertion (Oppenheimer & Leader, 1990), the operational capacity of the valve is not the likely cause. However, a prothesis that is too long may be "pistoning" (Blom & Singer, 1983) through the puncture.

"Pistoning" of the Prosthesis in the TE Puncture

During digital occlusion a long prosthesis may push into the esophagus so that the valve becomes imbedded in the posterior esophageal tissue. Pistoning which results in voice production difficulty, may be noted more often with duckbill valves as opposed to prostheses with internalized valves and a beveled tip. Should pistoning occur, valve operation may be disrupted. The clinician can assess this possibility by manually evaluating prosthesis movement

in the puncture site. The patient should also attempt voicing using less digital (closure) pressure on the stoma during airway occlusion. In some instances, excessive digital pressure may force the prosthesis into the esophageal wall, impeding valve operation (Blom & Singer, 1983; Bosone, 1986). If the prosthesis is too long, the clinician should consider changing the prosthesis to the next shorter length. The clinician must not, however, *underfit* the patient. Upon removal of the first prosthesis, the speech-language pathologist needs to inspect it to ensure that mucus is not blocking the airflow valve (Bosone, 1986). If the next shortest prosthesis is too short, the clinician should return to the original length device.

If a change of prosthesis does not result in an appreciable change in voice production, the speech-language pathologist should remove the prosthesis and again ensure that voicing is achieved through the open port. Successful voicing should be followed by re-insertion of a catheter or dilator prior to refitting the prosthesis. An unsuccessful attempt at voicing through the open port may indicate that some partial closure may be occurring (Bosone, 1986; Singer & Blom, 1980). This will require dilation to maintain patency of the port.

Instructions to the Patient

Once initial fitting has been successfully completed, the clinician should reiterate what has occurred and how the prosthesis functions. If at all possible, repeated insertion and removal of the prosthesis should be avoided in the initial session as it will be less traumatic to the tissue surrounding the fistula. The patient should be asked not to remove the prosthesis prior to a return visit to the speech-language pathologist. The patient must, however, be informed that should the prosthesis be coughed-out or extruded, he or she must reinsert the catheter to maintain patency of the puncture site. Patients should not attempt to reinsert the prosthesis themselves, but only insert a catheter. Urgent attempts at prosthesis insertion often result in tissue irritation and consequential swelling that makes insertion more difficult. The speech-language pathologist must ensure that the patient understands the potential consequences of repeated attempts at reinserting a prosthesis.

Initial Fittings by the Patient

Because a sufficient amount of information is given to the patient during the initial postoperative fitting session, it may not be appropriate for the patient to attempt the first prosthesis insertion at this time. This can typically wait until the second session. The procedure followed for insertion of a prosthesis should be identical to that presented and demonstrated by the clinician during the first session. Prior to training, the speech-language pathologist must confirm that the patient is able to insert a catheter should problems be encountered during prosthesis insertion. Training may be augmented by diagrams and/or the use of teaching aids (Smith et al., 1985).

Several issues are of importance in facilitating the patient's ability to successfully insert a voice prosthesis. A summary of these issues is provided in Table 12–3. If the clinician is able to provide clear direction and feedback to the patient, the chance of success will be increased. Although most patients demonstrate some degree of difficulty with prosthesis insertion during initial sessions, this is a normal process and further practice will likely reduce problems in the future.

Modifying Instructions

The clinician should always adapt levels of instruction to the patient's intellectual/cognitive abilities. This goal can be achieved with several simple adjustments. Patients unable to absorb standard amounts of information should be provided with less information in each session. If possible, multiple sessions can be arranged over the course of a day; for example, rather than a single 1-hour session in the morning, two half-hour sessions may be scheduled. Redundancy is essential and, when possible, written and/or diagrammatic materials should be provided. The clinician must also remember that many patients are now dealing with a substantial amount of new information and associated responsibility if they undergo TE puncture and choose to use a voice prosthesis. This is most apparent with patients who receive primary voice restoration because they must adjust to substantial anatomical, physiological, and psychological changes. Thus, adapting to each patient's unique capabilities at any given time will improve the chance of early success; this will hopefully have carryover to more advanced levels of training.

Common Clinical Problems and Their Solutions

Information provided in the literature suggests that several problems may be observed with use of a TE puncture voice prosthesis. An excellent summary of common problems and their clinical solutions

---

TABLE 12–3.
Preliminary Skills Required for TE Puncture.

1. Patient must be able to insert a catheter or dilation stent.
2. Patient must be able to visualize tracheostoma and TE puncture site.
3. Patient must demonstrate adequate manual skills that permit insertion of catheter and TE puncture voice prosthesis into port.
4. Patient must be able to place prosthesis on insertion device.
5. Patient must have cognitive ability and mental awareness to identify problems should they occur.

has been provided by Bosone (1986). These problems are best classified as generalized problems with either (1) the TE puncture site, (2) the voice prosthesis, or (3) the sound generator (PE segment) or a combination of these factors (Bosone, 1986). The manifestation of these problems may result in a variety of clinical observations. For example, leakage may occur through a prosthesis that is worn out, or around the prosthesis. These examples are a result of changes in the prosthesis and fistula, respectively.

Leakage through a prosthesis indicates that the prosthesis needs replacement. On average the patient should be able to use a prosthesis for about 12 weeks prior to replacement. Leakage always requires replacement of the prosthesis. While variability in prosthesis life may be specific to each patient dependent on their use, a "short life" of a prosthesis suggests candida growth on the prosthesis. This problem may be eliminated or reduced through regular disinfection using hydrogen peroxide (Blom & Singer, 1986).

Leakage around the prosthesis suggests several possible causes. Pistoning of the prosthesis within the TE puncture may expand its diameter, thus permitting leakage around the device. The speech-language pathologist must pay careful attention to such leakage to ensure that it is not the result of an expanding or migrating puncture site. Puncture expansion may indicate development of an extended fistula which must be brought to the immediate attention of the surgeon. If an extended fistula is not present, the clinical solution to the problem involves shrinking the puncture. Shrinkage permits a tighter seal between the circumference of the prosthesis (regardless of prosthesis size) and the walls of the puncture, thus eliminating leakage.

The best method of shrinking the puncture is to insert a catheter that is slightly smaller into the puncture. By doing so, the puncture will close around the catheter. This may require several days

for adequate shrinkage in some patients; however, shrinkage usually occurs quite quickly. Once the catheter is removed the prosthesis can be replaced in the puncture. If this proves to be unsuccessful electrocautery (Singer & Blom, 1980; Singer et al., 1981) may be recommended by the surgeon.

One final problem reported by some patients involves coughing out a voice prosthesis. While this problem was not uncommon with the early generations of voice prostheses, it has become infrequent with the introduction of the retention collar (Bosone, 1986). In those infrequent instances where a patient does cough out the prosthesis, he or she will have already been instructed in the ability to reinsert a catheter or the prosthesis.

Tracheostoma Breathing Value

Tracheoesophageal speakers have the option of using two methods to occlude the tracheostoma for speech production. Initially, patients were required to manually occlude the airway by sealing the tracheostoma with a finger. Despite success associated with digital closure, it could be observed by a listener, hence, it drew attention to the patient during communication. It was additionally noted that digital closure required unusual posturing of the arm. In such cases, this also might be disruptive to communication on a more global scale. Finally, some general issues regarding contact of the fingers and hand with the tracheostoma were raised; thus, general hygiene concerns emerged in relation to airway closure.

In response to these concerns, Blom et al. (1982) developed what was termed the *tracheostoma breathing value*. This valve was designed to be used in conjunction with the TE puncture voice prosthesis. Briefly, the tracheostoma breathing valve is a device which can be affixed to the tracheostoma to eliminate the patient's need for digital closure. The valve is comprised of a housing which is affixed directly to the skin around the tracheostoma and an adjustable airflow-sensitive diaphragm housing. Once the housing is affixed to the peristoma skin via double-faced tape and liquid adhesive, the airflow-sensitive diaphragm housing can be placed within the housing (Blom et al., 1982; Blom & Singer, 1983).

During quiet breathing the tracheostoma breathing valve remains open therefore, no disruption in the breathing cycle occurs. The diaphragm assembly, however, is designed so that on expiration of sufficient magnitude (i.e., for the purpose of speech production), it will close off and "seal" the airway. However, the valve needs to be fitted so that it will not close during increased respiration associated with normal physical activity (e.g., climbing stairs). Should some unusual physical activity occur which results in undesired closure of the valve, the patient can easily remove the diaphragm assembly from the housing. It can then be replaced once breathing returns to normal.

In situations where verbal communication is desired, the valve permits rapid closure of the airway for speech purposes and then "returns" to its open position when the patient again needs to inhale. When the seal is complete, exhalatory air is then diverted through the TE puncture voice prosthesis similar to that initiated following digital closure of the airway. In early devices the sensitivity of the diaphragm could be modified by changing it to one of several levels of resistance/compliance. That is, the diaphragm could be removed and replaced with one that offered the most appropriate resistance. On newer valves, the resistance can be modified by adjusting the aperture of the breathing valve so that more or less of the airflow-sensitive diaphragm can be utilized.

Overall, the tracheostoma breathing valve is well accepted by patients and appears to be relatively free of complications. The most significant problem noted clini-cally has been related to difficulty associated with maintenance of an adequate seal between the valve housing and the peristomal skin. This has been most notable in instances were patients present with irregular configurations of the stoma due to surgery. Because of these anatomical irregularities, some portions of the valve housing may exhibit incomplete contact with the tracheostomal skin. Insufficient bonding, even with use of tape and adhesive, may result in shorter periods of a complete seal. When the seal is disrupted, air begins to leak from under the housing when the diaphragm assembly is closed. Leakage of air further promotes loss of a complete seal in addition to creating air turbulence which is often disruptive to communication.

Several authors have reported clinical procedures to eliminate valve housing seal problems related to anatomical variations. Cantu, Shagets, Fifer, Andres, and Newton (1986) described a procedure in which "customized" housings could be fabricated for patients demonstrating this problem. Although it appeared that Cantu et al.'s (1986) procedure was successful, it was a multistep process that was time-consuming. It also required the professional expertise of a maxillofacial prosthetist, and care needed to be exercised when the fabrication material was being applied around the patient's airway.

Because of the concerns associated with the method reported by Cantu et al. (1986), Doyle, Grantmyre, and Myers (1989) presented a simplified clinical modification for customizing valve housings. Doyle et al.'s technique involved the heating of the housing with a prosthetic air gun, and then stretching and reforming sections of the housing to conform to the patient's anatomical irregularities. This procedure was done in graduated steps so that exact customization was facilitated. Results indicated that seal times increased from approximately 20 minutes to 2–3 hours in the first week. Follow-up of the patient indicated that at 6 months a seal was maintained for approximately 10–14 hours. This procedure has been used in additional patients with similar results.

Since the reports of Cantu et al. (1986) and Doyle et al. (1989) several additional products have become available commercially that may help to eliminate problems associated with tracheostoma valve sealing. The first is a rather aggressive, double-faced tape that is similar to that used for ostomy care. These tape rings are also thicker than the original tape rings. As such, they conform to small irregularities quite well. Finally, the valve housing itself is now available in two sizes. Although the internal diameter of the housing (for placement of the diaphragm assembly) remains unchanged, the outside diameter has been increased. This larger size housing permits potential for greater surface contact with the skin, and this may increase seal times. This larger housing may also compensate for poor skin contact in regions very close to the tracheostoma, such as those areas that exhibit bony structures in the sternoclavicular region. Thus, the addition of more aggressive adhesive disks and the availability of larger size valve housings may help to eliminate several sealing problems related to tracheostoma breathing valve use.

Prosthetic Considerations

Fungal Colonization

One problem observed early by some patients who used a TE puncture voice prosthesis was that the "life" of the prosthesis appeared to vary. It was generally believed that most patients could expect at least 3 months usage from a voice prosthesis. As more individuals chose to pursue the TE puncture voice restoration method, clinical information suggested that most patients could expect about 4–5 months usage from a single prosthesis provided care was taken to extend prosthesis life. In

some TE puncture patients, clinicians observed that prosthesis life was quite short, often considerably less that 1 month. Thus, questions were raised about the cause of this reduction.

Evaluation of this problem revealed that in some patients, their upper aerodigestive pathway exhibited rather substantial colonies of a yeastlike fungi *candida albicans*. Although this yeast is normally found on skin and in the oral cavity, as well as in other anatomical regions, some patients who had undergone laryngectomy appeared to exhibit a prolifery of this flora (Izdebski, Ross, & Lee, 1987; Mahieu, van Saene, Rosingh, & Schutte, 1986).

Mahieu et al. (1986) provided information obtained from both cultures and scanning electron microscopy evaluation of silicone TE puncture voice prostheses. They documented that candida growth occurred on the external surface of the voice prosthesis and that the yeastlike growth appeared to penetrate the material of the prosthesis (in this case a Groningen button). Based on their comprehensive assessment of the TE puncture prostheses, Mahieu et al. (1986) stated that "Candida organisms seem to possess a high affinity for silicone, resulting in adherence, cleaving, and invasive growth into the button." Although a "colonization index" suggested that candida was prevalent in "extremely high" concentrations both on the voice button and in the TE fistula, it is interesting to note that Mahieu et al. did not observe a predominance of "clinical manifestations of an infection" that might normally be found with such colonization.

Based on their findings, it was clear that the invasive growth pattern of the candida organism not only penetrated the prosthesis itself, but more importantly resulted in a build up of material on the esophageal flange of the valve. These deposits reduced the valving capacity of the prosthesis and permitted leakage through the prosthesis. To reduce this problem Mahieu et al. suggested a combined approach to reduced the overall presence of candida organisms found in the oropharyngeal region. This was accomplished through use of lozenges (amphotericin B) that reduced the presence of candida in the oropharynx. The second goal involved coating the prosthesis with *antimycotic agents* which could essentially resist penetration of the prosthesis by the candida organism.

The observations of Mahieu et al. (1986) have also been confirmed in a brief report by Blom and Singer (1986). Blom and Singer (1986) reported that in two TE puncture patients, penetration of the silicone material comprising the TE puncture voice prosthesis was observed to occur within 1 week of use. Further, they reported that "proliferation [of candida albicans] interfered with valve function" within 3 to 4 weeks of use. It would then appear that shortened life expectancy of a TE puncture voice prosthesis may in large part be due to the influence of the candida organism that exists in the upper aerodigestive path (Izdebski et al., 1986).

In contrast to the more elaborate procedures for reducing candida growth on the voice prosthesis, Blom and Singer (1986) recommended a simple approach to remedy the problem. They suggested that decontamination of the prosthesis could be performed in an ongoing, continuous fashion. That is, patients who demonstrated problems associated with candida were asked to interchange two TE voice prostheses. This involved having the patient remove the prosthesis after three days of use and replace it with the second device. The prosthesis that was removed was rinsed in water and then treated with hydrogen peroxide or nystatin. After soaking the prosthesis in the disinfecting solution for at least 1 day, the prosthesis was rinsed for later replacement. Blom and Singer reported that use of this protocol was successful in reducing the growth of candida albicans on the TE voice prosthesis. Follow-up of these two patients also indicated that the original prostheses were still functioning at 3 months. Based on the use of this protocol in these two patients,

Blom and Singer (1986) used this decontamination protocol for all patients by recommending that they "decontaminate" their prosthesis at least once a week to eliminate candida growth, hence, increasing prosthesis life.

Voice and Speech Treatment

Once the patient has been successfully fitted with the voice prosthesis, and he or she has been fully informed regarding its use and function, therapeutic emphasis can be directed toward direct communication goals. Because the patient has access to pulmonary air, many aspects of voicing require refinement rather than direct training. Given the rapid nature of TE voice restoration, the most important clinical goal from a speech perspective is to reduce the presence of behaviors that may ultimately become a problem. That is, while specific goals may be established and emphasized clinically, more global aspects of communication may require monitoring as they can be very disruptive to the communicative process.

Modifying Loudness and Effort Levels

Increased vocal loudness is common with TE speech production (Robbins et al., 1984). However, increased loudness and increased effort levels appear to exist in many patients. These two aspects of voice production offer an excellent opportunity to address both areas with several isolated tasks. Due to the relationship between loudness and effort, considerable attention should focus on reducing the effort level used for TE speech. Excessive effort is clearly perceptible as "strain" or "harshness" in the voice, and while this draws attention during communication, for some patients it may be quite fatiguing. If patients can be taught to exert only that amount of effort required to generate voicing, many aspects of voice quality may be improved to some degree. It is, therefore, essential to work on reducing effort levels before they become habitual for a patient.

Therapy that seeks to reduce excessive effort during speech production may be pursued effectively using several tasks. The first task requires the patient to speak in a soft voice. Because the PE segment requires a particular level of airflow to generate its vibration, a task that centers on reducing loudness often manifests in less effortful voice. The clinician is able to directly monitor this change in both intensity and effort. Specific feedback to patients on their success (or lack thereof) is often sufficient to meet this goal. However, at times patients who exhibit some degree of hearing loss may be less able to monitor this change. In such instances, more salient feedback may be required.

For patients who require additional methods of feedback in order to reduce their loudness/effort level, visual feedback can be very useful. If available, the Visi-Pitch can be used to provide ongoing feedback to the patient on relative levels of intensity. By establishing a "target window" for production levels on the Visi-Pitch, the patient can continuously monitor his or her production. To facilitate the patient's understanding of this goal, sustained vowels can be used in early steps of training.

Using a temporal window of about 6–8 seconds on the computerized version of the Visi-Pitch, the patient is requested to sustain a vowel for several seconds. This level should then be systematically decreased until the target level is identified by the clinician. If the original (loud) trial and the target trial are saved sequentially, a performance window can be generated. That is, a high and low level can be visually represented on the computer screen.

By employing the cursor function on the computer, repeated trials of vowels can be produced while the clinician drops the upper level of the window. This is accomplished by placing a horizontal cursor on

the screen or using a grease pencil to mark the decreasing levels. It is important to maintain the relative short duration of the production because increased length of utterance may result in increased effort levels. Once a specific criterion is achieved over at least two to three sets of trials, the task can be converted to a less artificial speech task.

Following success at the vowel level, the task can now be replicated with phrase and sentence level materials. Although a variety of materials are available to the clinician, construction of a simple set of materials may have utility for many patients. Specifically, the clinician should develop a set of phrases and sentences which vary from three to eight words in length. Each word must be a monosyllable however, thereby maintaining the syllabic length of the utterance. Phonetic construction does not necessarily need to be controlled.

Once materials are generated, the patient is requested to produce these materials beginning with three-word (syllable) constructions. Similar to the sustained vowel task, a criteria should be established and met prior to advancing to the next level (four words), as well as later levels. The goal of this task is again to have the patient maintain a loudness level within the established window. It is essential to note that some tolerance for excursions out of the window must exist. This is due to changes in intonation contour, phonetic contexts, and so forth. If the patient can successfully move through this series of sentences, habituation to an acceptable level of loudness will likely be achieved. As a consequence of this reduction, effort levels will also most likely be observed to decrease.

Monitoring Length of Utterance

It is not uncommon to observe TE speakers to generate extremely lengthy utterances. This is particularly evident early in therapy. While this behavior may not be unusual for a given patient (i.e., this behavior may have been exhibited prior to surgery), it may result in two negative by-products.

First, as utterance length increases the patient may feel the need to "press" a bit. This might then result in increasing levels of vocal effort that may be viewed negatively by the listener. Thus, effort level may increase with utterance length. The clinician must monitor this variable and bring it to the patient's attention before it becomes more difficult to modify.

The second by-product of increased length of utterance relates to the potential increase in overall speech rate. If speech rate increases substantially, general acceptability of speech may be reduced. However, and perhaps most importantly, increased speech rate may reduce the TE speaker's overall speech intelligibility. This may have dramatic consequences on communication and, therefore, requires monitoring throughout early treatment.

Reductions in speech rate may be accomplished quite easily by employing tasks frequently used in fluency protocols. Unfortunately, many of these tasks imposed a rather strict temporal period for production which has the potential to break the "cadence" of speech. Rate controls can also be accomplished through use of oral reading tasks provided materials are appropriate for the patient. Newspaper articles can often be adapted for this purpose, and the vocabulary is appropriate for patients who are able to read but who may not have extensive educational backgrounds.

If addressing speech rate, the emphasis should not be placed on lengthening phonetic elements within words, but on phrasal breaks. Many TE speakers disregard the opportunity for such breaks which results in more temporally compressed speech. Patients should be encouraged to monitor their speech output with particular attention paid to proceeding in a slow and easy manner.

Improving Speech Intelligibility

Because TE speech is characterized by a more normal speech flow, a patient's speech intelligibility may appear relatively good although, in fact, it may be reduced. This is a result of contextual influences that offer the listener cues to the content of the intended message. Thus, while specific words may be missed by the listener, he or she is able to interpret the message via identification of other words and the associated contextual aspects of the message.

All TE speakers should be evaluated for general levels of speech intelligibility. This can be accomplished through use of single word materials of which numerous lists are available in the literature. If specific classes of phonemes are determined to be problematic, specific treatment protocols can be established in hope of improving their production. Drillwork that emphasizes exaggerated articulation may offer sufficient improvement in many patients level of intelligibility.

Summary

This chapter has addressed a variety of issues related to tracheoesophageal puncture (TE) and use of the TE puncture voice prosthesis. An overview of this alaryngeal method, the surgical procedure required, and the general clinical findings have been presented. Based on information provided in the literature, TE speech offers the patient who undergoes a total laryngectomy a viable rehabilitative option in addition to esophageal and artificial laryngeal methods of alaryngeal communication. However, TE speech may not be suitable for all patients; consequently, the topic of patient candidacy and preoperative evaluation have also been discussed. Information relating to fitting, patient instruction, as well as voice and speech production have been reviewed. Finally, numerous issues pertaining to clinical troubleshooting and problem solving during the clinical process have been presented. Collectively, these issues form a critical element which enhances the patient's and clinician's ability to understand this alaryngeal method and, hopefully, enhances the patient's chance for successful use TE speech.

Comparative Performance by Esophageal, Artificial Laryngeal, and Tracheoesophageal Speakers

CHAPTER

Over the years a number of investigators have provided information on a variety of parameters associated with alaryngeal speech. Information has been gathered on laryngectomized speakers who use the three primary postsurgical alaryngeal methods (esophageal, tracheoesophageal, and artificial laryngeal speech). Parameters assessed most often include basic acoustic aspects of alaryngeal speech, particularly those of frequency, and intensity and related features which may signal linguistic contrasts such as intonation, stress, and juncture. A majority of this work has focused on intrinsic methods of alaryngeal speech. Additional information has been provided on temporal features associated with alaryngeal speakers. This work includes information from both descriptive and comparative studies.

Additional investigations on alaryngeal speakers have also addressed speech intelligibility for each alaryngeal mode. Similar to acoustic investigations, some of these studies have been conducted to describe the intelligibility of a particularly method of alaryngeal speech whereas others have been undertaken with a comparative focus. Intelligibility studies have varied substantially in regard to stimuli used (e.g., phoneme, word, or sentence level) and proficiency levels of speakers, and characteristics or expertise of the listener group (e.g., differences in age, level of sophistication relative to alaryngeal speech by the listener, hearing abilities, etc). Several investigators have also evaluated comparative performance of alaryngeal speakers who used more than a single method of alaryngeal communication. Finally, some studies have addressed broader issues of alaryngeal speech proficiency by evaluating listener judgments of gender identification and speech acceptability.

Thus, the purpose of this chapter is to present an overview of data from some of the more frequently referenced sources. To facilitate a basic understanding of the effects of alaryngeal speech on components of speech production, an overview of specific speech parameters will be provided. Information related to frequency and intensity, speech rate, intelligibility, and prosodic features, as well as that related to general issues of acceptability and gender identification will be presented.

Vocal Frequency

Data related to frequency characteristics of alaryngeal speakers is long-standing in the literature. Early studies of esophageal speakers identified mean fundamental frequency (F_0) values which ranged from 50 to 100 Hz (Damste, 1958; van den Berg and Moolenaar-Bijl, 1959). Snidecor and Curry (1959) reported a mean F_0 of 62.8 Hz (median = 93.27 Hz), a level almost one octave below that of the normal adult male speakers (Baken, 1987). Snidecor and Curry (1959) also reported a low F_0 value of 17.2 and a high of 135.5 Hz. Esophageal speakers have been reported to demonstrate a total range of frequencies of 13.2 tones, 2.8 tones greater than that exhibited by normal speakers (Snidecor & Curry, 1959; 1960). Snidecor and Curry (1960) stated it was "very doubtful that the average fundamental frequency level can be raised much, if any, above 66–70 cycles per second." Their doubts related directly to the limited airflow generated during esophageal phonation, therefore, limiting the functional duty cycle of the pseudoglottis.

Curry and Snidecor (1961) identified mean F_0 values ranging from 50.9 Hz to 76.7 Hz with a mean value of 62.8 Hz and a median of 63.3 Hz. These data compare favorably with those reported by Hoops and Noll (1969) for 22 male esophageal speakers. Hoops and Noll reported mean F_0 values ranging from approximately 43 to 86 Hz (M = 65.59 Hz). These data confirm the suggestion of Snidecor and Curry (1960) regarding the limited capacity for esophageal speakers to raise F_0 above

70 Hz. Curry and Snidecor (1961) also reported the total range of frequency associated with esophageal speech to vary between 12.1 and 14.7 tones. The "effective range" (median 90% of the frequencies produced) varied from 4.7 to 7.8 tones (M = 6.5).

Shipp (1967) reported mean F_0 values of 64.7 to 84.4 for low- and high-rated esophageal speakers, respectively. Effective range measurements (90% range) were found to be 8.0 and 7.6 tones for low- and high-rated speakers, respectively. Although no mean effective range for Shipp's (1967) entire series of speakers was provided, the mean for the six best speakers was 8.75 tones compared to 6.5 tones reported for "superior" speakers by Curry and Snidecor (1961). Shipp (1967) interpreted these data to support the notion that higher overall F_0s for esophageal speech result in higher ratings of speaker proficiency. The closer F_0 is to that of a normal speaker the greater the chance of being judged as more *acceptable* by the listener. However, additional acoustic components of esophageal voice (frequency perturbation, percent phonation time, etc.) may also influence overall voice quality with a corresponding influence on judgments of acceptability (Smith, Weinberg, Feth, & Horii, 1978), as well as those that may have a differential influence between men and women (Weinberg & Bennett, 1971, 1972).

Weinberg and Bennett (1972) investigated acoustic characteristics of 15 female and 18 male esophageal speakers. Results indicated that female speakers exhibited a mean F_0 of 87 Hz compared to a mean of 69 Hz for male speakers. While the mean F_0 values were found to be significantly different between males and females, other acoustic measures of vocal F_0 (e.g., standard deviation and range in semitones, 90% range) or durational measures related to periodic or aperiodic phonation, percent silence or percent phonation time were not. Thus, while lowered F_0 values are commonly found for esophageal phonation, differences between males and females was confirmed. This was interpreted by Weinberg and Bennett (1972) to suggest that perceptually salient correlates of gender identification were based in this acoustic difference (Weinberg & Bennett, 1971).

The most comprehensive comparative acoustic investigation to date was conducted by Robbins (1984) and Robbins et al. (1984). Comparative acoustic measures were gathered from three groups of speakers: 15 esophageal, 15 TE, and 15 laryngeal speakers. Results obtained for a reading task showed that speakers exhibited mean F_0 values of approximately 103 Hz, 102 Hz, and 77 Hz, for normal, TE, and esophageal speakers, respectively. The only statistically significant difference in F_0 existed between normal and esophageal speakers. Although the mean F_0 for TE speech closely approximated that of normal speakers, greater variability was demonstrated. A summary of comparative frequency measures reported by Robbins (1984) and Robbins et al. (1984) is presented in Table 13–1.

In summary, information of vocal fundamental frequency in the alaryngeal speaker indicates that this acoustic parameter is reduced substantially from that of the normal speaker. This is true for esophageal, TE, and artificial laryngeal speech. Although general trends in measures of vocal F_0 for each alaryngeal mode have been identified, variation is found between speakers. It also appears that reductions in voice F_0 have a direct impact on listener assessments of speaker proficiency.

Vocal Intensity

Data on intensity characteristics of alaryngeal speech have been reported by several authors. Hyman (1955) reported on three groups of alaryngeal speakers (normal, esophageal, and electrolaryngeal) and found relative mean sound pressure levels (SPLs) of 29 dB, 23 dB, and 33 dB, respectively. The intensity range for esophageal speakers was 11 dB. Although no comparative

TABLE 13–1.
Comparative Mean (*M*) Values for Frequency Measures Obtained From Normal, Laryngeal (*N* = 15), Esophageal (*N* = 15), and Tracheoesophageal (TE) (*N* = 15) Speakers During Sustained Vowel Phonation and Oral Reading Tasks.

	Sustained Vowel Phonation		
	Normal	**Esophageal**	**TE**
M F_0*	103.4	65.3	82.8
F_0 range*	5.8	73.9	39.9
M jitter*	0.1	4.1	0.7
Jitter ratio	7.7	182.5	51.4
Directional jitter	54.3	58.7	63.4
	Oral Reading		
	Normal	**Esophageal**	**TE**
M F_0*	102.8	77.1	101.7
F_0 range*	85.9	118.1	142.3

Source: From Robbins et al. (1984). A comparative acoustic study of normal, esophageal, and tracheoesophageal speech production. *Journal of Speech and Hearing Disorders, 49,* 202–210. American Speech-Language Hearing Association, reprinted with permission.
*In Hertz

range of intensity was presented for normal speakers, it is clear that a majority of esophageal speakers exhibit a restricted range in which intensity can be manipulated. The relationship between aerodynamic driving capacity and intensity of voice production is critical to the understanding of these reduced values (Isshiki, 1964). However, factors directly related to the vibratory source (tissue impedance and compliance) also influence vocal intensity.

Snidecor and Isshiki (1965) presented intensity data from a single superior esophageal speaker who produced a maximum intensity of 85 dB during vocalization of the vowel /a/. This is about 10 dB less than that typically observed for normal speakers (Baken, 1987). This esophageal speaker averaged approximately 20 dB for both upward and downward sweeps. These results compare favorably with those reported by van den Berg and Moolenaar-Bijl (1959) and Damste (1958) for esophageal speakers.

Further analysis of Snidecor and Isshiki's (1965) data revealed a mean "peak" value of 77 dB for propositional speech. According to Snidecor and Isshiki (1965), measurement of peak values may have "slightly exaggerated" intensity values in continuous speech, while relative values remain "stable and dependable."

Regardless of this superior esophageal speaker's close approximation to a normal talker's intensity, Snidecor and Isshiki noted that esophageal speech is characterized by an extremely limited dynamic range. However, those speakers exhibiting higher F_0 values are likely to exhibit greater intensity due to the physical relationship between these two parameters (Curry & Snidecor, 1961).

The comparative study reported by Robbins (1984) and Robbins et al. (1984) also obtained measures of intensity on their three groups of speakers (esophageal, TE, and laryngeal). Data indicate that TE speakers produced vocal intensities that were approximately 10 dB more intense than those of the normal speakers. However, vocal intensity for TE speakers was approximately 20 dB more intense than that of esophageal speakers. A summary of comparative acoustic findings provided by Robbins et al is presented in Table 13–2.

The increased intensity observed for TE speakers (Robbins, 1984; Robbins et al. 1984) is most likely a result of several interactive factors. Specifically, the interplay between aerodynamic driving pressures due to the TE speakers' access to a pulmonary air source and that associated with

TABLE 13-2.
Comparative Mean (M) Values for Intensity Measures Obtained From Normal, Esophageal, and Tracheoesophageal Speakers During Sustained Vowel and Oral Reading Tasks.

	Sustained Vowel Phonation		
	Normal	**Esophageal**	**TE**
M Intensity*	76.9	73.8	88.1
M Shimmer*	0.3	1.9	0.8
Directional shimmer (in %)	52.5	53.9	62.2
	Oral Reading		
M Intensity**	69.3	59.3	79.4

Source: From Robbins et al. (1984). A comparative acoustic study of normal, esophageal, and tracheoesophageal speech. *Journal of Speech and Hearing Disorders, 49,* 202–210. American Speech-Language Hearing Association, reprinted with permission.
*In dB SPL; **In dB/A

tissue compliance/resistance of the pharyngoesophageal (PE) segment has direct effects on both frequency and intensity (Robbins, 1984; Robbins et al., 1984). This interpretation has been supported by Weinberg et al. (1982) who demonstrated that esophageal airway resistance is indeed greater than that offered by the normal larynx during voice production.

Data presented by Robbins (1984) and Robbins et al. (1984) are also quite consistent with those presented by Weinberg, Horii, and Smith (1980). Weinberg et al. (1980) investigated long-time spectral characteristics and distributional properties associated with speech intensity during oral reading by 10 esophageal and 5 normal speakers. Esophageal speech was found to be reduced from that of normal speech on the order of 10 dB. Weinberg et al. (1980) reported mean dB SPLs which ranged from 61.9 to 69.0 (M = 65.1). This compared to a group mean for the normal speakers of 74.5 dB SPL.

In regard to the distributional properties of intensity during continuous discourse, Weinberg et al. (1980) found that "lower level speech output" was common to esophageal speakers. In fact, the modal intensity level noted by Weinberg et al. was 67 dB SPL for esophageal speakers while normal speakers exhibited modal levels of 82 dB SPL.

Data obtained by Weinberg et al. (1980) on average spectral levels also revealed that esophageal speakers demonstrated substantially reduced spectra from that of normal speakers. Specific reductions in the esophageal spectra were observed in the frequency range of 0–3000 Hz where the average spectrum was reduced by about 10 dB and in the range of 6000–9000 Hz with reductions of about 7 dB.

In summary, variation in the intensity of alaryngeal speech output has been reported for alaryngeal speakers. For intrinsic methods of alaryngeal speech, namely esophageal and TE speech, levels have been shown to be quite different from those of the normal speaker. Esophageal speech is typically less intense than normal speech while TE speech is more intense than that of the normal laryngeal speaker. In contrast, artificial laryngeal speech may vary in its intensity dependent upon the type of device and volume setting. These intensity differences would appear to influence speech intelligibility, particularly in situations of competing noise.

Temporal Features of Alaryngeal Speech

Snidecor and Curry (1959) reported "superior" esophageal speakers spoke at rates ranging from 85 to 129 words per minute (wpm). When reading a brief segment (59 words) of the Rainbow Passage (Fairbanks, 1960) speech rates ranged from 108 to 137 wpm (median = 122.5).

Snidecor and Curry (1959, 1960) found that none of six esophageal speakers they studied were able to count to greater than 10 (11 syllables) during a single air insufflation. This is sufficiently reduced from that of a normal speaker following a single breath. This difference results from the limited capacity (volume) of the esophageal reservoir used for esophageal speech and has an obvious influence on speech rate.

Snidecor and Curry (1959) presented data on mean pause time and mean duration for air-charging (insufflation). Measures ranged from 0.42 to 0.80 seconds for pause time and from 1.00 to 2.25 seconds mean duration for a group of six esophageal speakers. These measures explain critical differences that exist in the prosody of esophageal speech. That is, the need to re-insufflate the esophagus following several syllables breaks the normal rhythm and flow of speech production (DiCarlo et al., 1955; Gardner, 1971; Snidecor, 1978a). For example, Snidecor and Isshiki (1965) reported the speech rate of a single superior speaker to be 153 wpm. This speaker spent only slightly more than 50% of his total oral reading time in phonation due to the need to frequently re-insufflate the esophagus prior to initiating voice.

Robbins (1984) and Robbins et al. (1984) also reported temporal data gathered from three speaker groups. During a reading task, rates (in words per minute) of approximately 173 wpm, 127 wpm, and 99 wpm were exhibited by normal, TE, and esophageal talkers, respectively. A statistically significant difference in rate was found only between normal and esophageal speakers. Robbins (1984) and Robbins et al. (1984) also observed a doubling of the mean total pause time between normal and TE speakers (6.3 seconds vs. 11.6 seconds) and then again between TE and esophageal speakers (11.6 seconds vs. 22.9 seconds). Thus, both increased airway resistance (Weinberg et al., 1982) and differences in the driving capacity appear to have a rather dramatic effect on temporal aspects of intrinsic alaryngeal speech production. Although TE speakers have access to a large air source they must also produce substantially high flow rates through the PE segment in order to produce voicing. Thus, similarities in air supply between normal and TE speakers is offset by the increased resistance of the PE segment (Weinberg et al., 1982). A summary of temporal data presented by Robbins et al. (1984) is shown in Table 13–3.

In summary, temporal features associated with alaryngeal speech are influenced by several factors. For esophageal speakers, rate measures are influenced by the speech of esophageal air insufflation, the volume of the esophageal reservoir, and the resultant duration of the spoken utterance. Thus, speech rate is influenced by temporal intervals required for "recharging" the system and the decreased capacity of the power source. In contrast, TE speech is able to utilize a pulmonary power supply which eliminates frequent pauses for reinsufflation of the esophageal reservoir. Consequently, speech rate in TE speech is primarily a function of articulatory rate. Although limited data are available of artificial laryngeal speakers, duration characteristics are similar to those of the normal speaker due to an entirely external power supply and vibrator source.

Speech Intelligibility

The intelligibility of alaryngeal speech has been addressed by numerous investigators using various stimuli. DiCarlo et al., (1955) conducted the first comprehensive investigation of esophageal speech intelligibility. Using phonetically balanced (PB) words, multiple-choice sentences, and paragraph materials, DiCarlo et al. (1955) assessed the intelligibility of 15 esophageal speakers and that of normal speakers. Intelligibility judgments were made by both trained and lay listeners. Results indicated

TABLE 13–3.
Comparative Mean (M) Values for Durational Measures Obtained From Normal, Laryngeal, Esophageal, and Tracheoesophageal Speakers.

	Normal	Esophageal	TE
Words per minute*	172.8	99.1	127.5
Total pause time* (in seconds)	6.3	22.9	11.6
Total number of pauses*	9.7	35.4	13.0
M pause time* (in msec)	624.7	649.1	891.2
M MPT** (in secs)	21.8	1.9	12.2

Source: From Robbins et al. (1984). A comparative acoustic study of normal, esophageal, and tracheoesophageal speech. *Journal of Speech and Hearing Disorders, 49,* 202–210. American Speech-Language Hearing Association, reprinted with permission.
*Derived from oral reading task; **Derived from sustained phonation task

that consonant errors accounted for the greatest percentage of errors. Consonant errors also differed between esophageal speakers judged as either good or poor speakers.

DiCarlo et al. (1955) reported overall consonant intelligibility for high- and low-rated speakers was 93.1% and 64.7%, respectively. Although substantial differences between good and poor esophageal speakers was noted, similar intelligibility scores for production of voiced and voiceless consonants were demonstrated by the high-rated speakers (95.0% vs. 91.0%) and low-rated speakers (64.7% vs. 64.7%). Speakers also exhibited differences in their ability to produce consonants within specific phonetic classes (e.g., stops, fricatives, etc.). A summary of these data as reported by DiCarlo et al. (1955) are presented in Table 13–4. DiCarlo et al.'s data reveal that fricatives were consistently judged as of low intelligibility compared to other manner classes. The relative intelligibility of consonants by manner class did differ substantially between high- and poor-intelligibility speakers.

Since specific consonant classes differ significantly in relation to aerodynamic characteristics (Isshiki & Ringel, 1964; Subtelny, Worth, & Sakuda, 1966) changes in driving capacity (pressure and flow) and the alaryngeal source used influences consonant production along a variety of dimensions (Christensen, Weinberg, & Alphonso, 1978; Doyle et al., 1988; Sacco, Mann, & Schultz, 1966). It is also impor-tant to note that the PE segment is not an adductor-abductor mechanism and, therefore, is likely to influence the ability of esophageal an TE speakers to signal the voice-voiceless distinction (Christensen et al., 1978; Gomyo & Doyle, 1989; McKnight & Doyle, 1991). Consonants which normally require reduced aerodynamic flows (e.g., glides, nasals) are also voiced. Thus, consideration of the voicing distinction (cognate pairs) may be related in part to specify aerodynamic/intelligibility relationships in esophageal (and tracheoesophageal) speakers (Connor et al., 1985; Doyle et al., 1988; Doyle & Haaf, 1989; Gomyo & Doyle, 1987; Haaf & Doyle, 1987; Robbins, Christensen, & Kempster, 1987).

Hyman (1955) investigated the comparative intelligibility of esophageal, artificial laryngeal, and normal speakers. Multiple-choice word lists were recorded by speakers and then presented to listeners. Intelligibility judgments were obtained under five sound-field conditions: (1) the speaker with the least intense sound level was presented at 68 dB with other talkers being presented at relatively higher intensities; (2) esophageal speakers with the modal sound level for their group were presented at 68 dB with remaining speakers presented at relative greater intensities; (3) artificial laryngeal speakers with the modal sound level were presented at 68 dB with others in their group presented at relatively lower intensities; (4) all speakers were presented at 78 dB; and (5) all

TABLE 13–4.
Intelligibility of Consonant Classes Produced in PB Words by High- and Low-Rated Esophageal Talkers.

Manner Class	High Rated (%)	Low Rated (%)	Overall–All Talkers (%)
Glides	100.0	91.3	95.1
Nasals	96.1	32.5	62.9
Stop-Plosives	95.3	73.7	82.9
Laterals	92.9	79.5	85.7
Fricatives	88.4	43.9	67.1

Source: Adapted from DiCarlo et al. (1955).

speakers were presented at 78 dB with a background white noise competitor of 73 dB. In any condition a speaker's intelligibility score was based on the percentage of words correctly identified.

As anticipated, data obtained by Hyman (1955) revealed that in the first four conditions tested normal speakers were significantly more intelligible than either esophageal or artificial laryngeal speakers. Significant differences did not exist between esophageal and artificial laryngeal speakers and no significant differences were found between speaker groups in the white noise condition. Esophageal speakers' intelligibility ranged from approximately 35% to 56% (dependent on condition). In contrast, artificial laryngeal speakers' mean scores ranged from approximately 33% to 48%; normal speakers never exceeded a mean intelligibility of 73%.

In a second phase of Hyman's (1955) study each speaker produced 58 monosyllables. Stimuli consisted of 21 consonants which were represented in either the pre- or postvocalic position. Sixteen isolated vowels and diphthongs were also produced by each speaker. Results from this phase of Hyman's (1955) study indicated that normal speakers were significantly more intelligible than alaryngeal speakers. Vowels were identified with greater accuracy than consonants for all three groups of speakers. For esophageal speakers voiced consonants were identified more often than voiceless consonants; however, this pattern was reversed for both artificial laryngeal and normal speakers. Overall, prevocalic consonants were identified correctly more often than their postvocalic counterparts for all three speaker groups. Intelligibility was best for affricates, followed by glides, nasals, stop-plosives, and fricatives for esophageal speakers and for affricates, followed by nasals, fricatives, glides, and plosives for artificial laryngeal speakers. Both speaker groups exhibited particular difficulty producing interdental consonants and the glottal /h/. Intelligibility for normal speakers was also best for

affricates, followed by plosives, nasals, glides, and fricatives. Although order of intelligibility was similar between esophageal and normal speakers, absolute intelligibility percentages differed significantly between groups.

Shames, Font, and Matthews (1963) evaluated the intelligibility of 118 esophageal and 35 artificial laryngeal speakers. PB words were used to assess single word intelligibility. Speakers also recorded a standard paragraph. Every third speaker also recorded a 20-item sentence list (31 esophageal and 12 artificial laryngeal speakers). Intelligibility judgments for single words and sentences were obtained from five listeners who transcribed their responses. Scoring of sentence materials was based on identification of five "key words" in each sentence.

As a second part of the word intelligibility analysis conducted by Shames et al. (1963) three additional listeners transcribed their responses. Articulation distortions, substitutions, and omissions perceived by listeners were then assessed and quantified. During this phase of the investigation three judges agreed (i.e., reliability) on 71.8% of the perceived phonemes (whether correct or incorrect). Only 2.7% of judgments were in complete disagreement though specific errors were not provided.

Shames et al. (1963) reported that word and sentence intelligibility measures were highly correlated for each speaker group. Voiced/voiceless phoneme errors were significantly different between the esophageal and artificial laryngeal speakers with esophageal speakers demonstrating better intelligibility. Overall, esophageal speakers exhibited significantly higher mean intelligibility scores, as well as a significantly lower mean number of voiced/voiceless errors (Doyle et al., 1988) when compared to artificial laryngeal speakers. Esophageal talkers ($N = 107$) were judged to correctly produce a mean of 66% of consonants in words. A mean of 58% was identified for artificial larynx group.

Esophageal speakers were judged to produce a mean of 54.9% of PB words correctly compared to 35.5% by artificial laryngeal speakers. Voiced/voiceless confusions accounted for slightly less than 6% of the esophageal speakers errors, whereas they accounted for 8.5% of errors noted for the artificial laryngeal speakers.

Based upon these data, Shames et al. (1963) suggested that the results demonstrated the superiority of esophageal speech over artificial laryngeal speech. This assumption was judged to be correct in terms of "articulation, phonation, and intelligibility" (Shames et al., 1963, p. 282) even though speakers varied in speech proficiency. However, no significant differences were observed between esophageal and artificial laryngeal speakers for sentence intelligibility measures. Contextual influences could account for better intelligibility during a sentence task (Miller, Heise, & Lichten, 1971).

McCroskey and Mulligan (1963) studied the relative intelligibility of esophageal and artificial laryngeal speakers. Five esophageal and five artificial laryngeal speakers produced speech stimuli. Stimuli were comprised of each speaker's recording of a multiple-choice intelligibility list (Black, 1957) each composed of nine groupings of three words each. Intelligibility judgments were made by both sophisticated and naive listeners. Three groups of 10 adults each served as listeners; groups were composed of experienced speech pathologists, graduate students with some exposure to alaryngeal speech, and naive listeners without previous exposure to alaryngeal communication. All speech stimuli were presented to listeners in the sound-field at an intensity level of 74 dB SPL. Listeners were required to identify the stimulus from four choices offered in the response set.

McCroskey and Mulligan's (1963) results revealed mean intelligibility scores for esophageal speech of 66.8%, 62.9%, and 58.2% for professional, student, and naive listeners, respectively. Comparatively, the mean intelligibility of artificial laryngeal speech was 57.9%, 56.2% and 60.3%, again for the professional, student, and naive groups, respectively. Whereas general agreement for intelligibility judgments was found between professional and student listener groups, naive listeners judged esophageal speech to be substantially less intelligible (Doyle, Haaf, & Swift, 1989; Williams & Watson, 1985). Naive listeners also judged artificial laryngeal speech to be slightly more intelligible than either professional or student listeners. This finding may reflect two possible areas of listener bias. First, sophisticated listeners may be better listeners because of their training and, therefore, may judge the degraded alaryngeal speech signal with greater overall accuracy (Doyle et al., 1988). Second, sophisticated listeners may also possess an alaryngeal mode bias to some degree. That is, an intrinsic mode of alaryngeal speech (esophageal) may be judged as more acceptable than the less natural extrinsic form of alaryngeal speech (i.e., artificial larynx) and this may influence judgments of intelligibility.

Tikofsky (1965) assessed the comparative speech intelligibility of 9 esophageal and 10 normal speakers. All speakers recorded word lists comprised of (1) 50 consonant-syllable nucleus-consonant (CNC) words (Lehiste & Peterson, 1959), (2) 60 monosyllables with initial and/or final consonant clusters, and (3) 50 randomly selected spondaic words. In total, 570 normal-hearing young adults served as listeners; 19 groups of 30 listeners each were presented stimuli from a single speaker. Tikofsky's (1965) data analysis revealed that esophageal speakers were 49.7%, 54.9%, and 86.1% intelligible for CNCs, clusters, and spondees, respectively. Overall, normal speakers were judged to be 89.1%, 91.5%, and 97.9%, intelligible, again for CNC, cluster, and spondees, respectively.

Based on Tikofsky's (1965) findings and comprehensive statistical analyses, significantly poorer intelligibility for all speech materials was demonstrated by esophageal speakers. Tikofsky also found that reliability between the three types of speech stimuli for each speaker was highly correlated. That is, a given speaker's rank in comparison to others in their respective group remained consistent regardless of stimuli. Absolute intelligibility differences between individual speakers were, however, significantly greater for esophageal speakers. This finding highlights the fact that greater overall variability in speech intelligibility may be demonstrated by esophageal speakers. Tikofsky (1965) interpreted these data to support the assumption that:

Changes in the speech signals produced by esophageal speakers which effect a reduction in intelligibility appear to result from modifications of production other than just those introduced by the use of a different sound producing mechanism. (p. 29)

Based on this statement, Tikofsky (1965) directly addressed the possibility that productive speech differences exhibited by esophageal speakers in his and past research may have been influenced by nonphonatory (e.g., articulatory) aspects (Diedrich & Youngstrom, 1966). Tikofsky noted that inspection of the raw intelligibility data for the esophageal speakers indicated some stimulus words were better discriminators of intelligibility than others. Unfortunately, a summary of these data was not presented. It does appear possible, however, that poorer intelligibility was demonstrated for materials of particular phonetic construction related to the parameters of voicing, manner, or place of articulation (DiCarlo et al., 1955; Diedrich & Youngstrom, 1966; Nichols, 1976, 1977). Multiple interactions of these phonetic aspects also cannot be discounted. Tikofsky's (1965) data may have provided the first detailed opportunity to address intelligibility differentiation between normal and esophageal speakers, as well as distinctions between individual esophageal speakers.

Creech (1966) investigated 48 esophageal speakers who varied in speech proficiency and reported intelligibility scores ranging from 31% to 81% for multiple choice intelligibility materials. Eleven naive listeners served as judges and a mean intelligibility score of 62.2% was reported. Creech suggested that mean intelligibility scores for each speaker compared favorably with speaker proficiency ratings based on an equal-appearing-interval scale. Although a sufficiently wide range of speaker intelligibility was observed (i.e., difference score = 50%), Creech (1966) suggested that a judgment of 60% intelligibility for single words is a "good" level of proficiency for the traditional esophageal speaker. This confirms the rather striking degree of variability which exists between esophageal speakers.

Sacco, Mann, and Schultz (1967) were the first to investigate and present the intelligibility of esophageal speakers through use of perceptual confusion matrices. Nineteen speakers produced 16 English phonemes in consonant-vowel (CV) combinations which were then presented to 10 speech pathology students for perceptual judgment. Responses were then collapsed into confusion matrices for further analyses based Sacco et al.'s (1967) modifications in the distinctive feature system proposed by Miller and Nicely (1955). An overall intelligibility of 42% was reported.

Sacco et al.'s (1967) results indicated that intelligibility was best for nasals, followed by stop-plosives, and fricatives. As expected, the predominant perceptual errors occurred for phonemes that differed in voicing. Listeners correctly identified voiceless sounds with 60% accuracy as compared to voiced cognates (76%). This finding is noteworthy since esophageal speakers would be expected to exhibit greatest difficulty producing voiceless consonants due to the PE segment not being an abductor-adductor mechanism (Christensen et al., 1978).

Analysis by manner of articulation (Sacco et al., 1967) showed a similar intelligibility (range = 73–78%) across the three manner classes studied. It was also found that listeners misperceived fricatives as plosives and plosives as fricatives similarly. However, plosives and fricatives were infrequently identified as a nasal consonant; yet, when nasals were misperceived, listeners almost equally judged them to be either a plosive or a fricative.

Analysis of the affrication feature (termed "frication" by Sacco et al., 1967) was conducted to identify perceptual differences associated with an open or closed articulatory posture. Results indicated that relatively high intelligibility exists for both fricatives and plosive-nasal phonemes. However, a fricative was about twice as likely to be misidentified as a plosive-nasal than the opposite (27% vs. 15%). A durational analysis revealed that consonants of long duration (/s, ʃ, z, and ʒ/) were perceived as shortened in duration (24%), yet the opposite was infrequently observed (3%). This suggests that reduced aerodynamic driving capacity of the esophageal reservoir results in some articulatory adjustment (compensation) by the speaker (Diedrich & Youngstrom, 1966). Such adjustments in shortening duration may augment reduced vocal tract pressures during esophageal speech production (see Doyle et al., 1988; Robbins, Christensen, & Kempster, 1986).

Results from a study similar in design to that of Sacco et al. (1967) using a single esophageal speaker and a single TE speaker judged as "highly proficient" was reported by Doyle and Danhauer (1986). Prior to participating in the study, several tasks were undertaken in an attempt to ensure that these two speakers were well-matched in their intelligibility (< 1% difference). Speakers were required to produce consonant-vowel (CV) and vowel-consonant (VC) stimuli using 16 consonants and 5 vowels. Both professional and naive listeners phonetically transcribed their responses using an open response format. The overall intelligibility for the esophageal speakers was judged to be 85% and 79% for professional and naive listeners, respectively. In contrast, the TE speaker was judged to be 94% and 89% intelligible by professional and naive listeners, respectively. Doyle and Danhauer (1986) also found that voiced consonants were correctly perceived from 3–5% more often for the esophageal speaker and from 7–11% more often for the TE speaker. Results were interpreted to be indicative of the influence of a higher capacity (pulmonary) driving source in TE speakers upon phoneme production.

Hoops and Curtis (1971) evaluated the speech intelligibility of 28 male esophageal speakers. This study also sought information on the possible relationship of listener intelligibility scores to judgments of overall esophageal speech proficiency. According to Hoops and Curtis (1971) speakers represented "a wide range of speaking ability from poor to superior." Speech stimuli consisted of four sentence lists. Listeners were required to identify low redundancy "key words" for each sentence. Recordings of the Rainbow Passage (Fairbanks, 1960) were used for proficiency judgments. Listeners were 21 speech pathologists, divided into seven groups of three listeners each for intelligibility assessments. Seventy-five naive college students served as judges of the speakers' overall speech proficiency.

Listeners were presented the speakers' stimuli at approximately 70 dB SPL; the average ambient noise level was 50 dB SPL. Each listener group was presented sentences produced by four speakers, and no listener group heard the same speaker or word list during the experiment. Listeners transcribed their "best estimate" of key words they heard. Each listener's score for sentence materials was averaged for each speaker to determine mean intelligibility. In the proficiency phase of the study, listeners judged speakers over three sessions and were instructed to rate speakers on a 7-point equal-appearing-interval scale (1 = low proficiency, 7 = high proficiency). No instructions on characteristics of "good or bad" esophageal speech were provided.

Intelligibility scores presented by Hoops and Curtis (1971) ranged from 21.6% to 96.0% (mean 75.13%). Again, it is clear that esophageal speakers vary substantially in their intelligibility (Creech, 1966; Sacco et al., 1967). Similarly, judgments of speech proficiency ranged from a mean of 1.1 to 6.6. Statistical analyses of intelligibility and proficiency indicated a correlation of 0.376. Although the correlation exceeded a 0.05 level of confidence (for a zero-order correlation), other factors may weigh heavily on judgments of speech proficiency. In particular, judgments of sentence materials may provide an advantage to more fluent speakers. That is, a speaker capable of achieving a greater proportion of time in phonation may be judged more favorably (Shipp, 1967, 1970; Snidecor, 1978; Weinberg et al., 1982), these speakers may also have the capacity to generate higher vocal tract pressures which may influence articulatory proficiency.

Horii and Weinberg (1975) investigated the effects of broadband masking noise on the intelligibility of superior esophageal speech. Two highly proficient esophageal speakers recorded consonant rhyme stimuli (House, Williams, Hecker, & Kryter, 1965) and vowel rhyme stimuli (Horii, 1969). Consonant lists contained 50 monosyllabic words each with word-initial and word-final consonants represented equally. Vowel stimuli consisted of 24 monosyllables with 12 vowels represented twice each. Sixteen normal-hearing young adults served as listeners. Data were gathered over multiple sessions using a closed set (six choice) response paradigm. Esophageal stimuli were presented at four signal-to-noise (S/N) ratios (–9, –5, –1, and +3 dB) in addition to a no noise (quiet) condition. Vowel stimuli were presented under three S/Ns (–9, –5, and –1 dB). Horii and Weinberg (1975) used comparative intelligibility values for normal talkers obtained in a prior investigation (Horii, House, & Hughes, 1971) in order to assist interpretation of the esophageal data.

Results presented by Horii and Weinberg (1975) revealed that the overall intelligibility of esophageal vowel rhyme words perceived in quiet was about 98%. In the noise condition, overall functions revealed a descending slope of approximately 5% per dB, for consonants, and 4% per dB for vowels. Comparing esophageal to normal speech, vowel functions were essentially the same. However, consonant intelligibility for the esophageal speakers' stimuli was poorer in the more severe S/N ratios (–9, –5, and –1 dB). Differences in overall consonant intelligibility varied approximately 12% to 14% between normal and esophageal speakers for the two most adverse listening conditions (–9 and –5 dB) and were most pronounced for liquid-glides and nasals. When comparing normal and esophageal speakers' productions, however, fricative intelligibility was similar between the speakers under the highest noise conditions.

Viewing the Horii and Weinberg (1975) data in their entirety, esophageal consonant intelligibility is greatest for liquid-glides, followed by nasals, stop-plosives, and fricatives. These findings are consistent with those reported by Sacco et al. (1967). However, negligible intelligibility differences occurred between these consonant classes at any given S/N with overall intelligibility being remarkably similar between classes for esophageal speech. Findings were similar across word-initial and word-final productions of consonants. Finally, whereas normal speakers produced voiced consonants with greater overall effectiveness than voiceless consonants (69% vs. 47%), esophageal speakers demonstrated only a slight advantage for voiced consonant intelligibility (54% vs. 51%).

Horii and Weinberg's (1975) data suggest that masking did not differentially effect esophageal consonant intelligibility. This finding is not consistent with previous research (Miller & Nicely, 1955) which showed consonant intelligibility for a normal speaker's signal under conditions of masking to be altered as a function of consonant power spectra (Weinberg, Horii, & Smith, 1980). However, white noise did influence overall intelligibility of esophageal speakers compared to normals. This reduction ranged from 12% to 14%. These data confirm the difficulties frequently encountered by esophageal speakers in competing noise environments (Diedrich & Youngstrom, 1966; Gardner, 1971; Snidecor, 1978).

Kalb and Carpenter (1981) investigated the relative intelligibility of five esophageal and five artificial laryngeal speakers. In addition, five speakers capable of producing both methods of alaryngeal communication were also evaluated. All speakers were judged to be highly proficient in their respective mode(s) of communication. Using this paradigm, Kalb and Carpenter sought to identify possible effects that an individual speaker's variability may have on overall intelligibility in group comparisons.

In the experimental phase of Kalb and Carpenter's (1981) investigation, all speakers recorded one 50-item PB word list (Egan, 1948). A single normal speaker also produced stimuli in order to evaluate the listeners' discrimination of normal target stimuli. Thirty naive listeners transcribed the stimuli during the perceptual phase of the study. Speech stimuli were presented in the sound-field at a comfortable listening level.

Results indicated that the mean intelligibility score for the normal speakers was 98.4% with scores of 78.6% and 61.8% for esophageal and artificial laryngeal speakers, respectively. The third group of speakers, those who produced both modes of alaryngeal speech, were perceived as being 67.3% intelligible in the esophageal mode and 70.7% intelligible in the artificial laryngeal mode. Although the overall ranges of intelligibility for individual speakers in each group were similar, greater variation existed for the esophageal mode. Whereas a statistical difference in intelligibility was observed between esophageal and artificial laryngeal speaker groups, only minimal (and non-significant) differences were demonstrated for the comparative speech samples of those

who produced both modes of alaryngeal speech. This observation led Kalb and Carpenter (1981) to suggest that individual speaker variation may sufficiently influence data obtained using group designs. That is, the group design appeared to be strongly influenced by productive capabilities of individual speakers. Although prior comparisons of different modes of alaryngeal speech may have demonstrated significant differences between groups evaluated, differences related to individual speaker variation rather than collective differences between a particular method of alaryngeal speech may have also been reflected. Past research may then be confounded to some degree by the effects of individual speaker variation. These findings have critical bearing upon the validity of group designs in intelligibility studies with alaryngeal speakers, and always must be considered when evaluating such data.

Weiss and Basili (1985) evaluated perceptual confusions of listeners to word stimuli (primarily CVCs) produced by laryngectomized subjects using two methods of artificial alaryngeal speech (Western Electric and Servox). Six experienced listeners directly transcribed the speakers' productions. Intelligibility for words resulted in a mean group score of 33% for the Western Electric device and 36% for the Servox. Individual speaker scores ranged from 16% to 54% with the Western Electric and from 19% to 55% for the Servox. Weiss and Basili noted that while considerable difference existed across their laryngectomized speakers, individual speakers exhibited remarkable similarity in their intelligibility across devices. Difference scores across devices ranged from 1% to 11%. Weiss and Basili (1985) further analyzed their perceptual data to define patterns of perceptual confusions related to manner of production and voicing, as well as phonetic position (i.e, word-initial and word-final). A summary of these data segmented by type of artificial larynx is shown in Table 13–5.

As can be seen, phonetic position and manner of production did influence the

TABLE 13–5.
Percent Intelligibility Segmented by Initial and Final Phonetic Position and Manner Class for Speakers Using the Western Electric and Servox Artificial Larynx.

	Western Electric Artificial Larynx	
	Phonetic Position	
Manner Class	Initial	Final
Stops	49	60
Fricatives	30	50
Nasals	74	59
Affricates	53	75
Liquid/Glides	84	79
Servox Artificial Larynx		
Stops	52	69
Fricatives	36	54
Nasals	80	48
Affricates	61	88
Liquid/Glides	90	80

Source: From Weiss, M. S. & Basili, A. R. (1985). Electrolaryngeal speech produced by laryngectomized subjects: Perceptual characteristics. *Journal of Speech and Hearing Research, 28,* 294–300. American Speech-Language Hearing Association, reprinted with permission.

overall intelligibility. In regard to voicing distinctions, similar patterns of errors were noted regardless of artificial laryngeal device. Weiss and Basili (1985) observed that the most common perceptual error for voiceless stops in the initial position was that of identification of the voiced cognate. In contrast, when initial voiced stops were intended, generally high levels of intelligibility (i.e., from 64% to 90%) were exhibited. When voiceless stops were produced in the final phonetic position, higher intelligibility scores were always greater than those observed for word-initial productions. Slight reductions in intelligibility were, however, typically observed for final voice stops when compared to those produced in the initial position. When confusion data for fricatives were assessed, initial voiceless targets were generally found to be more intelligible than their cognates. This was also true of final consonants with the exception of interdental fricatives. Although some differences for fricatives in the pattern of perceptual confusions between the two artificial laryngeal devices

used were noted, a specific trend was not identified. Weiss and Basili (1985) interpreted these combined data to indicate that speech intelligibility does not appear to be influenced by artificial device type. Rather, individual speaker differences must be addressed (Kalb & Carpenter, 1981). Consequently, Weiss and Basili recommended that treatment programs for artificial laryngeal speakers be structured so that emphasis is placed on articulation skills that would facilitate improved voiced and voiceless consonant production (Duguay, 1983).

Dudley, Robbins, Singer, Blom, and Fisher (1981) were the first to evaluate the intelligibility of TE speakers. They assessed the intelligibility of nine TE speakers using monosyllabic stimuli. Twelve listeners were individually presented stimuli at a level of 65 dB SPL. However, to assess effects of noise on the intelligibility of TE speech, six of the speakers' stimuli were recorded with a noise competitor (12 person multitalker complex). Competing noise was presented at two signal-to-noise ratios (+3 and +5 dB). Intelligibility in the two noise conditions and a third, quiet condition were evaluated. Listeners identified the word by choosing one of two minimally contrasting word choices. Results from the Dudley et al. (1981) study showed that average intelligibility ranged from approximately 72% to 83% for the three listening conditions (Horii & Weinberg, 1975). As would be expected, intelligibility in quiet was superior to the noise conditions.

An additional aspect of Dudley et al.'s (1981) study was an analysis conducted on errors for the +3 dB and quiet conditions. Comprehensive analyses of these errors revealed that in quiet, voicing errors accounted for 21% of the errors, followed by place (14%) and manner errors (12%). The remaining errors (53%) were multiple interactions of place, manner, and voicing. In the competing noise condition, voicing errors were greatest (32%) followed by manner errors (30%) and place errors (24%). Thus, the addition of a noise competitor resulted in the greatest increases in errors for manner (18%), followed by place (10%), and then voicing (9%). Competing noise would appear to alter the intelligibility of TE speech by reducing manner cues. It is interesting, however, that in analysis of these data, 86% of the all errors were single feature errors (Dudley et al., 1981), a 33% increase from that noted in the quiet condition.

Overall, the findings of Dudley et al. (1981) revealed that TE speech intelligibility in competing noise parallels that of normal speech masked by continuous noise (Miller & Nicely, 1955). Specifically, nasals and glides were more resistant to noise competition than stops or fricatives. These data are in some disagreement with those of Horii and Weinberg (1975) for esophageal speakers. This may be due to several influences that derive directly from the noise itself and, therefore, may affect perception quite differently (e.g., composition of competing noise, white noise vs. multitalker noise). Characteristics of the noise must also be considered with the acoustic characteristics of the signal with which it competes. Thus, combined influences of the primary signal and the competition must be considered.

Finally, Dudley et al. (1981) analyzed voice/voiceless distinctions. They found that in quiet twice as many voiceless consonants were perceived as voiced, as voiced consonants were perceived as voiceless. Equal opportunity for identification existed for both voiced and voiceless targets. These data are consistent with those of Sacco et al. (1967) obtained from esophageal talkers. In noise, voiced-for-voiceless errors occurred approximately 25% more often (Horii & Weinberg, 1975). The number of correctly identified voiceless consonants was quite similar in quiet and in noise. This suggests that the voicing feature, whether it be esophageal or TE, is sensitive to disruption by noise competition.

Clark and Stemple (1982) used synthetic sentence (SSI) materials (Jerger, Speaks, & Trammell, 1968) to assess intelligibility in single laryngeal, artificial laryngeal, esophageal, and TE speakers. All four speakers were judged as "above average" for their respective mode of communication. Synthetic sentences were chosen because they do not contain linguistically redundant, predictable lexical items within the constructions. Clark and Stemple, therefore, believed intelligibility could be assessed in a more natural context, while at the same time reducing the inherent, linguistically bound influences on judgments of intelligibility.

Twenty young adult listeners were presented speaker stimuli at one of three message-to-competition ratios (MCRs), either 0, –5, or –10 dB. The competing signal was an ongoing monologue produced by a normal speaker. Stimuli were presented at 70 dB SPL. Results revealed no significant differences between the normal laryngeal, artificial laryngeal, esophageal, or TE speakers at the 0 MCR.

Significant differences in SSI intelligibility were observed at the –5 and –10 MCRs. The mean intelligibility for the esophageal speaker was 28%, 85%, and 98% for the –10, –5, and 0 dB MCRs, respectively.

The TE speakers' scores were 12%, 76%, and 99% for the same three MCRs. At the –5 MCR, the artificial laryngeal speaker's intelligibility was significantly better than that of the esophageal speaker. The normal laryngeal, artificial laryngeal, and esophageal speaker's speech were all judged to be significantly more intelligible than that of the TE speaker at this level. For the –10 MCR, speech intelligibility for the normal laryngeal, artificial laryngeal, and esophageal speakers was significantly better than the TE speaker.

The Clark and Stemple (1982) study was a significant departure from past intelligibility investigations of alaryngeal speech. Specifically, they attempted to approximate "real life" listening situations (i.e., sentence stimuli and noise competition). Compared to previous research, SSI materials appeared to offer a favorable method of assessment. However, several issues in the Clark and Stemple (1982) study are important.

First, only a single speaker using each alaryngeal method recorded stimuli. As a result, individual differences may have affected judgments to an even greater extent than group data (Kalb & Carpenter, 1982). As such, generalizations cannot be safely made from the data. An additional concern relates to the SSI stimulus materials. Although these sentences eliminated linguistic redundancy, the closed set response paradigm (10 choices) may spuriously indicate intelligibility of an entire sentence even if only single words are identified. If listeners had transcribed each sentence word-for-word, intelligibility may have been more accurately evaluated. Such considerations would be of importance in future assessments of alaryngeal speech intelligibility.

In a follow-up study, Clark (1985) compared the intelligibility of the same alaryngeal speakers' productions of synthetic sentences between two groups of listeners. Eleven normal-hearing young adults and ll older individuals with high-frequency presbycusic hearing losses

served as listeners. Speech stimuli were those used previously (Clark & Stemple, 1982) as were the MCRs investigated. Results revealed differences both in the intelligibility of alaryngeal speech modes and between the young and older listening groups. At the –5 MCR, normal speech intelligibility was significantly different between listener groups. Esophageal speech intelligibility was also judged as significantly different between groups at this MCR. Both listener groups found normal speech intelligibility to be significantly better than either esophageal or TE speech intelligibility.

At the –10 MCR, a significant difference was again identified between listener groups for the normal talker. Both listener groups judged TE speech to be significantly less intelligible than normal, esophageal, or artificial laryngeal speech. Surprisingly, however, older listeners judged the artificial laryngeal talker's speech intelligibility to be significantly better than that of the normal talker. Thus, degree and configuration of hearing loss would appear to be a critical factor to consider in the intelligibility judgments of alaryngeal speakers. Although the artificial laryngeal speech likely had a more consistent energy spectrum, and more stable intensity than that of the normal speaker, it is interesting that an obviously degraded speech signal was perceived as more intelligible. Whether Clark's (1985) findings were due to the differential amplification of particular speech sounds via the artificial laryngeal device, or as a result of a degraded normal speech signal is unknown. Another reason for this finding may relate to the fact that the normal speakers' productions were in competition with a normal talker's monologue. Perhaps this similarity made a clear intelligibility distinction more difficult for listeners with a hearing loss.

Tardy-Mitzell, Andrews, and Bowman (1985) evaluated the acceptability and intelligibility of 15 TE speakers (10 males and 5 females). All were videotaped and included: (1) each speaker's description of his or her home environment, (2) counting, (3) reading of The Grandfather Passage (Darley, Aronson, & Brown, 1975), and (4) a 50-item word list.

Forty-six naive listeners served as judges for the samples, and all acceptability and intelligibility judgments were made from videotaped recordings. Speaker acceptability was rated on a l-to-7 equal-appearing interval scale with "l" being least acceptable and "7" being most acceptable. Criteria for these judgments were based on a speaker's fluency, speech rate, inflection, and pleasantness of quality. Intelligibility judgments were based on speech samples from the word lists. Listeners identified the word spoken from six choices differing only in a single consonant. Thus, intelligibility was defined as the overall intelligibility, or percent correct, for the 50-item word list. Scores were collapsed into an overall mean intelligibility score for each TE speaker.

The results obtained by Tardy-Mitzell et al. (1985) indicated that for acceptability ratings only two of 15 talkers were given overall ratings of less than 4.0. Four speakers were rated as 4.0, six as 5.0, and three as 6.0. No significant differences in acceptability ratings were found between male and female speakers. Judgments of intelligibility ranged from 80.7% to 97.5% with a mean of 93.0%, a median of 94.5%, and a mode of 96.0%. Although no significant difference was identified between males and females, the overall female group intelligibility score was 4.6% higher than males.

The findings of Tardy-Mitzell et al. (1985) reveal that their TE speakers were highly intelligible to naive listeners and, further, were judged as being of relatively high acceptability. The overall intelligibility findings are sufficiently better than those reported previously for esophageal and TE speakers (Dudley et al., 1981; Kalb & Carpenter, 1981; Shames et al., 1963). Regarding TE speakers in particular, Tardy-Mitzell et al.'s mean intelligibility score was approximately 10% higher than

that reported by Dudley et al. (1981). This is interesting since Dudley et al.'s listeners were only required to identify the target stimuli from a two-choice response format. This would appear to offer a higher probability of listener identification of the target stimuli and, subsequently, a higher judged intelligibility.

Williams and Watson (1985) investigated differences in speech proficiency among 12 esophageal, 12 TE, and 12 artificial laryngeal talkers. An additional dimension of this study compared ratings of three groups of judges who varied in knowledge and exposure to laryngectomized speakers. Listener groups consisted of (1) naive judges without prior exposure to laryngectomized individuals, (2) informed judges with some exposure, and (3) expert judges who had several years experience with laryngectomized speakers. Judgments were made for each speaker's recording of (1) stating their name and counting to 10; (2) reading of words, sentences, and paragraphs; (3) a picture description; and (4) conversation.

Listeners rated speech samples on eight variables: vocal quality, pitch, speech rate, loudness, intelligibility, visual presentation during speech, extraneous speech noise (stoma noise), and overall communicative effectiveness. Upon factor analysis, many variables clustered together and were thus redefined as (1) pitch and quality, (2) visual presentation during speech, (3) speech rate, (4) extraneous noise, (5) loudness, and (6) intelligibility and overall communicative effectiveness.

The results of Williams and Watson's (1985) study revealed naive listeners' judgments of TE speakers' speech rate to be significantly better than that of esophageal speakers and that TE loudness was significantly better than for electrolaryngeal speakers. For ratings of intelligibility and overall communicative effectiveness, TE speakers were judged to be significantly better than electrolaryngeal speakers but significant differences were not found between esophageal and TE groups.

Judgments by the informed listener group revealed judgments of TE speech were significantly better than either esophageal or electrolaryngeal speech on all variables except speech rate. Judgments showed that esophageal speakers were significantly better than electrolaryngeal speakers. For the variable of rate, both the TE and electrolaryngeal speakers were significantly better than the esophageal speakers.

The expert group of listeners judged TE speech as superior to that of the other two speaker groups. Specifically, TE speakers were judged significantly better on all variables except pitch, quality, and loudness. No other significantly different findings among the speaker groups were noted.

Based on the findings by Williams and Watson (1985) it appears that the sophistication of listeners can significantly alter perceptual judgments of alaryngeal speech. Sophisticated (trained or professional) listeners may reveal better scores than untrained naive listeners. Thus, use of naive listeners may provide a more accurate index of speech intelligibility. Williams and Watson's (1985) results also demonstrate the critical relationship that multiple factors play in judgments of alaryngeal speech.

Blom et al. (1986) conducted a prospective study of TE speech intelligibility. They evaluated 47 patients (14 females, 33 males) prior to and four days following TE puncture. Evaluations conducted before TE puncture and use of the voice prosthesis were done in the speaker's primary mode of communication (i.e., esophageal speech, electrolaryngeal speech, or whispered speech). All speakers recorded speech stimuli (Modified Rhyme Test materials) which were then evaluated by naive listeners. Preoperative assessment of intelligibility resulted in a group mean score of 78.15% compared to a postoperative score of 91.51%. Of the 47 speakers assessed, 74% ($N = 35$) exhibited significantly improved speech intelligibility using TE speech. Of those patients who did

not show significant improvements in their intelligibility using TE speech ($N = 12$), 7 of them had pre-TE puncture intelligibility scores $\geq 90\%$. Improvements were also observed in listener judgments of speech acceptability.

Doyle et al. (1988) presented data on consonantal intelligibility of three well-matched esophageal and three TE speakers and a single speaker who was proficient in both modes. All speakers generated multiple productions of all 24 English consonants in the intervocalic loci of a nonsense (CVCVC) production. These productions were then presented to 15 listeners who were requested to transcribe the intervocalic consonant. Based on data obtained, Doyle et al. reported that overall intelligibility scores for the esophageal speakers ranged from approximately 52% to 62%. The TE speakers demonstrated intelligibility scores that ranged from approximately 59% to 72%. For the speaker proficient in both modes (i.e., "dual-mode speaker"), an esophageal mode score of approximately 42% was obtained while a score of approximately 71% was obtained in the TE mode. Doyle et al. (1988) also reported that while voicing errors were frequently observed, TE speakers exhibited a tendency toward "voicing" regardless of whether a voiced or voiceless consonant was intended. A similar trend was also seen with the dual-mode speaker in the TE mode. When data were analyzed by manner of production, TE speakers demonstrated significantly greater intelligibility for all manner classes except affricates where identical scores across alaryngeal mode were noted.

In summary, numerous studies of speech intelligibility have been conducted over the years. Unfortunately, no two studies have utilized similar designs and, consequently, comparison of these data is difficult. This difficulty is further compounded by the effects of individual speaker variation on measures of speech intelligibility. This appears to be a significant factor that is commonly observed when individual data are evaluated. Thus, while alaryngeal speech can be globally viewed as a degraded speech signal, intelligibility differences across speakers within and between alaryngeal modes may be substantial. This has direct clinical implications in that a clear picture of which alaryngeal mode is most likely to result in the best overall intelligibility (when considered independently from other perceptual attributes) is currently unspecified.

Perceptual Attributes: Listener Preference and Acceptability

Several investigations have assessed a variety of perceptual attributes related to alaryngeal speech. These studies have typically varied in their outcome, and some inconsistencies have been noted. Bennett and Weinberg (1973) provided one of the more comprehensive lists of factors which may influence why alaryngeal speakers are judged to be "nonnormal" speakers. The most frequently noted reasons underlying the unacceptability of esophageal speech are (1) voice quality does not sound normal, (2) speech is too slow, and 3) pitch is too low (Bennett & Weinberg, 1973). For electrolaryngeal speech, the reasons cited were (1) quality does not sound normal, (2) speech sounds mechanical, (3) speech is too slow, and (4) voice is monotonous (Bennett & Weinberg, 1973). Thus, while listeners may provide an indication that specific parameters of speech are not normal (e.g., rate, pitch, etc.), the most frequently occurring judgments are related to judgments which entail a broader assessment of verbal communication (Smith, Weinberg, Feth, & Horii, 1978; Weinberg & Bennett, 1971). Unfortunately, well-defined and comprehensive studies which address the influence of both isolated and combined features of alaryngeal speech on listener judgments are sorely lacking. As such, future research into this important area is worthy of attention.

Clark and Stemple (1982) found that while TE speech may be less intelligible in competing noise situations, it was judged to be most "pleasant" when compared to esophageal and artificial laryngeal speech. Many perceptual features of importance in judging the overall quality of alaryngeal have been obtained as secondary or indirect components of studies which have focused on other aspects of voice or speech production (Shipp, 1967). Based on data presented in the literature, there is really no clear indication of what type of speech is best or most preferred.

The reason for this lack of clarity is that while particular features of speech may be judged independently in a relative manner, it is the multidimensional nature of speech which ultimately provides the listener with the best "feel" for what constitutes better or more acceptable speech. One feature which does appear to carry considerable weight in the perceptual domain is that of speech rate. Slow speech, particularly as a result of frequent pauses, appears to have a rather substantial impact on the listener (Shipp, 1967). Thus, listener judgments appear to be influenced by productive speech rate (in words per minute), the length of phrases produced, as well as the rhythm with which it is produced (DiCarlo et al., 1955; Diedrich & Youngstrom, 1966). This does not, however, exclude the salience of other perceptual features on judgments of alaryngeal speech (Smith et al., 1978).

Findings by Clark and Stemple (1982) have suggested that TE speech is less intelligible in noise conditions than esophageal, artificial laryngeal (Servox), or normal speech. However, Clark and Stemple's (1982) listeners also judged TE speech to be the most pleasant of the three alaryngeal modes evaluated. Fifty-five percent of the listeners ($N = 20$) preferred TE speech over artificial laryngeal (25%) and esophageal speech (20%). When the same listeners were asked to judge which mode was least pleasant to listen to, 60% indicated esophageal, with 20% indicating artificial laryngeal, and 20% indicating TE speech.

Blom et al. (1986) evaluated speech acceptability as part of their prospective study of TE speech. Listeners were asked to rate speech samples obtained prior to and 4 days following TE puncture using a 5-point scale (1 = least acceptable, 5 = most acceptable). Based on listener assessments of acceptability as a group, significant improvements in judgments were observed following TE puncture (i.e., $M = 2.01$ vs. $M = 3.41$). When individual speaker data were evaluated, 30 of 47 speakers demonstrated "very" significant improvements in judged acceptability with TE speech, 5 patients demonstrated "mildly" significant improvement, with 12 patients exhibiting no statistically significant change following TE puncture. These data indicated that TE speech was characterized by improved listener judgments of speech acceptability in approximately 75% of the speakers evaluated. Given the short interval that followed TE puncture and subsequent ratings (i.e., 4 days), improved levels of acceptability may be achieved with greater experience using the TE voice prosthesis.

Trudeau (1987) compared listener judgments of speech acceptability between groups of esophageal and TE speakers who were judged to be good or excellent in their proficiency and those of normal laryngeal speakers. Both male and female speakers were included. Initial classification of subjects into proficiency groups was done by having experienced speech-language pathologists rate speech samples. All speakers provided speech samples of oral reading (Rainbow Passage) which were then presented to naive listeners. Listeners were asked to rate each speaker using a 5-point equal-appearing interval scale which pertained to how "pleasant" the speech was judged to be. Overall results indicated that those females who were judged to be excellent speakers by the speech-language pathologists were judged by naive listeners to be better speakers than excellent male speakers. For the good speakers, the opposite was noted. It was interesting to note, however, that mode of

alaryngeal speech did not appear to have any affect on judgments of acceptability.

Sedory, Hamlet, and Connor (1989) sought to evaluate the relationship of perceptual and acoustic characteristics inherent in excellent esophageal and TE speech. Speakers were requested to produce the first three sentences from the Rainbow Passage, and these samples were then presented to listeners who made judgments using a paired-comparison paradigm. A sustained vowel production in the form of a maximum phonation time (MPT) task was also obtained. The sustained vowel task primarily served as an temporal index of extended phonation. Listeners were asked to identify which sentence from two was most acceptable to listen to. Based on the combined acoustic measure obtained from the sustained phonation Sedory et al. (1989) found that TE speakers demonstrated significantly longer mean extended phonation times, increased intensity, and more syllables per breath.

In regard to perceptual judgments, while very high levels of agreement between listeners in their rating of speech samples were noted, no significant difference was identified between the excellent esophageal and TE speakers (Sedory et al., 1989). Finally, no significant correlations between acoustic measures and perceptual rank of the speakers investigated were noted. These data clearly suggest that while several acoustic variables may differ across esophageal and TE speech modes, they do not appear to influence listener judgments of preference. Although Sedory et al. (1989) noted that listeners frequently stated that speech samples presented were "too similar to make a preference judgment," listeners did acknowledge that some perceptual features did influence how they judged samples. Specifically, "smoothness," "clarity of speech," and "more normal sounding voice" appeared to be salient features in relation to preferred speakers. This suggests that overall voice quality, intelligibility, and naturalness may be important perceptual dimensions for distinguishing speakers both within and across alaryngeal mode. In contrast, listeners indicated that "nonspeech noises," "audible inhalations or injections," "slurring of words," and poor control of "loudness and rate" were judged as unacceptable features of speech. This suggests that extraneous noise, intelligibility, as well as temporal features may characterize poorer speakers.

Prosodic Characteristics

As a result of total laryngectomy and the use of nonnormal voicing systems (whether intrinsic or extrinsic), considerable reductions exist in the laryngectomized speaker's ability to manipulate frequency, intensity, and duration. In normal laryngeal speakers, the ability to volitionally manipulate these acoustic parameters is believed to underlie the speaker's ability to signal a variety of linguistic contrasts. Thus, the inability for alaryngeal speakers to signal linguistic (suprasegmental) markers such as stress, intonation, juncture, and duration may be observed. Yet the physiologic limitations exhibited by certain types of alaryngeal talkers may result in differences in their ability to code such prosodic elements.

Gandour and Weinberg (1982) investigated the ability of alaryngeal talkers to produce "contrastive stress." Generally, data revealed that with the exception of several users of the Servox artificial larynx, esophageal, TE, and users of the Western Electric device were able to successfully signal contrastive stress. Two studies (Gandour & Weinberg, 1983; Gandour et al, 1983) have addressed questions pertaining to intonational and lexical stress contrasts. Due to the fact that alaryngeal speakers communicate via nonconventional source excitation, air supplies, and articulatory mechanisms, Gandour and Weinberg (1983) investigated questions relating to which alaryngeal speakers can produce specific linguistic contrasts. Gandour and Weinberg (1983) studied five groups of speakers (normal, esophageal,

TE, Western Electric and Servox users) while they produced stimuli in question and statement formats (e.g., "Bev loves Bob? and "Bev loves Bob!"). Forty naive adult listeners identified alaryngeal productions using a two-interval-forced-choice procedure. Results indicated that normal, esophageal, and TE speakers produced the respective intonational contrasts in a highly effective manner (means = 99.7%, 98.3%, and 90.0%, respectively); however, no significant differences existed between these three groups. Gandour and Weinberg suggested that these findings indicate TE and esophageal speakers are able to control and regulate F_0 to assure the production of contrastive intonation.

Using the same subjects in a follow-up study, Gandour et al. (1983) investigated alaryngeal speakers' ability to produce lexical stress (i.e, OBject vs. obJECT, etc.). As found with the previous study on contrastive stress (Gandour and Weinberg, 1983), normal, esophageal, and TE speakers were all able to produce lexical stress with a high degree of success. However, users of the artificial larynx (Western Electric and Servox) exhibited considerably more difficulty. These findings highlight the ability of esophageal and TE speakers to control and regulate critical elements of linguistic emphasis, regardless of their use of a nonnormal phonatory source (Gandour et al., 1983). This appears to be quite apparent in esophageal speakers who are rated as being highly proficient alaryngeal speakers (McHenry et al., 1982).

Scarpino and Weinberg (1981) also assessed the ability of highly proficient esophageal speakers to encode junctural patterns which are used to separate word boundary (e.g., "seem able" vs. "see Mable"). Overall, it appears that esophageal speakers are extremely successful at marking such boundaries. Thus, a variety of linguistic contrasts appear to be effectively coded by alaryngeal speakers. This is particulary true for those individuals who use esophageal or TE speech.

Summary

Measures of frequency, intensity, speech rate, and intelligibility are important parameters in defining and differentiating alaryngeal from normal laryngeal speakers. Many alterations in these parameters are specifically related to anatomic, physiologic, and aerodynamic changes subsequent to total laryngectomy. Data presented provides a general comparative foundation from which alaryngeal methods can be evaluated. Clearly all alaryngeal speakers will exhibit some reductions in a variety of parameters from those of the normal speaker. This is due primarily to the loss of the normal voicing source, the larynx. While an abnormal voicing source has sufficient potential to influence acoustic, temporal, and intelligibility measures, it also has a substantial effect on listener perceptions of the individual speaker. Specifically, a listener's perception of multidimensional aspects of the individual's voice and speech (e.g., voice quality) would appear to have a considerable effect on its acceptability.

Finally, while some studies have focused on describing the characteristics of a single population others have employed a comparative format across the different modes of alaryngeal speech. Unfortunately, adherence to strict defining criteria have not always been apparent in studies of alaryngeal speakers. Even within a specific group of alaryngeal speakers (e.g., esophageal, TE, artificial laryngeal) vast individual differences in productive capabilities have been observed. Although data generally indicate that specific trends exist for a given alaryngeal mode it is clear that alaryngeal speakers exhibit performance characteristics that extend over a considerable range. It is, however, important to note that performance may differ substantially between poor, average, and superior speakers for any given mode. Thus, substantial heterogeneity has been observed and is to be expected both within and across alaryngeal speech modes.

Long-Term Counseling of the Patient

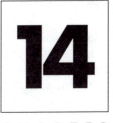

14

CHAPTER

The nature of cancer as a disease process typically requires prompt and generally aggressive treatment. This is also true for patients with laryngeal cancer. In such circumstances, the elapsed time between the diagnosis of cancer, application of the primary treatment modality, and confrontation with the consequences of medical management may be a matter of several days (Reed, 1983a; Salmon, 1986a, 1986b). The patient's adjustment to the diagnosis of a malignancy, its management, and the subsequent disability is not, however, a short-term phenomenon (Blood, Luther, & Stemple, 1992; Gunn, 1984).

Adjustment is indeed a continuing process. Although numerous patient factors influence the degree and speed with which adjustment occurs, patients will always recognize "new" limitations as time goes on. Many of these limitations may be specific to the individual. The purpose of this chapter is to address this particular concern, namely, that patients will often need additional information, insights, and counseling well after formal voice and speech therapy has been discontinued. In doing so, several issues pertaining to need for timely access to additional information will be outlined. An overview of how long-term counseling and information provision can be facilitated is also presented.

The Process of Adaptation Following Laryngectomy

In most instances, the patient's early concerns following laryngectomy usually pertain to issues that are the most salient to that specific point in time. That is, immediate needs typically take priority for the patient and members of his or her family. This "hierarchy" of importance is clearly acknowledged by the clinician who structures counseling to address the most

247

salient changes first. In the patient who undergoes total laryngectomy, this involves coverage of those areas related to primary anatomic and physiologic changes, as well as the loss of normal laryngeal speech.

In contrast, those changes that are more subtle in character are frequently not acknowledged early in the postoperative period unless the patient or a member of his or her family specifically requests such information. Similarly, many of the more subtle consequences of laryngectomy may not be fully acknowledged or realized by the patient until sometime following discharge from regular, formal voice and speech treatment. During voice and speech treatment the patient is usually focusing attention and energy on basic aspects of acquiring functional alaryngeal verbal communication.

It is not uncommon nor unexpected to have patients focus their attention on the most conspicuous changes and associated problems early in the rehabilitative process. Once an understanding of this problem is addressed, they may shift their focus to the next most conspicuous problem. All patients who have had a laryngectomy will need to address several identical problems (e.g., anatomical and physiologic changes postoperatively) (Blood et al., 1992; Reed, 1983a; Salmon, 1986a, 1986b), yet each patient will also eventually encounter problems that will be unique to him or her as an individual (Burish, Meyerowitz, Carey, & Morrow, 1987; Gates, Ryan, Cantu, & Hearne, 1982; Gates, Ryan, & Lauder, 1982; Gunn, 1984). This realization by the patient must be met with an opportunity to seek information and if possible identify a solution to the problem.

difficulty, the ability to discuss this with others is usually of great value. Those whom the patient might speak with include the speech-language pathologist, other professionals, or other individuals who have undergone laryngectomy and/or members of their family (Salmon, 1986a, 1986b, 1986c). While professional sources offer specific perspectives that the patient will likely find helpful, input from other laryngectomized individuals appears to provide an invaluable source of information should the patient desire such contact (Reed, 1983; Salmon, 1986c). It is, therefore, necessary for the speech-language pathologist to consider potential sources for such continuing "counseling" services and, ideally, to determine how the patient's (and members of his or her family) needs can best be attended to in a timely and efficient manner (Blood, Simpson, Dineen, Kauffmann, & Raimondi, 1993; Reed, 1983a).

Unfortunately, the domain of clinical speech-language pathology usually carries with it considerable caseload demands in relation to direct patient contact hours. This trend has increased dramatically over the past few years. As a result of this increase in the number of patients seen, the associated time demands (preparation, report writing, etc.) have also increased. The demand to see an increased number of patients as part of a "desired" caseload has many significant drawbacks; the most important appears related to the speech-language pathologist's generalized inability to conduct long-term follow-up with patients. This limitation poses a real and significant threat to the successful long-term rehabilitation of the laryngectomized patient and members of the family.

The Continuing Need for Information

Although many patients are extremely resourceful, and in fact often devise methods to solve a specific problem or area of

Addressing the Void

The lack of proper follow-up with patients who have been treated for laryngeal cancer poses numerous problems. Rehabilitation of the patient who undergoes treatment for laryngeal cancer is a long-term phenomenon (Darvill, 1982; Salmon, 1986b). Thus, limiting the clinician's ability to formally or informally interact and work with the patient and members of the family or significant others in the period well after discharge appears contrary to the ultimate goals of the patient's rehabilitation. Formal follow-up services provided by the speech-language pathologist are just as important as the follow-up sessions necessary to monitor the patient's medical status. The patient's ultimate capacity for adjustment (physical and psychological) may hinge in part on such follow-up (Blood et al., 1992).

While it is not unreasonable to expect that regular follow-up on at least a monthly basis for the first few months following discharge from therapy can occur, the speech-language pathologist is frequently confronted with an inability to do so at regular intervals beyond the "initial" period following discharge from therapy. Regular contacts between the patient and the speech-language pathologist offer substantial advantages to both the patient and members of his or her family. The process of being diagnosed with laryngeal cancer, and consequently undergoing some method of medical management, certainly carries with it the potential for substantial changes over time. These changes cross physical, psychological, and social boundaries.

Individuals who are diagnosed early and receive appropriate conservative methods of treatment have an excellent prognosis not only in eliminating the cancer (Bailey, 1985a) but in their ability to return to a normal life. These individuals frequently undergo few changes in their lifestyle, whether it be vocational or avocational. However, individuals who undergo more aggressive methods of treatment, particularly those with extensive surgical resections, must adapt considerably (Gates, Ryan, & Lauder, 1982; Gunn, 1984). This requirement for adaptation comes on two fronts.

The first of these relates to the individual's ability to adjust to and accept dramatic anatomical and physiological limitations. Activities that were simple prior to surgery (e.g., showering) may now require substantial adaptation, motivation, and tolerance (Morozink, 1986). Even common household tasks may be problematic for some patients. Additional limitations related to surgery (e.g., neck dissection) may also present substantial physical disability and discomfort (Schutt, 1986). Issues related to care of the tracheostoma, covering it from the view of others (Kelly, 1986; Lauder, 1989), and other questions are of great importance to the patient. Particular problems may be encountered by the female patient (Gardner, 1966; Stack, 1986).

Second, the patient's awareness of many "other" consequences of medical treatment is often particularly evident in the first 6 months following therapy. This may coincide with the patient's attempts to return to work, resume "old" social activities, and so forth. (Darvill, 1983; Goldberg, 1975; Mellette, 1985; Sanchez-Salazar & Stark, 1972; Shanks, 1986). Although some of the problems encountered by patients may have their basis in anatomical and physiologic changes, the healing process, and compensation, many of these problems may center around the psychosocial impact of laryngectomy on the patient (Amster et al., 1972; Gilmore, 1974, 1986; Smith & Lesko, 1988). The acknowledgment of these problems and their effects on the patient's social, and hence psychological, well-being may be significant.

The patient's awareness of the full spectrum of changes may be equally as overwhelming as the initial diagnosis and anticipation prior to treatment. Some patients cope better than others with this type of continuing challenge (Lauder, 1989; Shanks, 1986b; Snidecor, 1978). Yet as the time posttreatment increases, the impact of postsurgical changes may also continue to be confronted in more natural contexts. That is, each patient will experience limitations particular to his or her given lifestyle, interests, and family, vocational, or avocational demands. Changes in family dynamics, particularly between the patient and his/her spouse or companion are frequently observed. Issues related to sexuality are often of concern to patients and their spouse or partner. Family roles may change dramatically following laryngectomy. Patients must have the opportunity to verbalize their concerns, express their thoughts, fears, and desires, and have the chance to work through difficulties they encounter. Adjustment to such significant changes in one's life cannot be a passive process.

The opportunity for the patient to address these problems with the speech-language pathologist may offer valuable insights that might facilitate either modifications or adaptations to eliminate or reduce the problem, or possibly offer strategies for coping with the acknowledged loss. Clearly, long-term counseling involves an individual-oriented approach in order to meet each patient's specific needs and inquiries. Addressing these problems, however, may be best provided via a support system comprised of individuals who are truly empathetic to the needs of the laryngectomized individual and members of the family. The "Laryngectomee Group" has the potential to meet this need.

The Laryngectomy Group

The "laryngectomy group" is best viewed as a support group for patients and members of their family. These support groups may manifest in varied forms dependent on the locale. In larger metropolitan areas laryngectomy groups may be conducted through local cancer agencies, rehabilitation centers, clinics, community colleges, or universities, whereas in smaller centers they may be offered directly through the speech clinic where therapeutic services were provided. The American Cancer Society and the Canadian Cancer Society, as well as the International Association of Laryngectomees (IAL) are the best known organization for broad-based networks of support.

Regardless of the organization involved or the setting, support groups have the potential to offer patients and members of their family excellent access to information. Information provided also has the value of being viewed through a "patient's eyes." As a result of this patient-oriented approach to information provision, participation may be easier for some patients. In regard to "Laryngectomee Clubs," Darvill (1982) has stated:

> The emotional and social readjustments necessary for a laryngectomee are made easier in the positive and encouraging atmosphere of a club which can act as a valuable bridge between therapy and the return to an active social life. Many helpful practical hints are handed on and firm friendships made. (p. 213)

The general goal of the laryngectomy groups is to provide a knowledgeable resource to the patient and family. This support network may also offer the patient a "sounding board" for a variety of concerns, worries, and complaints. It also serves a dual purpose in that the opportunity for socialization that may otherwise be avoided by the patient is facilitated. In some settings, continued voice and speech therapy may be provided by both professional and lay teachers of alaryngeal speech. Thus, both formal and informal methods of support and secondary education are usually offered via the laryngectomy group.

Community Resources

Those centers that perform a substantial number of laryngectomies each year should formally seek to establish a support group for patients. Ideally, the groups should be established in conjunction with community agencies that share a common interest. The local cancer society is likely to be supportive of endeavors of this nature and in some instances may be able to provide facilities for such meetings. They may also assist in identifying possible participants in the community.

Although it is extremely valuable to have active participation by both the community-based cancer agency and speech-language pathology community in these support groups, the group's mission should be devised and guided by those who are members of the group. Thus, the support group is encouraged to be self-sufficient in developing objectives, encouraging participation, and affiliating itself with hospitals and clinics. The success of these groups is generally judged to be fulfilling to most patients and appears to offer easy and regular access to information that may not be formally provided by the speech-language pathologist. It is essential to note, however, that the speech-language pathologist must be accessible to all laryngectomized patients should the patient require professional input.

Summary

Once patients are discharged from formal therapy, they will confront a variety of obstacles that impact on their full recovery and rehabilitation. Efforts to decrease limitations that are noted by patients is essential in this postdischarge period. Thus, some opportunity for long-term counseling efforts is extremely important. Although the speech-language pathologist and other professionals may serve as a valuable resource to the patient, support groups may be more appropriate avenues for problem solving by the laryngectomized patient and his or her family. The support group also offers the patient the opportunity for social reintegration that may assist adjustment and acceptance following laryngectomy.

Quality of Life and Laryngeal Cancer

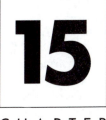

15

CHAPTER

Not every illness can be overcome. But, . . . there is always a margin within which life can be lived with meaning and even with a certain measure of joy, despite illness. (Cousins, 1979, p. 149)

The diagnosis and treatment of illness is often viewed in a rather myopic manner, wherein treatment itself is perceived as the "end result" in patient care. Contemporary viewpoints now place increased importance on what occurs in the postdiagnosis and treatment period. Medical treatment, therefore, is most appropriately viewed as the initial stage of the rehabilitation process, and it is the period *following treatment* that may comprise the essential elements that constitute the success or failure of treatment.

A patient's outcome following treatment for a specific illness can be defined along a number of dimensions. This is likely true for the majority of diseases and illnesses, although the dimensions which define a patient's posttreatment outcome may vary. For example, although the disease itself may be ameliorated via treatment, the diagnosis and/or treatment may result in significant changes that affect the patient's physical, psychological, social,

and psychosocial well-being. This is particularly evident when treatment entails recognizable physical disfigurement.

In this realm, questions concerning the patient's survival of serious illness or disease and the individual's desire to again enter his or her previous milieu are frequently raised. These questions specifically focus on the quality of one's life. The purpose of this chapter is to provide information on the potential effects of laryngeal cancer and its treatment on the quality of the patient's life. Issues addressed herein are not to be interpreted as all-inclusive but, rather, as an overview of the patient's physical, psychological, and psychosocial well-being.

Understanding the Problem

The term "quality of life" may in many respects be viewed as a solely subjective

253

construct. Quality of life may, however, also be delineated along several objective dimensions. Records, Tomblin, and Freese (1992) have defined quality of life using both subjective and objective indices. Specifically, Records et al. (1992) have stated that quality of life:

> Includes a person's objective status in various life domains (e.g., occupation, marital status), as well as the person's subjective perceptions of well-being. (p. 44)

According to Records et al.'s (1992) review of the literature on the construct of quality of life, measures of an individual's subjective well-being are influenced by dimensions of "positive affect" (i.e., happiness), "negative affect" (i.e., stress or worry), and "satisfaction" (i.e., expectations vs. reality) (Records et al., 1992). Thus, quality of life cannot be viewed as a unitary or unidimensional phenomenon. Using the definition provided by Records et al. (1992), one set of criteria that constitutes inherent features for quality of life cannot be generalized to all individuals. Quality of life is indeed best defined within the "eyes of the beholder," and it is consequently influenced by factors specific to a given individual. When these issues are considered within the context of health and illness, treatment success may be best determined via qualitative features.

A diagnosis of serious illness challenges even the strongest individual. This challenge may be found to exist across many dimensions dependent on the nature of the diagnosis. This is of particular importance in those who exhibit a chronic disease (Shook, 1983; Smith, 1981). In many instances, the diagnosis of serious illness is accompanied by emotional responses that are similar to those associated with the death of a loved one (i.e., denial, fear, anger, etc.) (Kubler-Ross, 1969, 1975; Square, 1986b). Thus, a grieving process is commonly observed in such situations. Leder (1990) has stated that:

> To fall ill is not simply to undergo a physiologic transformation, but a transformation of one's experiential world . . . the future grows uncertain, habitual roles are abandoned. (p. 2)

Thus, the acknowledgment of illness offers the individual a unique perspective into what qualitative dimensions define health.

Regardless of anatomical site, the individual's response to the diagnosis of cancer clearly conforms to a pattern of emotional upheaval and grieving observed with other chronic diseases (Smith, 1981). Yet serious illness challenges more than just one's physical health; perhaps more importantly, a patient's emotional and psychological well-being is contested and jeopardized. A patient's ability to cope with numerous changes following cancer treatment may at specific periods in the posttreatment process seem insurmountable. The patient must also confront the stigmata that commonly surround a diagnosis of malignant disease.

Stigmatization and Laryngeal Cancer

As with any type of treatment for laryngeal cancer, particularly treatments that require surgery, three basic elements are of extreme importance following partial or total laryngectomy: (1) control of the malignancy, (2) adaptation to anatomical and physiological alterations resulting from treatment, and (3) psychological and social adjustment. Although postoperative recovery and survival is generally high with laryngeal cancer (American Cancer Society, 1990; Bailey, 1985a; UICC, 1987), significant anatomic and physiologic changes are typically unavoidable. In patients with laryngeal cancer, however, these problems are often complicated by the loss of the patient's primary mechanism of verbal communication. Yet the patient's need to accept and adapt to these changes is not the only area that impacts on recovery and the quality of life in the postoperative period. The patient must also cope with the often subtle stigma that is frequently associated with cancer.

An additional factor that complicates the individual's resolution to laryngeal cancer, as well as his or her adaptation to physiological changes and the loss of oral communication, relates to the secondary consequences of resulting social isolation. Thus, the stigmatizing character of cancer as a disease class and laryngectomy as the method of treating the malignancy, as well as the patient's own disruption of self-concept and body-image have a profound impact on recovery and rehabilitation (Dropkin, 1989). This stigmatization may also cross multiple boundaries. For example, "aesthetic" concerns may emerge for both the patient's physical appearance and his or her communication.

The pervasive effects of laryngec-tomy on the patient, from both social and communicative perspectives, have been aptly characterized by Goffman (1963) in his book *Stigma: Notes on the Management of a Spoiled Identity*. Although Goffman addresses disorder, disability, and handicap in a global sense, the essence of his treatise is particularly applicable to those with laryngeal cancer. Goffman (1963) states that:

> Society established the means of categorizing persons and the compliment of attributes felt to be ordinary and natural for members of each of these categories. (p. 2)

Thus, it is society that establishes the criteria that underlie normality and abnormality. Further, Goffman (1963) suggests that from these preconceived standards which define "ordinary and natural," society is "transforming them into normative expectations, into righteously presented demands" (p. 2). Expectation, therefore, serves to provide a societal construct from which comparison and evaluation will evolve. Individuals "who *do not* depart negatively from the particular expectations at issue" (Goffman, 1963, p. 5) are considered to be "*normal.*" Those who do not conform to society's expectations possess attributes which ultimately serve to "discredit" one's social identity; the individual is ostensibly devalued as a person. Consequently, an individual's social identity is judged relative to the preconceived expectations of a society, what Goffman has termed "virtual social identity," and that which the individual truly possesses, one's "actual social identity" (Goffman, 1963, p. 2). Patients who undergo laryngectomy may then be seen to possess a variety of "attributes" which may then stigmatize them within a society. The notions underlying stigma culminate in whether the individual will be accepted by society in lieu of those "negative" attributes he or she possesses.

The stigmata associated with laryngectomy are minimally three-fold in our society. That is, three specific factors, each and of themselves highly stigmatizing, would appear to have the potential to affect the laryngectomized patient's postsurgical adjustment and, ultimately, the quality of life. First, the laryngectomized individual must deal with aesthetic and cosmetic expectations of society. That is, physical appearance is highly valued in most societies, particularly in Western cultures. Not only does the laryngectomized patient need to cope with social standards regarding physical appearance, but he or she must do so under many surgically imposed restrictions. Second, the loss of one's larynx results in rapid and profound communicative limitations. Third, cancer is frequently viewed negatively by others and, hence, has the potential to be in and of itself a highly stigmatizing disease. Although each of these three factors can be viewed as independent elements, they are indeed interdependent.

Physical Factors

Similar to other cancer patients, laryngectomized patients must cope with and adjust to significant physical changes. Although these changes require requisite physical adaptation, the associated cosmetic change may result in a need for social adaptation. In many instances, the physical consequences of laryngectomy and associated treatment are difficult to disguise in their entirety. The presence of the tracheostoma, changes in neck structure due to concomitant dissection, presence of scar tissue due to reconstruction, as well as a host of other physical features cannot always be hidden from others.

Coping with physical disfigurement which results from laryngectomy has not been addressed comprehensively in the literature. It does appear that disruption in one's self-concept in relation to body image is a direct outgrowth of such disfigurement (Dropkin, 1981). Observable defects in one's physical appearance draws attention to the patient. This reduces his or her ability to "blend in" in addition to providing a basis for stigmatization. Physical appearance, therefore, has a direct impact on one's ability to again be fully integrated into his or her respective social milieu.

For some, this disfigurement does not appreciably disrupt their ability to move through recovery, rehabilitation, and eventual social re-entry. For others, however, the degree of disfigurement provides a real and significant obstacle to recovery (Dropkin, 1991; Dropkin & Scott, 1983). Loss of normal verbal communication and discernable physical disfigurement demands that the even the most stoic patient garner all possible resources to attempt re-entry to society at large. Quality of life has a clear potential to be affected by both of these features following laryngectomy. Patients who are unable (or unwilling) to confront the most direct consequences of laryngectomy, or those who are unable to acknowledge their handicap (Blood & Blood, 1982), are at risk for exhibiting reclusive behavior and becoming isolated from others.

Communicative Factors

It is well documented that laryngectomy results in profound changes in the individual's communicative abilities. This includes changes in frequency, intensity, speech rate, prosody, and intelligibility. Therefore, an alaryngeal method which "normalizes" these features may in turn alter the communicators' *pragmatic* behaviors. Thus, social interactions may become enhanced not only due to the adequacy of verbal communication, but through the associated characteristics inherent to the alaryngeal speech signal. When considered with Goffman's (1963) concepts of "normal expectations," one can see the social importance of achieving acceptable behaviors, both communicatively and socially (Bennett & Weinberg, 1973; Prutting, 1982).

Even if laryngectomy existed without its physical deformities, removal of the larynx would not go unnoticed in our society due to the profound communication deficit which it epitomizes. Van Riper's (1978) classic definition of speech deviancy characterizes the loss of one's larynx quite aptly:

> Speech is abnormal when it deviates so far from the speech of other people that it calls attention to itself, interferes with communication, or causes the speaker or his listeners to be distressed. (p. 43)

Prutting (1982) has stated that it is communicative behavior which serves as a vehicle for initiating, maintaining, and terminating relations with other people. Specifically, Prutting (1982) suggested that, "It is one's social identity that is often affected by having a speech, language, and/or hearing disorder." In addition to the communicative limitations related to laryngectomy, social identity and competence may be destroyed as a result of objectional behaviors which accompany the production of alaryngeal speech. The concomitant behaviors found to be objectionable during the production of esophageal speech have been succinctly reported by Van Riper (1978):

> The gulping sound as air is injected into the esophagus, the weakness of the sound produced; the very low pitch, the hoarse quality; the contortions such as lip squeezing or extending the neck with the head thrown back; the whoosh of air through the opening in the neck that accompanies the speech attempt and causes the little gauze apron covering the hole to flap; the abdominal distention when the air is swallowed; and finally, the borborygmus that may occur. (pp. 343–344)

Despite the dramatic, even somewhat theatrical description by Van Riper (1978), the pervasive effect of verbal and nonverbal behaviors on communicative competence is not inaccurate. Thus, when such behaviors are considered, it is readily seen that all methods of alaryngeal speech production may be characterized by a number of these objectionable behaviors. It might then be inferred that when esophageal, TE, and artificial laryngeal speakers are compared, verbal and/or nonverbal characteristics associated with a particular alaryngeal method may more negatively affect any given communicative interaction.

Based on data offered by Blood et al. (1992), however, the type of alaryngeal speech used (esophageal, TE, or artificial laryngeal) does not appear "to interfere with overall adjustment, self-esteem, or general well-being" (p. 67). Thus, despite the limitations associated with all methods of alaryngeal communication, the mode of speech does not appear to have a significant impact on the patient's self-perception of important intrinsic features.Clearly, rehabilitative efforts that will allow "normal" speech production patterns to be more closely approximated, will also likely afford the laryngectomized patient a social advantage. Blood et al. (1992) have reported that a laryngectomized patient's ratings of self-esteem and general well-being are closely correlated with listener judgments of voice acceptability. This factor may, at least to some degree, outweigh the stigmata associated with physical deformity. However, structural and functional changes subsequent to laryngectomy are still likely to be stigmatizing to the patient.

Finally, the impact of losing a means of effective communication is of extreme importance from an emotional standpoint. As noted, many patients diagnosed with laryngeal cancer will undergo treatment procedures that either significantly disturb or eliminate normal verbal communication (Blood, 1993; Blood et al., 1994). Without a means of verbal communication, a reasonable communicative vehicle for addressing emotional stress is unavailable. This has the significant potential to disrupt communication among family members, hence, reducing the interactive component so common to effective support systems. Coping and psychological adjustment to cancer as an illness almost certainly finds its foundation in having the capacity to communicate one's fear, anxiety, and anticipation. When one undergoes laryngectomy, this capacity may be altered substantially.

Disease Factors

As a diagnostic entity, "cancer" is perhaps the most feared diagnosis of all. Yet many patients diagnosed with malignant disease may indeed "beat the odds" and survive at least 5 years postdiagnosis and treatment (UICC, 1987). Survival has traditionally been determined in relation to whether malignant disease has recurred subsequent to the initial, primary malignancy and the elapsed period of time until the patient succumbed to disease. These "survival" data segmented by site of cancer origin, age of onset, gender, race and/or ethnic origin, cancer subtype, and numerous other parameters are then used as global predictors of the prognosis for new patients. The statistical nature of these data is, unfortunately, sorely lacking in the capacity to "quantify" treatment effectiveness or success. That is, survival has traditionally been characterized as a durational phenomena.

The use of durational-based data as a prognostic indicator does indeed have value in the clinical domain. However, the temporal period which transpires post-diagnosis and treatment for cancer is not always the best metric of survival. Survival clearly encompasses more than "how long" one lives. For example, a patient who survives for 1 year following a diagnosis of cancer does not necessarily experience a less complete or fulfilling life than another patient who survives for 3 years postdiagnosis and treatment. It is what constitutes any given period of time that ultimately serves as a measure of treatment "success" and subsequent survival. Survival must, therefore, be assessed across a variety of dimensions.

When a malignancy is diagnosed, aggressive forms of treatment may not be uncommon. In individuals diagnosed with cancer of the larynx, the time elapsed from pathological confirmation to treatment is frequently quite brief. When a diagnosis of cancer occurs, treatment is seldom elective.[1] Due to this, the patient may still be attempting to cope with the shock of his or her diagnosis, while at the same time confronting changes resulting from treatment (e.g, altered physical function, loss of speech communication). A diagnosis of cancer demands prompt treatment, yet the patient is frequently unable to fully grasp what has and will occur over both the short- and long-term posttreatment period. Emotional responses to the disease are compounded by the necessity and sequelae of treatment.

The urgency of medical intervention with many cancers including those of the larynx is not the final step in the patient's journey through illness (i.e., diagnosis, treatment, recovery, rehabilitation). As with all forms of malignant disease, questions related to the best method of controlling the cancer and the likelihood of its recurrence are primary from the patient's perspective. However, both the patient and his or her loved ones and the physician who diagnoses the cancer know that only time will provide an answer to the second question. Outside of patients diagnosed with advanced metastatic cancer, the patient's ultimate period of survival is unknown. This places further stress on the patient and members of his or her family over the course of the posttreatment period (Reed, 1983a). The fear of recurrent disease is an inevitable burden that all patients diagnosed with cancer must confront. It is hoped that this fear is not so oppressive as to disable the patient from living normally in the presence of the diagnosis and treatment.

Survival and the Quality of One's Life

Welch-McCaffrey, Hoffman, Leigh et al. (1989) have identified a variety of psychological, physiological, and social responses of individuals to cancer diagnosis and treatment. Many of the responses identified have a direct relationship to the unknown question of what the future holds. That is, survival following a diagnosis of cancer is placed within the context of continuing uncertainty about one's health in relation to malignant disease (Mullan, 1984). Survival, therefore, cannot be evaluated in only a quantitative manner. It is not only the continuation of life and the patient's perseverance in the presence of illness that is at the center of one's survival,

---

[1]Patients do, however, have the ultimate right to determine the treatment they will receive and/or the right to refuse treatment. Discussion of these issues have been presented by Myers (1991b), Ward (1989), and others.

but the ability to experience a quality of life that is close to that which existed pre-treatment. The *quality of one's life* in the posttreatment period will best define the patient's survival in the broadest sense.

Questions related to quality of life in cancer patients is not a new area of inquiry or clinical concern. Despite the acknowl-edgment of the importance of quality of life and its suspected relationship to method of treatment, assessment of such qualitative aspects are limited (O'Young & McPeek, 1987). Until recently, there has been a considerable void of clinical data in the area of quality of life for those with laryngeal cancer (Blood et al., 1992; Myers & Baird, 1991). What constitutes a good or acceptable quality of life is a uniquely per-sonal perspective. Perhaps it is the defini-tional limitations of what constitutes quality of life that poses the major im-pediment to such inquiry. In regard to this definitional limitation Aaronson (1991) has stated:

> Just as cancer is a collective term for some 100 forms of disease, so is quality of life an omnibus term summarizing a range of related, interacting dimensions. In-deed, attempts at establishing boundaries around the quality of life construct have proven difficult. (p. 846)

Quality of life would, however, appear to be characterized by a sense that life is worth living and that living has meaning to both the patient and others. Communi-cation is the essence of a person's personal and social identity. As a result, rehabilita-tive efforts must also consider the social consequences of the disorder. As noted previously, the central feature of the stig-matized individual's situation in life re-volves around the question of one's "acceptance" by society. This acceptance, when combined with a communication deficit, weights heavily on the laryn-gectomized patient's social competence (Prutting, 1982).

As previously described, the stigma associated with laryngeal cancer is likely to be multifaceted. If some aspect of the patient's condition (e.g., the disease he or she suffers from, the physical changes subsequent to treatment, the loss of nor-mal verbal communication, etc.) is stigma-tizing, then the ability to live a "normal" life is restricted from a societal perspec-tive. Such restriction has substantial po-tential for creating added emotional dis-tress which further complicates rehabili-tation and social re-entry. If re-entry does not occur, quality of life will certainly be diminished.

Summary

This chapter has addressed issues related to the stigma associated with laryngeal cancer and quality of life following its treatment. Cancer of the larynx results in significant changes in one's physical and psychological well-being. These changes have the potential to substantially impact on the individual's psychosocial well-be-ing. Although traditional views of rehabili-tation have centered on the medical treatment and the concurrent durational aspects of survival, survival is character-ized by numerous qualitative dimensions. Several issues pertaining to the stigmatiz-ing effects of laryngeal cancer have placed survival within a different and uniquely human context. Specifically, laryngec-tomized patients must confront limitations due to cancer management, the percep-tion of cancer as a disease entity, and the communication deficits that occur follow-ing treatment. These limitations influence the patient's acceptance following treat-ment and ultimately their social identity. Clearly, qualitative features of the post-treatment period and the interaction of these features with societal expectations must be considered jointly with traditional therapeutic regimens. By doing so rehabili-tation will be improved considerably, and patients will be better prepared to re-en-ter society.

Final Comments: Can We Better Serve the Patient?

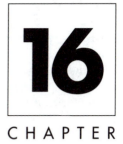

16

CHAPTER

> Illness is the night-side of life, a more onerous citizenship. Everyone who is born holds dual citizenship, in the kingdom of the well and in the kingdom of the sick. Although we all prefer to use only the good passport, sooner or later each of us is obliged, at least for a spell, to identify ourselves as citizens of that other place. (Sontag, 1978, p. 3)

This introductory passage from *Illness as Metaphor* (Sontag, 1978) so elegantly describes the unique character of life. Illness is a normal process that all individuals encounter at some point during their lives. When the illness is serious, however, the individual will always experience the added burden of coping with the concomitant emotional crisis related to the type of disease, its diagnosis, and prognosis (Lewis, Gottesman, & Gurstein, 1979), and its effects on loved ones. Although the response of the individual who is diagnosed with cancer may vary from person to person, all individuals fear the worst—loss of life.

For most individuals under these circumstances, the illness they suffer from and experience first-hand does not restrict their ability to verbally express their emotions to others. For individuals diagnosed with a laryngeal malignancy, treatment will frequently limit and potentially eliminate this communicative capacity. When the ability to communicate is lost, the pro-cess of recovery and rehabilitation may often be influenced appreciably.

Within previous chapters of this text information related to laryngeal cancer has been presented in substantial detail. Much of the information presented and discussed was done so in a rather technical and perhaps sterile manner. This format for presentation of information related to cancer as a disease process, its diagnosis, modalities of treatment (primary and secondary), and the consequences of treatment, as well as other areas provides a framework from which laryngeal cancer can be better understood by the speech-language pathologist. It is believed that much of the information outlined and discussed will serve to guide the clinician in the methods and techniques of voice and speech rehabilitation following either conservation or radical cancer surgery. Rehabilitation efforts that are grounded in a more global understanding of what changes have occurred as a result of treatment will permit development of clinical programs that are more individualized.

The importance of information concerning laryngeal cancer as a diagnostic entity does not, however, offer a comprehensive view of factors that will underlie the patient's "true" rehabilitation. Although the speech-language pathologist must exhibit an understanding of anatomic and physiologic sequelae of medical treatment, the clinician must also develop an awareness for other factors that ultimately influence the success of rehabilitative efforts.

For example, a diagnosis of "cancer" may distance some friends and family members from the patient, thereby reducing the patient's access to a support network. The loss of "normal" verbal communication may further isolate some patients from re-entering a variety of activities. If alaryngeal communication, regardless of mode, is not truly functional from an intelligibility perspective, the patient will be unable to successfully meet important communicative needs. The patient's inability to meet these communicative needs not only impacts on the patient directly, but on loved ones as well. Family relationships may be strained due to laryngeal cancer, its treatment, and consequences. The emergence of such difficulties in family dynamics has the potential to limit the patient's most significant source(s) of emotional support. Laryngectomy may result in job loss and subsequent economic difficulties; it may impact one's social well-being. The effects of laryngeal cancer on one's life are indeed far-reaching. Thus, the speech-language pathologist must view the patient's rehabilitation, and most specifically, the resultant communication deficit in an expanded and more human context.

Comprehensive rehabilitation of the patient with laryngeal cancer ideally requires consideration of numerous factors and input from a multidisciplinary team of professionals. The speech-language pathologist must play a key role in the patient's rehabilitation, but the speech-language pathologist cannot effectively function alone. At the minimum a comprehensive program of rehabilitation includes speech-language pathologists, physicians, nurses, physical therapists, occupational therapists, social workers, and access to psychological counseling services for both the patient and family members.

In many settings, a broad base of professional resources with specific expertise in the rehabilitation of those diagnosed with laryngeal cancer may be limited. Sources that are available must then cooperatively strive to provide the best and most comprehensive care possible to the patient and members of his or her family. However, the success of the rehabilitation program will most certainly hinge on the patient's ability to communicate. Thus, beyond the diagnosis of laryngeal cancer and its formal medical treatment, the speech-language pathologist will be in the position to significantly influence the patient's quality of life.

Rehabilitation following laryngectomy should be guided by one primary goal: to provide the patient with the greatest opportunity for returning to as normal a life as possible. This goal will always be at the core of successful rehabilitation. All patients will endure some level of change and/or restriction following treatment for laryngeal cancer. Yet in most cases, an awareness and understanding of the problem will culminate in active efforts to make necessary adjustments. This is equally true whether the underlying changes are of an anatomic, physiologic, psychologic, or social nature. With proper support and encouragement, most individuals have the ability to adapt in times of crisis and significant change (Mullan, 1984). As stated by Gunn (1983):

> Cancer, like any serious life problem, can develop qualities in people that they never knew they possessed. Maturing experiences are seldom pleasant, but the effects they have on character are very often positive . . . while it is difficult to portray a cancer diagnosis in a positive light, a patient's reaction or the reaction

of the family can be something of great value. (p. 3)

If the rehabilitation journey for those diagnosed with laryngeal cancer is viewed as a collaborative, dynamic process between the patient and the clinician, the capacity to meet the primary goal of rehabilitation will be strengthened and the patient's life will almost certainly be enhanced.

In closing, the patient as a person can never be forgotten. The speech-language pathologist has the opportunity to expand rehabilitation efforts so that the patient's life can be fulfilling, regardless of the amount of time that remains. There is no doubt that retaining one's social identity is critical to successful postlaryngectomy rehabilitation. Based on this need, social validation studies would appear to offer unique insights into the nature of laryngectomy as a social/communicative disorder. Such studies might include the assessment of laryngectomized patients' self-perceptions of their communicative competence, as well as perceptions by others. Additionally, interactional studies that would include analysis of nonverbal and paralinguistic behaviors such as body contact, posture, gaze, facial and gestural movements, and turn-taking would most definitely assist the comprehensive rehabilitation effort. Data from such investigations may then serve to elucidate the range of effects that result from laryngectomy and for particular alaryngeal speech methods. Finally, data from these types of studies would serve to enhance the success of postlaryngectomy speech rehabilitation; for without it, voice and speech rehabilitation is incomplete.

References

Aaronson, N.K. (1991). Methodologic issues in assessing the quality of life of cancer patients. *Cancer, 67,* 844–850.

Amatsu, M. (1978). A new one-stage surgical technique for post-laryngectomy speech. *Archives of Otorhinolaryngology, 220,* 149–152.

American Cancer Society. (1984). *Cancer facts and figures—1990.* Atlanta, GA: American Cancer Society.

American Cancer Society. (1990). *Cancer facts and figures—1990.* Atlanta, GA: American Cancer Society.

American Cancer Society. (1991). *Cancer facts and figures—1990.* Atlanta, GA: American Cancer Society.

American Cancer Society. (1993). *Cancer facts and figures—1993.* Atlanta, GA: American Cancer Society.

American Joint Committee for Cancer Staging and End Results Reporting: Clinical Staging System for Cancer of the Larynx. (1962). Chicago: American Joint Committee.

American Joint Committee for Cancer Staging and End Results Reporting: Clinical System for Staging Carcinoma of the Larynx (Revised). (1978). In O.H. Beahrs, D.T. Carr, & P. Rubin (Eds.), *Manual for staging of cancer 1978.* Chicago: Whiting Press.

American Joint Committee for Cancer Staging and End-Results Reporting. (1983). In O.H. Beahrs & M.H. Myers (Eds.), *Manual for staging cancer.* Philadelphia: J.B. Lippincott.

American Speech-Language-Hearing Association. (1989). AIDS/HIV: Implications for speech language pathologists and audiologists. *Asha, 31,* 46–48.

American Speech-Language-Hearing Association. (1990). Report updates. AIDS/HIV: implications for speech language pathologists and audiologists. *Asha, 32,* 46–48.

Amster, W.W. (1986). Advanced stage of teaching alaryngeal speech. In R.L. Keith & F.L. Darley (Eds.), *Laryngectomee rehabilitation* (pp. 177–192). San Diego: College-Hill Press.

Amster, W. W., Love, R. J., Menzel, O. J., Sandler, J., Sculthorpe, W. B., & Gross, F. M. (1972). Psychosocial factors and speech after laryngectomy. *Journal of Communication Disorders, 5*, 1–18.

Andrews, J.C., Mickel, M.D., Monahan, G.P., Hanson, D.G., & Ward, P.H. (1987). Major complications following tracheoesophageal puncture for voice rehabilitation. *Laryngoscope, 97*, 562–567.

Angermeier, C.B., & Weinberg, B. (1981). Some aspects of fundamental fequency control by esophageal speakers. *Journal of Speech and Hearing Research, 46*, 85–91.

Anthony, W.A. (1984). Societal rehabilitation: changing society's attitudes toward the physically and mentally disabled. In R. Marinell & A. Dell Orto (Eds.), *The psychological and social impact of physical disability* (2nd ed., pp. 194–205). New York: Springer-Verlag.

Aronson, A.E. (1980). *Clinical voice disorders*. New York: Thieme Stratton.

Aronson, A.E. (1985). *Clinical voice disorders* (2nd ed.). New York: Thieme Stratton.

Atkinson, M., Kramer, P., Wyman, S., & Ingelfinger, F.J. (1957). The dynamics of swallowing: I. Normal pharyngeal mechanisms. *Journal of Clinical Investigation, 36*, 518–558.

Auerbach, O., Hammond, E.C., & Garfinkel, L. (1970). Histologic changes in the larynx in relation to smoking habits. *Cancer, 25*, 92–104.

Bailey, B.J. (1985a). Glottic carcinoma. In B.J. Bailey & H.F. Biller (Eds.), *Surgery of the larynx* (pp. 257–278). Philadelphia: W.B. Saunders.

Bailey, B.J. (1985b). Management of carcinoma in situ and microinvasive carcinoma of the larynx. In B.J. Bailey & H.F. Biller (Eds.), *Surgery of the larynx* (pp. 229–241). Philadelphia: W.B. Saunders.

Bailey, B.J. (1985c). Glottic reconstruction. In B.J. Bailey & H.F. Biller (Eds.), *Surgery of the larynx* (pp. 279–292). Philadelphia: W.B. Saunders.

Baken, R.J. (1987). *Clinical measurement of speech and voice*. San Diego: College-Hill Press.

Baker, H.W. (1985). Staging: Introduction. In P.B. Chretien, M.E. Johns, D.P. Shedd, E.W. Strong, & P.H. Ward (Eds.), *Head and neck cancer: Volume 1* (pp. 87–89). Philadelphia: B.C. Decker.

Barney, H.L. (1958). A discussion of some technical aspects of speech aids for postlaryngectomized patients. *Annals of Otology, Rhinology, and Laryngology, 67*, 558–570.

Barney, H.L., Haworth, F., & Dunn, H. (1959). An experimental transistorized artificial larynx. *Bell System Technical Journal, 38*, 1337–1356.

Barton, R.T. (1965). Life after laryngectomy. *Laryngoscope, 75*, 1408–1415.

Batsakis, J.G. (1979). *Tumors of the head and neck: Clinical and pathological considerations* (2nd ed.). Baltimore: Williams & Wilkins.

Becker, G.D. (1989). Surgery for advanced primary or recurrent cancer of the head and neck. In A.R. Kagan & J. Miles (Eds.), *Head and neck oncology: Clinical management* (pp. 96–100). New York: Pergamon.

Beckett, R.L. (1969). Pitch perturbation as a function of subjective vocal constriction. *Folia Phoniatrica, 21*, 416–425.

Bennett, S., & Weinberg, B. (1973). Acceptability ratings of normal, esophageal, and artificial larynx speech. *Journal of Speech and Hearing Research, 16*, 608–615.

Berkowitz, J.F., & Lucente, F.E. (1985). Counseling before laryngectomy. *Laryngoscope, 95*, 1332–1336.

Berger, G., van Nostrand, A.W.P., Harwood, A.R., & Bryce, D.P. (1985). Failure analysis of T1 glottic carcinoma treated with radical radiotherapy for cure with surgery in reserve. In P.B. Chretien, M.E. Johns, D.P. Shedd, E.W. Strong, & P.H. Ward (Eds.) *Head and neck cancer: Volume 1* (pp. 195–199). Philadelphia: B.C. Decker.

Bergman, A.B., Neiman, H.L., & Warpeha, R.L. (1979). Computed tomography of the larynx. *Laryngoscope, 89*, 812–817.

Berke, G.S., Gerratt, B.R., & Hanson, D.G. (1983). An acoustic analysis of the effects of surgical therapy on voice quality. *Otolaryngology Head and Neck Surgery, 91*, 502–508.

Berlin, C.I. (1963). Clinical measurement of esophageal speech: I. Methodology and curves of skill acquisition. *Journal of Speech and Hearing Disorders, 28*, 42–51.

Berlin, C.I. (1964). Hearing loss, palatal function, and other factors in post-laryngectomy rehabilitation. *Journal of Chronic Diseases, 17*, 677–684.

Berlin, C.I. (1965). Clinical measurement of esophageal speech: III. Performance of non-biased groups. *Journal of Speech and Hearing Disorders, 30*, 174–183.

Berry, W.R. (1978a). Indications for the use of artificial larynx devices. In S.J. Salmon &

L.P. Goldstein (Eds.), *The artificial larynx handbook* (pp. 17–23). New York: Grune & Stratton.

Berry, W.R. (1978b). Attitudes of speech pathologists and otolaryngologists about artificial larynges. In S.J. Salmon & L.P. Goldstein (Eds.), *The artificial larynx handbook* (pp. 35–41). New York: Grune & Stratton.

Biller, H.F. (1985). Conservation surgery of the larynx. In P.B. Chretien, M.E. Johns, D.P. Shedd, E.W. Strong, & P.H. Ward (Eds.), *Head and neck cancer: Volume 1* (pp. 206–207). Philadelphia: B.C. Decker.

Biller, H.F. (1987). Conservation surgery past, present, and future. *Laryngoscope, 97,* 38–41.

Biller, H.F., Ogura, J.H., & Pratt, L.L. (1971). Hemilaryngectomy for T2 glottic cancers. *Archives of Otolaryngology, 93,* 238–243.

Biller, H.F., & Som, M.L. (1977). Vertical partial laryngectomy for glottic carcinoma with posterior subglottic extension. *Annals of Otology, Rhinology, and Laryngology, 86,* 715–718.

Billroth, T. (1873). Ulber die erste durch Theodor Billroth am menschen ausgefuhrte kehldopf-extirpation und die auswendig einges kunstlichen kehlkopfes. *Archives Klinical Cheiroskopy, 17,* 343–354.

Bisi, R.H., & Conley, J.J. (1965). Psychologic factors influencing vocal rehabilitation of the postlaryngectomy patient. *Annals of Otology, Rhinology, and Laryngology, 74,* 1073–1078.

Black, J.W. (1957). Multiple-choice intelligibility tests. *Journal of Speech and Hearing Disorders, 22,* 213–235.

Blanchard, S.L. (1982). Current practices in the counseling of the laryngectomy patient. *Journal of Communication Disorders, 15,* 233–241.

Blaugrund, S.M., Gould, W.J., Haji, T., Meltzer, J., Block, C., & Baer, T. (1984). Voice analysis of the partially ablated larynx: A preliminary report. *Annals of Otology, Rhinology, and Laryngology, 93,* 311–317.

Blom, E.D. (1978). The artificial larynx: Past and present. In S.J. Salmon & L.P. Goldstein (Eds.), *The artificial larynx handbook* (pp. 57–86). New York: Grune & Stratton.

Blom, E.D, & Singer, M.I. (1983). Prosthetic voice restoration following total laryngectomy. In W.H. Perkins (Ed.), *Voice disorders* (pp. 137–145). New York: Thieme-Stratton.

Blom, E.D., & Singer, M.I. (1986). Disinfection of silicone voice prostheses. *Archives of Otolaryngology Head and Neck Surgery, 112,* 1303.

Blom, E.D., Singer, M.I., & Hamaker, R.C. (1982). Tracheostoma valve for postlaryngectomy voice rehabilitation. *Annals of Otology, Rhinology, and Laryngology, 91,* 576–578.

Blom, E.D., Singer, M.I., & Hamaker, R.C. (1985). An improved esophageal insufflation test. *Archives of Otolaryngology Head and Neck Surgery, 111,* 211–211.

Blom, E.D., Singer, M.I., & Hamaker, R.C. (1986). A prospective study of tracheoesophageal speech. *Archives of Otolaryngology Head and Neck Surgery, 112,* 440–447.

Blood, G.W. (1981). The interaction of amplitude and phonetic quality in esophageal speech. *Journal of Speech and Hearing Reseach, 24,* 308–312.

Blood, G.W. (1993). Development and assessment of a scale addressing communication needs of patients with laryngectomies. *American Journal of Speech-Language Pathology, 2,* 82–90.

Blood, G.W., & Blood, I.M. (1982). A tactic for facilitating social interaction with laryngectomees. *Journal of Speech and Hearing Disorders, 47,* 416–419.

Blood, G.W., Luther, A.R., & Stemple, J.C. (1992). Coping and adjustment in alaryngeal speakers. *American Journal of Speech-Language Pathology, 1,* 63–69.

Blood, G.W., Simpson, K.C., Dineen, M., Kauffmann, S.M., & Raimondi, S.C. (1993). Spouses of individuals with laryngeal cancer: Caregiver strain and burden. *Journal of Communication Disorders, 27,* 1–17.

Blood, G.W., Simpson, K.C., Raimondi, S.C., Dineen, M., Kauffmann, S.M., & Staggard, K.A. (1994). Social support of laryngeal cancer survivors: Voice and adjustment issues. *American Journal of Speech-Language Pathology, 3,* 37–44.

Bone, R.C. (1989). Surgical management of cancer of the supraglottic larynx. In A.R. Kagan & J. Miles (Eds.) *Head and neck oncology: Clinical management* (pp. 101–104). New York: Pergamon.

Boone, D.R., & McFarlane, S.C. (1988). *The voice and voice disorders* (4th ed.). Englewood Cliffs, NJ: Prentice Hall.

Bosone, Z.T. (1986). Tracheoesophageal fistulization for voice restoration: presurgical considerations and trouble-shooting procedures. In R.L. Keith & F.L. Darley (Eds.), *Laryngectomee rehabilitation*, (pp. 193–209). San Diego: College-Hill Press.

Bozymski, E.M., & Pharr, S.Y. (1972). Esophageal manometry and speech proficiency in post-laryngectomy patients. *Gastroenterology, 62*, 726.

Brewer, D.W., Gould, L.V., & Casper, J. (1974). Fiber-optic study of the post-laryngectomized voice. *Laryngoscope, 84*, 666–670.

Broders, A.C. (1926). Carcinoma. Grading and practical application. *Archives of Pathology, 2*, 376–381.

Bryce, D.P. (1985). Cancer of the larynx: introduction. In P.B. Chretien, M.F. Johns, D.P. Shedd, E.W. Strong, & P.H. Ward (Eds.), *Head and neck cancer* (pp. 194–195). Philadelphia: B.C. Decker.

Burch, J.D., Howe, G.R., Miller, A.B., & Semenciu, R. (1981). Tobacco, alcohol, asbestos, and nickel in the etiology of cancer of the larynx: A case-control study. *Journal of the National Cancer Institutes, 67*, 1219–1224.

Burish, T.G., Meyerowitz, B.E., Carey, M.P., & Morrow, G.R. (1987). The stressful effects of cancer in adults. In A. Baum and J.E. Singer (Eds.), *Handbook of pyschology and health, Volume 5: Stress* (pp. 137–173). Hillsdale, NJ: Lawrence Erlbaum.

Byles, P.L., Forner, L.L., & Stemple, J.C. (1985). Communication apprehension in esophageal and tracheoesophageal speakers. *Journal of Speech and Hearing Disorders, 50*, 114–119.

Byrne, J., Kessler, L.G., & Devesa, S.S. (1992). The prevelence of cancer among adults in the United States: 1987. *Cancer, 69*, 2154–2159.

Callaway, E., Truelson, J.M., Wolf, G.T., Thomas-Kincaid, L., & Cannon, S. (1992). Predictive value of objective esophageal insufflation testing for acquisition of tracheoesophageal speech. *Laryngoscope, 102*, 704–708.

Campbell, B.H., & Goepfert, H. (1989). Partial laryngectomy as a salvage procedure for radiation failure. In A.R. Kagan & J. Miles (Eds.), *Head and neck oncology: Clinical management* (pp. 91–95). New York: Pergamon Press.

Cann, C.I., Fried, M.P., & Rothman, P.H. (1985). Epidemiology of squamous cell cancer of the head and neck. *Otolaryngology Clinics of North America, 18*, 367–388.

Cantu, E., Shagets, F.W., Fifer, R.C., Andres, C.J., & Newton, A.D. (1986). Customized valve housing. *Laryngoscope, 96*, 1159–1163.

Carniol, P.J., & Fried, M.P. (1982). Head and neck carcinoma in patients under 40 years of age. *Annals of Otology, Rhinology, and Laryngology, 91*, 152–155.

Caruso-Herman, D. (1989). Concerns for the dying patient and family. *Seminars in Oncology Nursing, 5*, 120–123.

Casiano, R.C., Cooper, J.D., Lundy, D.S., & Chandler, J.R. (1991). Laser cordectomy for T1 glottic carcinoma: A 10-year experience and videostroboscopic findings. *Otolaryngology—Head and Neck Surgery, 104*, 831–837.

Chodosh, P.L., Giancarlo, H.R., & Goldstein, J. (1984). Pharyngeal myotomy for vocal rehabilitation postlaryngectomy. *Laryngoscope, 94*, 52–57.

Christensen, J. (1970). Patterns and origin of some esophageal responses to stretch and electrical stimulation. *Gastroenterology, 59*, 909–916.

Christensen, J.M., Weinberg, B., & Alphonso, P.J. (1978). Productive voice onset time characteristics of esophageal speech. *Journal of Speech and Hearing Research, 21*, 56–62.

Chu, W., & Strawitz, J.G. (1978). Results in suprahyoid, modified radical, and standard radical neck dissections for metastatic squamous cell carcinoma: Recurrence and survival. *American Journal of Surgery, 136*, 512–515.

Chung, C-T., & Sagerman, R.H. (1989). Radiation and surgery for advanced cancer of the larynx and pyriform sinus. In A.R. Kagan, & J. Miles (Eds.), *Head and neck oncology: Clinical management* (pp. 3–11). New York: Pergamon Press.

Clark, J.G. (1985). Alaryngeal speech intelligibility and the older listener. *Journal of Speech and Hearing Disorders, 50*, 60–65.

Clark, J.G., & Stemple, J.C. (1982). Assessment of three modes of alaryngeal speech with a synthetic sentence identification (SSI) task in varying message-to- competition ratio. *Journal of Speech and Hearing Research, 25*, 333–338.

Code, C.F. (1981). Normal esophageal function. In S. Stipa, R.H.R. Belsey, & A. Moraldi,

Medical and surgical problems of the esophagus. New York: Academic Press.

Conley, J. (1959). Vocal rehabilitation by autogenous vein graft. *Annals of Otology, Rhinology, and Laryngology, 68,* 990–995.

Conley, J.J. (1964). Swallowing dysfunctions associated with radical surgery of the head and neck. *Archives of Surgery, 80,* 602–612.

Conley, J. (1984). Changes in otolaryngology—head and neck surgery. *Acta Otolaryngologica, 97,* 387–391.

Conley, J., DeAmesti, F., & Pierce, M. (1958). A new surgical technique for the vocal rehabilitation of the laryngectomized patient. *Annals of Otology, Rhinology, and Laryngology, 67,* 655–664.

Connor, N.P., Hamlet, S.L., & Joyce, J.C. (1985). Acoustic and physiologic correlates of the voicing distinction in esophageal speech. *Journal of Speech and Hearing Disorders, 50,* 378–384.

Cousins, N. (1979). *Anatomy of an illness as perceived by the patient*. New York: W.W. Norton.

Cousins, N. (1983). *The healing heart: Antidotes to panic and helplessness*. New York: W.W. Norton.

Creamer, B., & Schlagel, J. (1957). Motor responses of the esophagus to distention. *Journal of Applied Physiology, 10,* 498–504.

Creech, H.B. (1966). Evaluating esophageal speech. *Journal of the Speech and Hearing Association of Virginia, 7,* 13–19.

Crile, G. (1906). Excision of cancer of the head and neck: With special reference to the plan of dissection based on one hundred and thirty-two operations. *Journal of the American Medical Association, 47,* 1780–1793.

Cullen, J.W. (1989). Principles of cancer prevention: tobacco. In V.T. DeVita, S. Hellman, & S.A. Rosenberg (Eds.), *Cancer: Principles and practice of oncology* (pp. 181–195). Philadelphia: J.B. Lippincott.

Curry, E.T., & Snidecor, J.C. (1961). Physical measurement and pitch perception in esophageal speech. *Laryngoscope, 71,* 415–424.

Damste, P.H. (1958). *Oesophageal speech after laryngectomy*. Groningen, Netherlands: Boedrukkefif Voorheen Grbroeders Hoitsema.

Damste, P.H. (1979). Some obstacles in learning esophageal speech. In R.L. Keith &

F.L. Darley (Eds.), *Laryngectomee rehabilitation* (pp. 49–61). San Diego: College-Hill Press.

Damste, P.H. (1986). Some obstacles to learning esophageal speech. In R.L. Keith and F.L. Darley (Eds.), *Laryngectomee rehabilitation*, (2nd ed., pp. 85–92). San Diego: College-Hill Press.

Damste, P.H., & Lerman, J.W. (1969). Configuration of the neoglottis: An x-ray study. *Folia Phoniatrica, 21,* 347–358.

Daou, R.A., Shultz, J.R., Remy, H., Chan, N.T., & Attia, E.L. (1984). Laryngectomee study: Clinical and radiologic correlates of esophageal voice. *Otolaryngology—Head and Neck Surgery, 92,* 628–634.

Darley, F.L. (1978). The case history. In F.L. Darley & D.C. Spriestersbach (Eds.), *Diagnostic methods in speech pathology* (2nd ed., pp. 37–60). New York: Harper and Row.

Darley, F.L., Aronson, A.E., & Brown, J.E. (1975). *Motor speech disorders*. Philadelphia: W.B. Saunders.

Darvill, G. (1983). Rehabilitation—Not just voice. In Y. Edels (Ed.), *Laryngectomy: Diagnosis to rehabilitation* (pp. 192–217). Rockville, MD: Aspen.

Davis, R.M. (1987). Current trends in cigarette advertising and marketing. *New England Journal of Medicine, 316,* 725–732.

Davis, R., Vincent, M., Shapshay, S., & Strong, M. (1982). The anatomy and complication of "T" versus vertical closure of the hypopharynx after laryngectomy. *Laryngoscope, 92,* 16–22.

Department of Health and Human Services (1980). *The health consequences of smoking for women: A report of the surgeon general*. Rockville, MD: Office on Smoking and Health, U.S. Department of Health and Human Services.

DeRienzo, D.P., Greenberg, D., & Araire, A.E. (1991). Carcinoma of the larynx: Changing incidence in women. *Archives of Otolaryngology—Head and Neck Surgery, 117,* 681–685.

DeSanto, L.W. (1974). Selection of treatment for in situ and invasive carcinoma of the glottis. In P.W. Alberti & D.P. Bryce, (Eds.), *Centennial conference on laryngeal carcinoma* (pp. 146–150). New York: Appleton-Century-Crofts.

DeSanto, L.W. (1985). Treatment options in early cancers of the larynx. In P.B.

Chretien, M.F. Johns, D.P. Shedd, E.W. Strong, & P.H. Ward (Eds.), *Head and neck cancer* (pp. 202–206). Philadelphia: B.C. Decker.

DeSanto, L.W., Holt, J.J., Beahrs, O.H., & O'Fallon, W.M. (1982). Neck dissection: Is it worthwhile? *Laryngoscope, 92,* 502–509.

DeSanto, L.W., Pearson, B.W., & Olsen, K.D. (1989). Utility of near-total laryngectomy for supraglottic, pharyngeal, base-of-tongue, and other cancers. *Annals of Otology, Rhinology and Laryngology, 98,* 2–7.

DeWeese, D.D., & Saunders, W.H. (1977). *Textbook of Otolaryngology* (5th ed.). St. Louis: C.V. Mosby.

Dey, F.L., & Kirchner, J.A. (1961). The upper esophageal sphincter after laryngectomy. *Laryngoscope, 7,* 99–115.

DiCarlo, L.M., Amster, W., & Herer, G. (1955). *Speech after laryngectomy.* Syracuse, NY: Syracuse University Press.

Diedrich, W.M. (1968). The mechanism of esophageal speech. *Annals of the New York Academy of Sciences, 155,* 303–317.

Diedrich, W.M. & Youngstrom, K.A. (1966). *Alaryngeal speech.* Springfield, IL: Charles C. Thomas.

Donegan, J.O., Gluckman, J., & Singh, J. (1981). Limitations of the Blom-Singer technique for voice restoration. *Annals of Otology, Rhinology, and Laryngology, 90,* 495–497.

Dorland's Illustrated Medical Dictionary (25th ed.). (1974). Philadelphia: W.B. Saunders.

Doyle, P.C. (1985). Another perspective on esophageal insufflation testing. *Journal of Speech and Hearing Disorders, 50,* 408–409.

Doyle, P.C., & Danhauer, J.L. (1986). Consonant intelligibility of alaryngeal talkers: Pilot data. *Human Communication Canada, 10,* 21–28.

Doyle, P.C., Danhauer, J.L., & Lucks Mendel, L. (1990). A SINDSCAL analysis of perceptual features for consonants produced by esophageal and tracheoesophageal talkers. *Journal of Speech and Hearing Disorders, 55,* 756–760.

Doyle, P.C., Danhauer, J.L., & Reed, C.G. (1988). Listeners' perceptions of consonants produced by esophageal and tracheo-esophageal talkers. *Journal of Speech and Hearing Disorders, 53,* 400–407.

Doyle, P.C., Grantmyre, A., & Myers, C. (1989). Clinical modification of the tracheostoma breathing valve for voice restoration. *Journal of Speech and Hearing Disorders, 54,* 189–192.

Doyle, P.C., & Haaf, R.G. (1989). Perception of pre-vocalic and post-vocalic consonants produced by tracheoesophageal speakers. *Journal of Otolaryngology, 18,* 350–353.

Doyle, P.C., Leeper, H.A., Houghton, C., Heeneman, H., & Martin, G.F. (1992, November). *Perceptual characteristics of hemilaryngectomized and near-total laryngectomized male speakers.* Paper presented at the Annual Convention of the American Speech-Language-Hearing Association, San Antonio, TX.

Doyle, P.C., Swift, E.R., & Haaf, R.G. (1989). Effects of listener sophistication on judgments of tracheoesophageal talker intelligibility. *Journal of Communication Disorders, 22,* 105–113.

Doyle, P.J., & Flores, A.D. (1977). Treatment of carcinoma in situ of the larynx. *Journal of Otolaryngology, 6,* 363–368.

Doyle, P.J., Flores, A.D., & Douglas, G.S. (1977). Carcinoma in situ of the larynx. *Laryngoscope, 87,* 310–316

Dropkin, M.J. (1981). Changes in body image associated with head and neck cancer. In L.B. Marino (Ed.), *Cancer nursing* (pp. 560–581). St. Louis: Mosby.

Dropkin, M.J. (1989). Coping with disfigurement and dysfuction after head and neck surgery: a conceptual framework. *Seminars in Oncology Nursing, 5,* 213–219.

Dropkin, M.J., & Scott, D.W. (1983). Body image reintegration and coping effectiveness after head and neck surgery. *Society of Otorhinolaryngology Head and Neck Nursing Journal, 2,* 7–16.

Dudley, B.L., Robbins, J.A., Singer, M.I., Blom, E.D., & Fisher, H.B. (1981, November). *An intelligibility study of tracheoesophageal speech.* Paper presented at the Annual Convention of the American Speech-Language-Hearing Association, Los Angeles, CA.

Duguay, M.J. (1966). Preoperative ideas of speech after laryngectomy. *Archives of Otolaryngology, 83,* 237–240.

Duguay, M.J. (1977). Esophageal speech. In M. Cooper and M.H. Cooper (Eds.), *Approaches to vocal rehabilitation* (pp. 346–381). Springfield, IL: Charles C. Thomas.

Duguay, M.J. (1978). Why not both? In S.J. Salmon & L.P. Goldstein (Eds.), *The artificial larynx handbook* (pp. 3–10). New York: Grune & Stratton.

Duguay, M. (1979). Special problems of the alaryngeal speaker. In R.L. Keith & F.L. Darley (Eds.), *Laryngectomee rehabilitation* (pp. 423–444). San Diego: College-Hill Press.

Duguay, M.J. (1980). The speech-language pathologist and the laryngectomized lay teacher in alaryngeal speech rehabilitation. *Asha, 22,* 965–966.

Duguay, M. (1983). Teaching use of an artificial larynx. In W.H. Perkins (Ed.), *Voice disorders* (pp. 127–135). New York: Thieme-Stratton.

Duguay, M.J. (1991). Esophageal speech training: The initial phase. In S.J. Salmon & K.H. Mount (Eds.), *Alaryngeal speech rehabilitation* (pp. 47–78). Austin, TX: Pro-Ed.

Edelman, F. (1984). Attitudes and practices regarding speech aid use following laryngectomy. *Journal of Speech and Hearing Disorders, 49,* 220–223.

Edels, Y. (1983). Pseudo-voice: Its theory and practice. In Y. Edels (Ed.), *Laryngectomy: Diagnosis to rehabilitation* (pp. 107–141). Rockville, MD: Aspen.

Egan, J.P. (1948). Articulation testing methods. *Laryngoscope, 58,* 955–991.

Ellis Jr., R.H. (1971). Upper esophageal sphincter in health and disease. *Surgical Clinics of North America, 51,* 553–565.

Elner, A., & Fex, S. (1988). Carbon dioxide laser as a primary treatment of T1S and T1A tumours. *Acta Oto Laryngologica, 449* (Suppl.), 135–139.

Endicott, J.N., Cantrell, R.W., Kelly, J.H., Neel, H.B., Saskin, G.A., & Zajtchuk, J.T. (1989). Head and neck surgery and cancer in aging patients. *Otolaryngology—Head and Neck Surgery, 100,* 290–291.

Ernster, V.L. (1988). Trends in smoking, cancer risk, and cigarette promotion. *Cancer, 62,* 1702–1712.

Evans, E. (1990). *Working with laryngectomees.* Bicester, Oxon, Great Britain: Winslow Press.

Fairbanks, G. (1960). *Voice and articulation drillbook.* New York: Harper & Row.

Falk, R.I., Pickle, L.W., Brown, L.M., Mason, T.J., Buffler, P.A., & Fraumeni, J.F. (1989). Effects of smoking and alcohol consumption on laryngeal cancer risk in costal Texas. *Cancer Research, 49,* 4024–4029.

Fee, W.E., & Goffinett, D.R. (1985). Treatment of early lesions of the head and neck. In P.B. Chretien, M.E. Johns, D.P. Shedd, E.W. Strong, & P.H. Ward (Eds.). *Head and neck cancer: Volume 1,* (pp. 140–143). Philadelphia, PA: B.C. Decker.

Feinmesser, R., Freeman, J.L., Noyek, A.M., & Birt, D.B. (1987). Metastatic neck disease: a clinical/radiographic/pathologic correlative study. *Archives of Otolaryngology—Head and Neck Surgery, 113,* 1307–1310.

Feinmesser, R., Freeman, J.L., Noyek, A.M., Birt, D.B., Gullane, P.J., & Mullen, J.B. (1990). MRI and neck metastasis: A clinical, radilogical, pathological correlative study. *Journal of Otolaryngology, 91,* 136–140.

Felton, B.J., Revenson, T.A., & Hinrichsen, G.A. (1984). Stress and coping in the explanation of psychological adjustment among chronically ill adults. *Society and Science in Medicine, 13,* 889–898.

Finkbeiner, E.R. (1978). Surgery and speech, the pseudoglottis and respiration in total standard laryngectomee. In J.C. Snidecor (Ed.), *Speech rehabilitation of the laryngectomized* (pp. 58–85). Springfield, IL: Charles C. Thomas.

Friedman, W.H., Katsantonis, G.P., Siddoway, J.R., & Cooper, M.H. (1981). Contralateral laryngoplasty after supraglottic laryngectomy with vertical extension. *Archives of Otolaryngology, 107,* 742–745.

Fyke, F.E., & Code, C.F. (1955). Resting and deglutition pressures in the pharyngoesophageal region. *Gastroenterology, 29,* 24–34.

Gandour, J., & Weinberg, B. (1982). Perception of contrastive stress in alaryngeal speech. *Journal of Phonetics, 10,* 347–359.

Gandour, J., & Weinberg, B. (1983). Perception of intonational contrasts in alaryngeal speech. *Journal of Speech and Hearing Research, 26,* 142–148.

Gandour, J., & Weinberg, B. (1984). Production of intonation and contrastive stress in electrolaryngeal speech. *Journal of Speech and Hearing Research, 27,* 605–612.

Gandour, J., & Weinberg, B. (1985a). Production of intonation and contrastive stress in esophageal and tracheoesophageal speech. *Journal of Phonetics, 13,* 83–95,

Gandour, J., & Weinberg, B. (1985b). Production of syntactic stress in alaryngeal speech. *Language and Speech, 28,* 295–306.

Gandour, J., Weinberg, B. & Garzione, B. (1983). Perception of lexical stress in alaryngeal speech. *Journal of Speech and Hearing Research, 26,* 418–424.

Gandour, J., Weinberg, B., & Petty, S.H. (1985). Production of lexical stress in alaryngeal speech. *Folia Phoniatrica, 37,* 279–286.

Gandour, J. Weinberg, B. & Kosowsky, A. (1982). Perception of syntactic stress in alaryngeal speech. *Language and Speech, 25,* 299–304.

Gardner, W.H. (1961). Problems of laryngectomees. *Rehabilitation Record, 2,* 15–19.

Gardner, W. H. (1966). Adjustment problems of laryngectomized women. *Archives of Otolaryngology, 83,* 31–42.

Gardner, W.H. (1971). *Laryngectomee speech and rehabilitation.* Springfield, IL: Charles C. Thomas.

Gately, G. (1976). Another technique for teaching the laryngectomized person to inject air for the production of esophageal tone. *Journal of Speech and Hearing Disorders, 42,* 311.

Gates, G.A. (1980). Upper esophageal sphincter: Pre- and post-laryngectomy—a normative study. *Laryngoscope, 90,* 454–464.

Gates, G.A., & Hearne, E.M. (1982). Predicting esophageal speech. *Annals of Otology, Rhinology, and Laryngology,* 454–457.

Gates, G.A., Ryan, W., Cantu, E., & Hearne, E. (1982). Current status of laryngectomee rehabilitation: II. Causes of failure. *American Journal of Otolaryngology, 3,* 8–14.

Gates, G.A., Ryan, W., & Lauder, E. (1982). Current status of laryngectomee rehabilitation: IV. Attitudes about laryngectomee rehabilitation should change. *American Journal of Otolaryngology, 3,* 97–103.

Gates, G.A., Ryan, W., Cooper, J.C., Lawlis, G.F., Cantu, E., Hayashi, T., Lauder, E., Welch, R.W., & Hearne, E. (1982). Current status of laryngectomee rehabilitation: I. Results of therapy. *American Journal of Otolaryngology, 3,* 1–7.

Gerhardt, D.C., Shuck, T.J., Bordeaux, R.A., & Winship, D.H. (1978). Human upper esophageal sphincter: Response to volume, osmotic, and acid stimuli. *Gastroenterology, 75,* 268–274.

Gibbs, H.W., & Achterberg-Lawlis, J. (1979). The spouse as facilitator for esophageal speech: A research perspective. *Journal of Surgical Oncology, 11,* 89–94.

Gilmore, S. I. (1974). Social and vocational acceptability of esophageal speakers compared to normal speakers. *Journal of Speech and Hearing Research, 17,* 599–607.

Gilmore, S.I. (1986). The psychosocial concomitants of laryngectomy. In R.L. Keith & F.L. Darley (Eds.) *Laryngectomee rehabilitation* (pp. 425–495). San Diego: College-Hill Press.

Goepfert, H. (1984). Are we making any progress? *Archives of Otolaryngology, 110,* 562–563.

Goepfert, H., Lindberg, R.D., & Jesse, R.H. (1981). Combined laryngeal conservations surgery and irradiation: Can we expand indications for conservation therapy? *Otolaryngology Head and Neck Surgery, 89,* 974–978.

Goffinet, D.R., Fee, W.E., & Goode, R.L. (1984). Combined surgery and postoperative irradiation in the treatment of cervical lymph nodes. *Archives of Otolaryngology, 110,* 736–738.

Goffman, E. (1963). *Stigma: Notes on the management of spoiled identity.* Englewood Cliffs, NJ: Prentice Hall.

Goldberg, R.T. (1975). Vocation and social adjustment after laryngectomy. *Scandinavian Journal of Rehabilitative Medicine, 7,* 1–8.

Goldstein, L.P. (1978a). The artificial larynx: Pro and con. In S.J. Salmon & L.P. Goldstein (Eds.), *The artificial larynx handbook* (pp. 11–15). New York: Grune & Stratton.

Goldstein, L.P. (1978b). Listener judgments of artificial larynx speech. In S.J. Salmon & L.P. Goldstein (Eds.), *The artificial larynx handbook* (pp. 27–33). New York: Grune & Stratton.

Goldstein, J., & Price, J. (1987). Rehabilitation of patients with tumors of the larynx. In S. Hawley & W. Panje (Eds.), *Comprehensive management of head and neck tumors* (pp. 1014–1023). London: W.B. Saunders.

Gomyo, Y., & Doyle, P.C. (1989). Perception of stop consonants produced by esophageal and tracheoesophageal speakers. *Journal of Otolaryngology, 18,* 184–188.

Gonnella, C., Parker, C. Hollender, J., Lowell, G., Petterson, P., & Miller, S. (1978). *Normative criteria for cancer rehabilitation.* Rehabilitation Research Monograph Series 1. Atlanta: Emory University.

Goodman, M. (1989). Managing the side effects of chemotherapy. *Seminars in Oncology Nursing, 5,* 29–52.

Gorenflo, C.W., & Gorenflo, D.W. (1991). The effects of information and augmentative communication technique on attitudes toward nonspeaking individuals. *Journal of Speech and Hearing Research, 34,* 19–26.

Graham, J. (1983). The course of the patient from presentation to diagnosis. In Y. Edels (Ed.), *Laryngectomy: Diagnosis to rehabilitation* (pp. 1–17). London: Aspen.

Graham, S., Mettlin, C., Marshall, J., Priore, R. Rzepka, T., & Shedd, D. (1981). Dietary factors in the epidemiology of cancer of the larynx. *American Journal of Epidemiology, 113,* 675–680.

Gray, J.R., Coldman, A.J., & MacDonald, W.C. (1992). Cigarette and alcohol use in patients with adenocarcinoma of the gastric cardia or lower esophagus. *Cancer, 69,* 2227–2231.

Green, G., & Hults, M. (1982). Preferences for three types of alaryngeal speech. *Journal of Speech and Hearing Disorders, 47,* 141–145.

Greene, J.S. (1947). Laryngectomy and its psychologic implications. *New York State Journal of Medicine, 47,* 53–56.

Greene, M.L.C. & Mathieson, L. (1989). *The Voice and its disorders* (5th ed.). Newark, NJ: Whurr Publishers Limited.

Griffith, J., & Miner, L.E. (1979). *Phonetic context drillbook.* Englewood Cliffs, NJ: Prentice-Hall.

Griffiths, C., & Love, J. (1978). Neoglottic reconstruction after total laryngectomy: A preliminary report. *Annals of Otology, Rhinology, and Laryngology, 87,* 180–184.

Guenel, P., Chastang, J.F., Luce, D., Leclerc, P., & Brugere, J. (1988). A study of the interaction of alcohol drinking and tobacco smoking among French cases of laryngeal cancer. *Journal of Epidemiology anc Community Health, 42,* 350–354.

Gunn, A.E. (1984). Cancer rehabilitation: An overview. In A.E. Gunn (Ed.), *Cancer rehabilitation* (pp. 1–22). New York: Raven.

Gussack, G.S., & Hudgins, P.A. (1991). Imaging modalities in recurrent head and neck tumors. *Laryngoscope, 101,* 119–124.

Guyatt, G.H., & Newhouse, M.T. (1985). Are active and passive smoking harmful? *Chest, 88,* 445–451.

Haaf, R.G., & Doyle, P.C. (1986, December). *Perceptual confusions in the speech of tracheoesophageal talkers.* Paper presented at the Fall Meeting of the Acoustical Society of America, Anaheim, CA.

Hamaker, R.C., Singer, M.I., Blom, E.D., & Daniels, H.A. (1985). Primary voice restoration at laryngectomy. *Archives of Otolaryngology, 111,* 182–186.

Hanks, J.B., Fisher, S.R., Meyers, W.C., Christian, K.C., Postlethwait, R.W., & Jones, R.S. (1981). Effect of total laryngectomy on esophagaeal motility. *Annals of Otology, Rhinology and Laryngology, 90,* 331–334.

Harris, L.L., & Smith, S. (1989). Chemotherapy in head and neck cancer. *Seminars in Oncology Nursing, 5,* 174–181.

Harrison, D. (1990). Moral dilemmas in head and neck cancer. *Laryngoscope, 100,* 1191–1193.

Harwood, A.R., Hawkins, N.V., Keane, T., Cummings, B. Beale, F.A., Rider, W.D., & Bryce, D.P. (1980). Radiotherapy of early glottic cancer. *Laryngoscope, 90,* 465–470.

Heatley, D.G., & Anderson, A.G. (1992). Tracheoesophageal puncture for speech rehabilitation after laryngectomy. *Laryngoscope, 102,* 581–582.

Henderson, R.D. (1983). *Esophageal manometry in clinical investigation.* New York: Praeger.

Henderson, R.D., Boszko, A., & van Nostrand, A.W.P. (1974). Pharyngoesophageal dysphagia and recurrent laryngeal nerve palsy. *Journal of Thoracic and Cardiovascular Surgery, 68,* 507–511.

Hendrickson, F.R. (1985). Radiation therapy treatment of larynx cancers. *Cancer, 55,* 2058–2061.

Henley, J., & Souliere Jr., C. (1986). Tracheoesophageal speech failure in the laryngectomee: The role of constrictor myotomy. *Laryngoscope, 96,* 1016–1020.

Hinds, M.W., Thomas, D.B., & O'Reilly, H.P. (1979). Asbestos, dental x-rays, tobacco, and alcohol in the epidemiology of laryngeal cancer. *Cancer, 44,* 1114–1120.

Hinton, C.D., & Myers, E.M. (1991). Larynx. In E.M. Myers (Ed.), *Head and neck oncology: Diagnosis, treatment, and rehabilitation* (pp. 281–298). Boston: Little, Brown and Company.

Hintz, B.L., Kagan, A.R., Nussbaum, H., Rao, A.R., Chan, P.Y.M., & Miles, J. (1981). A 'watchful waiting' policy for in situ carcinoma of the vocal cords. *Archives of Otolaryngology, 107,* 746–751.

Hirano, M. (1976). Technique for glottic reconstruction following vertical partial laryngectomy: A preliminary report. *Annals of Otology, Rhinology, and Laryngology, 85,* 25–31.

Hirano, M. (1981). *Clinical examination of voice.* New York: Springer-Verlag.

Hirano, M., & Bless, D.M. (1993). *Videostroboscopic examination of the larynx.* San Diego: Singular.

Hirano, M., Kurita, S., & Matsuoka, H. (1987). Vocal function following hemilaryngectomy. *Annals of Otology, Rhinology, and Laryngology, 96,* 586–589.

Ho, C.M., Wei, W.I., Lau, W.F., & Lam, K.H. (1991). Tracheoesophageal stenosis after immediate tracheoesophageal puncture. *Archives of Otolaryngology—Head and Neck Surgery, 117,* 662–664.

Hoasjoe, D.K., Martin, G.F., Doyle, P.C., & Wong, F.S. (1992). A comparative acoustic analysis of voice production by near-total laryngectomy and normal laryngeal speakers. *Journal of Otolaryngology, 21,* 39–43.

Hoops, H.R., Clark, W.M., & Martin, D.E. (1975). Description of a team approach to the rehabilitation of the laryngectomized speaker. *Laryngoscope, 85,* 559–564.

Hoops, H.R., & Curtis, J.F. (1971). Intelligibility of the esophageal speaker. *Archives of Otolaryngology, 93,* 300–303.

Hoops, H.R., & Noll, J.D. (1969). Relationship of selected acoustic variables to judgments of esophageal speech. *Journal of Communication Disorders, 2,* 1–13.

Hoover, L.A., Calcaterra, T.C., Walter, G.A., & Larrson, S.G. (1984). Preoperative CT scan evaluation for laryngeal carcinoma: correlation with pathological findings. *Laryngoscope, 94,* 310–315.

Horii, Y. (1969). *Specifying the speech-to-noise ratio: Development and evaluation of a noise with speech-envelope characteristics.* Unpublished doctoral dissertation: Purdue University.

Horii, Y., House, A.S., & Hughes, G.W. (1971). A masking noise with speech envelope characteristics for studying intelligibility. *Journal of the Acoustical Society of America, 49,* 1849–1856.

Horii, Y., & Weinberg, B. (1975). Intelligibility characteristics of superior esophageal speech presented under various levels of masking noise. *Journal of Speech and Hearing Research, 18,* 413–419.

Horn, D. (1962). Laryngectomee survey report. New York: *International Association of Laryngectomees.*

House, A.S., Williams, C.E., Hecker, M.H.L., & Kryter, K. (1965). Articulation testing methods: consonantal differention with closed-response set. *Journal of the Acoustical Society of America, 37,* 158–166.

Hunt, R.B. (1964). Rehabilitation of the laryngetomee. *Laryngoscope, 74,* 382–395.

Hurbis, C.G., Tiesenga, J.E., Goodman, D.A., & Wenig, B.L. (1991). A new instrument for the simplification of tracheoesophageal puncture. *Laryngoscope, 104,* 410–416.

Hyman, M. (1955). An experimental study of artificial larynx and esophageal speech. *Journal of Speech and Hearing Disorders, 20,* 291–299.

Isshiki, N. (1964). Regulatory mechanism of voice intensity variation. *Journal of Speech and Hearing Research, 7,* 17–29.

Isshiki, N. (1978). Air flow in esophageal speech. In J.C. Snidecor (Ed.), *Rehabilitation of the laryngectomized* (2nd). Springfield, IL: Charles C. Thomas.

Isshiki, N., & Ringel, R. (1964). Air flow during the production of selected consonants. *Journal of Speech and Hearing Research, 7,* 233–244.

Isshiki, N., & Snidecor, J.C. (1965). Air intake and usage in esophageal speech. *Acta Otolaryngologica, 59,* 559–574.

Izdebski, K., Ross, J.C., & Lee, S. (1987). Fungal colonization of tracheoesophgeal voice prosthesis. *Laryngoscope, 97,* 594–597.

Jackson, C., & Jackson, C.L. (1939). *Cancer of the larynx.* Phildelphia: W.B. Saunders.

Jerger, J., Speaks, C., & Trammell, J.A. (1968). A new approach to speech audiometry. *Journal of Speech and Hearing Disorders, 33,* 318–328.

Johns, M.E., & Cantrell, R.W. (1981). Voice restoration of the total laryngectomy patient: The Singer-Blom technique. *Otolaryngology—Head and Neck Surgery, 89,* 82–86.

Johnson, J.T., Barnes, E.L., Myers, E.N., Schramm, V.L., Borochovitz, D., & Sigler, B.A. (1981). The extracapsular spread of tumors in cervical node metastasis. *Archives of Otolaryngology, 107,* 725–729.

Johnson, J.T., Casper, J., & Lesswing, N.J. (1979). Toward the total rehabilitation of the alaryngeal patient. *Laryngoscope, 89,* 1813–1819.

Jung, T.T.K., & Adams, G.L. (1980). Dysphagia in laryngectomized patients. *Otolaryngology Head Neck Surgery, 88,* 25–33.

Kalb, M.B., & Carpenter, M.A. (1981). Individual speaker influence on relative intelligibility of esophageal speech and artificial larynx speech. *Journal of Speech and Hearing Disorders, 46,* 77–80.

Kallen, L.A. (1934). Vicarious vocal mechanisms. *Archives of Otolaryngology, 20,* 460–503.

Karim, A.B.M.F., Snow, G.F., Siek, H.T.H., & Njo, K.H. (1983). Quality of voice in patients irradiated for laryngeal carcinoma. *Cancer, 51,* 47–49.

Keane, T.J. (1985). Clinical staging of head and neck cancer. In P.B. Chretien, M.E. Johns, D.P. Shedd, E.W. Strong, & P.H. Ward (Eds.). *Head and neck cancer: Volume 1* (pp. 140–143). Philadelphia, PA: B.C. Decker.

Keane, T.J., & Cummings, B.J. (1986). Radiotherapy of head and neck cancers. *Clinics in Oncology, 5,* 557–573.

Keith, R.L. (1977). Teaching of esophageal speech. *Journal of the National Student Speech and Hearing Association, 7,* 8–12.

Keith, R.L., Leeper, H.A., & Doyle, P.C. (1993, November). *Long- and short-term voice characteristics of near-total laryngectomy.* Paper presented at the Annual Convention of the American Speech-Language-Hearing Association, Anaheim, CA.

Keith, R.L, & Pearson, B.R. (1987, November). *Speech rehabilitation after near total laryngectomy.* Paper presented at the Annual Convention of the American Speech-Language-Hearing Association, New Orleans, LA.

Keith, R.L., Pearson, B., Thomas, J.E., & Lipton, R.J. (1988, November). *Speech rehabilitation after near-total laryngectomy.* Paper presented at the Annual Convention of the American Speech-Language-Hearing Association, Boston, MA.

Keith, R.L., Thomas, J.E., & Pearson, B. (1987, November). *Speech rehabilitation after near total laryngectomy with reconstructed speech shunt.* Paper presented at the Annual Convention of the American Speech-Language-Hearing Association, New Orleans, LA.

Keith, R.L., Shane, H.C., Coates, H.L., & Devine, K.D. (1984). *Looking forward . . . A guidebook for the laryngectomee.* NY: Thieme-Stratton Inc.

Keith, R.L., & Shanks, J.C. (1983). Laryngectomee rehabilitation: Past and present. In N.J. Lass (Eds.), *Speech and language: Advances in basic research and practice,* Vol. 9 (pp. 103–152). New York: Academic Press.

Keith, R.L., & Shanks, J.C. (1986). Historical highlights: Laryngectomee rehabilitation. In R.L Keith & F.L. Darley (Eds.), *Laryngectomee rehabilitation* (pp. 3–53). San Diego, CA: College-Hill Press.

Keith, R.L., & Thomas, J.E. (1989). *Speech practice manual for dysarthria, apraxia, and other disorders of articulation.* Toronto: B.C. Decker.

Kelly, D. (1986). Appropriate covering for the tracheal stoma area. In R.L Keith & F.L. Darley (Ed.), *Laryngectomee rehabilitation,* (237–246). San Diego: College-Hill Press.

Kirchner, J.A. (1958). The motor activity of the cricopharyngeus muscle. *Laryngoscope, 68,* 1119–1151.

Kirchner, J.A. (1969). One hundred laryngeal cancers studied by serial section. *Annals of Otology, Rhinology, and Laryngology, 78,* 689–709.

Kirchner, J.A. (1970). Cancer at the anterior commissure of the larynx. *Archives of Otolaryngology, 91,* 524–525.

Kirchner, J.A. (1975). Growth and spread of laryngeal cancer as related to partial laryngectomy. *Laryngoscope, 85,* 1516–1521.

Kirchner, J.A. (1984). Invasion of the framework by laryngeal cancer. *Acta Otolaryngologica, 97,* 392–397.

Kirchner, J.A. (1985). Treatment of laryngeal cancer. In P.B. Chretien, M.E. Johns, D.P. Shedd, E.W. Strong, & P.H. Ward (Eds.). *Head and neck cancer: Volume 1* (pp. 199–210). Philadelphia: B.C. Decker.

Kirchner, J.A. (1989). What have whole organ sections contributed to the treatment of laryngeal cancer? *Annals of Otology, Rhinology and Laryngology, 98,* 661–667.

Kirchner, J.A., & Carter, D. (1987). Intralaryngeal barriers to the spread of cancer. *Acta Otolaryngologica, 103,* 503–513.

Kirchner, J.A., Cornog, J.L., & Holmes, R.E. (1974). Transglottic cancer. *Archives of Otolaryngology, 99,* 247–253.

Kirchner, J.C., Kirchner, J.A., & Sasaki, C.T. (1989). Anatomical foramina in the thyroid cartilage: Incidence and implications for the spread of laryngeal cancer. *Annals of Otology, Rhinology, and Laryngology, 98,* 421–425.

Kirchner, J.A., & Owen, J.R. (1977). Five hundred cancers of the larynx and pyriform sinus. *Laryngoscope, 87,* 1288–1303.

Kirchner, J.A., Scatliff, J., Dey, F.L., & Shedd, D.P. (1963). The pharynx after laryngectomy. *Laryngoscope, 73*, 18–33.

Kirchner, J.A., & Som, M.L. (1971a). Clinical significance of the fixed vocal cord. *Laryngoscope, 81*, 1029–1044.

Kirchner, J.A., & Som, M.L. (1971b). Clinical and histological observations on supraglottic cancer. *Laryngoscope, 81*, 638–645.

Kirchner, J.A., & Som, M.L. (1975). The anterior commissure technique of partial laryngectomy: Clinical and laboratory observations. *Laryngoscope, 85*, 1308–1317.

Kitzing, P., & Toremalm, N.G. (1970). The situation of the laryngectomized patient. *Acta Otolaryngologica, 263*, 119–123.

Kommers, M.S., & Sullivan, M.D. (1979). Wives' evaluation of problems related to laryngectomy. *Journal of Communication Disorders, 12*, 411–430.

Kommers, M.S., Sullivan, M.D., & Yonkers, A.J. (1977). Counseling the laryngectomized patient. *Laryngoscope, 87*, 1961–1965.

Koop, C.E. (1985). Is a smokeless society by 2000 attainable? *Archives of Internal Medicine, 145*, 1581.

Komorn, R. (1974). Vocal rehabilitation in the laryngectomized patient with a tracheoesophageal shunt. *Annals of Otology, Rhinology, and Laryngology, 83*, 445–451.

Koufman, J.A. (1986). The endoscopic management of early squamous carcinoma of the vocal cord with the carbon dioxide surgical laser: clinical experience and a proposed sub classification. *Otolaryngology Head and Neck Surgery, 95*, 531–537.

Kubler-Ross, E. (1969). *On death and dying*. New York: Macmillan.

Kubler-Ross, E. (1975). *Death, the final stage of growth*. Englewood Cliffs, NJ: Prentice Hall.

Lauder, E. (1968). The laryngectomee and the artificial larynx. *Journal of Speech and Hearing Disorders, 33*, 147–157.

Lauder, E. (1970). The laryngectomee and the artificial larynx—a second look. *Journal of Speech and Hearing Disorders, 35*, 62–65.

Lauder, E. (1989). *Self-help for the laryngectomee*. San Antonio, TX: Lauder Publishing.

Lawson, W., & Biller, H.F. (1985). Supraglottic cancer. In B.J. Bailey & H.F. Biller, *Surgery of the larynx* (pp. 243–255). Philadelphia: W.B. Saunders.

Lebrun, Y. (1973). *The artificial larynx*. Amsterdam: Swets & Zeitlinger.

Leder, D. (1990). Illness and exile: Sophocles' philoctetes. In P.W. Graham & E. Sewell (Eds.), *Literature and medicine* (pp. 1–11). Baltimore: Johns Hopkins University Press.

Lehiste, I., & Peterson, G.E. (1959). Linguistic considerations in the study of speech intelligibility. *Journal of the Acoustical Society of America, 131*, 250–286.

Leeper, H.A., Doyle, P.C., Heeneman, H., Martin, G.F., Hoasjoe, D.K., & Wong, F.S. (1993). Acoustic characteristics of voice following hemilaryngectomy and near-total laryngectomy. *Journal of Medical Speech-Language Pathology, 1*, 89–94.

Leeper, H.A., Heeneman, H., & Reynolds, C. (1990). Vocal function following vertical hemilaryngectomy: A preliminary investigation. *Journal of Otolaryngology, 19*, 62–67.

Levin, N.M. (1962). *Voice and speech disorders: medical aspects*. Springfield, IL: Charles C. Thomas.

Lewin, J.S., Baugh, R.F., & Baker, S.F. (1987). An objective method for prediction of tracheoesophageal speech production. *Journal of Speech and Hearing Disorders, 52*, 212–217.

Lewis, M.S., Gottesman, D., & Gutstein, S. (1979). The course and duration of crises. *Journal of Consultation in Clinical Psychology, 47*, 128–134.

Lindsay, J.R., Morgan, R.H., & Wepman, J.M. (1944). The cricopharyngeus muscle in esophageal speech. *Laryngoscope, 54*, 55–61.

Logemann, J. (1983a). *Evaluation and treatment of swallowing disorders*. San Diego: College-Hill Press Inc.

Logemann, J.A. (1983b). Vocal rehabilitation after extensive surgery for post-cricoid carcinoma. In Y. Edels (Ed.), *Laryngectomy: Diagnosis to rehabilitation* (pp. 233–248). Rockville, MD: Aspen.

Lopez, M.J., Kraybill, W., McElroy, T.H., & Guerra, O. (1987). Voice rehabiltation practices among head and neck surgeons. *Annals of Otology, Rhinology, and Laryngology, 96*, 261–63.

Lowry, L.D. (1981). Artificial larynges: A review and development of a prototype self-contained intraoral artificial larynx. *Laryngoscope, 91*, 1332–1355.

Lowry, L.D., Marks, J.E., & Powell, W.J. (1973). 260 laryngeal carcinomas. *Archives of Otolaryngology, 98*, 147–151.

Luboinski, B., Eschwege, F., & Stafford, N. (1989). Voice rehabilitation after laryngectomy: controversies. In A.R. Kagan & J. Miles (Eds.), *Head and neck oncology: Clinical management* (pp. 162–164). New York: Pergamon Press.

Lund, W.S., & Ardran, G.M. (1964). The motor nerve supply of the cricopharyngeal sphincter. *Annals of Otology, Rhinology, and Laryngology, 73*, 599–617.

Mafee, M.F., Schild, J.A., Valvassori, G.E., & Capek, V. (1983). Computer tomography of the larynx: correlation with anatomic and pathologic studies in cases of laryngeal carcinoma. *Radiology, 147*, 123–128.

Mahadevan, V., & Hart, I.R. (1990). Metastasis and angiogenesis. *Reviews in Oncology, 3*, 97–103.

Mahieu, H.F., van Saene, H.K.J., Rosingh, H.J., & Schutte, H.K. (1986). Candida vegetations on silicone voice prostheses. *Archives of Otolaryngology—Head and Neck Surgery, 112*, 321–325.

Mahieu, H.F., Annyas, A.A., Schutte, H.K., & van der Jagt, E.J. (1987). Pharyngoesophageal myotomy for vocal rehabilitation of laryngectomees. *Laryngoscope, 97*, 451–457.

Mancuso, A.A., Calcaterra, T.C., & Hanafee, W.N. (1978). Computed tomography of the larynx. *Radiology Clinics of North America, 16*, 195–208.

Mancuso, A.A., Hanafee, W.N., Juillard, G.J., Winter, J., & Calcaterra, T.C. (1977). The role of computed tomography in the management of cancer of the larynx. *Radiology, 124*, 243–244.

Mancuso, A.A., Maceri, D., Rice, D., & Hanafee, W.H. (1981). CT of cervical lymph node cancer. *American Journal of Radiology, 136*, 381–385.

Maniglia, A.J. (1982). Vocal rehabilitation after total laryngectomy: A flexible fiberoptic endoscopic technique for tracheoesophageal fistula. *Laryngoscope, 92*, 1437–1439.

Maniglia, A.J., Lundy, D.S., Casiano, R.C., & Swim, S.C. (1989). Speech restoration and complications of primary versus secondary tracheoesophageal puncture following laryngectomy. *Laryngoscope, 99*, 489–491.

Martin, D.E. (1986). Pre- and post-op anatomical and physiological observations in laryngectomy. In R.L. Keith & F.L. Darley (Eds.), *Laryngectomy rehabilitation* (pp. 221–225). San Diego: College-Hill Press.

Martin, H. (1963). Rehabilitation of the laryngectomy. *Cancer, 16*, 823–841.

Mathieson, C.M., Stam, H.J., & Scott, J.P. (1990). Psychosocial adjustment after laryngectomy: A review of the literature. *Journal of Otolaryngology, 19*, 331–336.

Maves, M.D., & Lingeman, R. (1982). Primary vocal rehabilitation using the Blom-Singer and Panje voice prosthesis. *Annals of Otology, Rhinology and Laryngology, 91*, 458–460.

McConnel, F.M.S., & Duck, S.W. (1986). Indications for tracheoesophageal puncture speech rehabilitation. *Laryngoscope, 96*, 1065–1068.

McCroskey, R.L., & Mulligan, M. (1963). The relative intelligibility of esophageal speech and artificial-larynx speech. *Journal of Speech and Hearing Disorders, 28*, 37–41.

McGarvey, S.D., & Weinberg, B. (1984). Esophageal insufflation testing in nonlaryngectomized adults. *Journal of Speech and Hearing Disorders, 49*, 272–277.

McGavran, M.H., Bauer, W., & Ogura, J.H. (1961). The incidence of cervical lymph node metastases from epidermoid carcinoma of the larynx and their relationship to certain characteristics of the primary tumor: A study based on the clinical and pathological findings for 96 patients treated by primary en bloc laryngectomy and radical neck dissection. *Cancer, 14*, 55–66.

McGuirt, F.W., & Koufman, J.A. (1987). Endoscopic laser surgery: an alternative in laryngeal cancer treatment. *Archives of Otolaryngology—Head and Neck Surgery, 113*, 501–505.

McHenry, M., Reich, A. & Minifie, F. (1982). Acoustical characteristics of intended syllabic stress in excellent esophageal speakers. *Journal of Speech and Hearing Research, 25*, 554–564.

MacKnight, C.A., & Doyle, P.C. (1992, November). *Idiosyncratic patterns of voice onset time in superior tracheoesophageal speakers.* Paper presented at the Annual Convention of the American Speech-Language-Hearing Association, San Antonio, TX.

McMinn, R.M.H., Hutchings, R.T., & Logan, B.M. (1981). *A colour atlas of head and neck anatomy.* London: Wolfe.

McNeil, B.J., Weichselbaum, R., & Pauker, S.G. (1981). Speech and survival: Tradeoffs between quality and quantity of life in laryngeal cancer. *The New England Journal of Medicine, 305*, 982–987.

McWilliams, J.A.O. (1991). History and physical examination. In E.M. Myers (Ed.), *Head and neck oncology: Diagnosis, treatment, and rehabilitation* (pp. 19–43). Boston: Little, Brown and Company.

Mellette, S.J. (1985). The cancer patient at work. *CA, 35*, 360–373.

Mellette, S.J. (1989). Rehabilitation issues for cancer survivors: Psychosocial challenges. *Journal of Psychosocial Oncology, 7*(4), 93–110.

Mendez, P., Maves, M.D., & Panje, W.R. (1985). Squamous cell carcinoma of the head and neck in patients under 40 years of age. *Archives of Otolaryngology, 111*, 762–764.

Meyer, G.W., & Castell, D.O. (1980). Current concepts in esophageal function. *American Journal of Otolaryngology, 1*, 440–446.

Mihashi, K. (1977). Investigations of phonatory function following vertical partial laryngectomy. *Otolaryngology Fukuoka, 23*, 786–806.

Miller, M.H. (1958). The responsibility of the speech therapist to the laryngectomized patient. *Archives of Otolaryngology, 70*, 213–219.

Miller, S., Harrison, L.B., Solomon, B., & Sessions, R.B. (1990). Vocal changes in patients undergoing radiation therapy for glottic cancer. *Laryngoscope, 100*, 603–606.

Miller, G.A., Heise, G.A., & Lichten, W. (1971). The intelligibility of speech as a function of the context of test materials. In I. Ventry, J. Chaiklin, & R. Dixon (Eds.), *Hearing measurement: A book of readings.* New York: Appleton-Century-Crofts.

Miller, G.A., & Nicely, P.E. (1955). An analysis of perceptual confusions among English consonants. *Journal of the Acoustical Society of America, 27*, 338–352.

Mintz, D.R., Gullane, P.J., Thomson, D.H., & Ruby, R.R.F. (1981). Perichondritis of the larynx following radiation. *Otolaryngology Head and Neck Surgery, 89*, 550–554.

Moolenaar-Bijl, A. (1953). Connection between consonant articulation and the intake of air in oesophageal speech. *Folia Phoniatrica, 5*, 212–216.

Moon, J.B., & Weinberg, B. (1987). Aerodynamic and myoelastic contributions to tracheoesophageal voice production. *Journal of Speech and Hearing Research, 30*, 387–395.

Moore, C. (1971). Cigarette smoking and cancer of the mouth, pharynx, and larynx. *Journal of the American Medical Association, 218*, 553–558.

Morbidity and Mortality Report (1986). Cigarette smoking in the United States. *Morbidity and Mortality Weekly Report, 36*, 581–585.

Morozink, N. (1986). Nursing care of the laryngectomee outside the hospital environment. In R.L. Keith & F.L. Darley (Eds.), *Laryngectomy rehabilitation*, pp. 323–330. San Diego, CA: College-Hill Press.

Morrison, M.D. (1988). Is chronic gastroesophageal reflux a causative factor in glottic carcinoma? *Otolaryngology—Head and Neck Surgery, 99*, 370–373.

Morrison, M.D., & Ogrady, M. (1986). Primary tracheo-esophageal puncture voice restoration with laryngectomy. *Journal of Otolaryngology, 15*, 69–74.

Mullan, F. (1984). Re-jentry: The educational needs of the cancer survivor. *Health Education Quarterly, 10*, 88–94.

Murrills, G. (1983). Pre- and early post-operative care of the laryngectomee and spouse. In Y. Edels (Ed.), *Laryngectomy: Diagnosis to rehabilitation*, (pp. 58–74). London, England: Aspen.

Murry, T., Bone, R.C., & Von Essen, C. (1975). Changes in voice production during radiotherapy for laryngeal cancer. *Journal of Speech and Hearing Disorders, 39*, 194–201.

Murry, T., & Singh, S. (1982). Acoustic and perceptual features of laryngeal cancer. In A. Sekey (Ed.), *Electroacoustic analysis and enhancement of alaryngeal speech* (pp. 119–134). Springfield, IL: Charles C. Thomas.

Muscat, J.E., & Wynder, E.L. (1992). Tobacco, alcohol, asbestos, and occupational risk factors for laryngeal cancer. *Cancer, 69*, 2244–2251.

Myers, C.L., & Baird, A.J. (1992, May). *Quality of life: Issues in communication disorders.* Paper presented at the annual conference of the Canadian Association of Speech-Language Pathologists and Audiologists, Saskatoon, Saskatchewan.

Myers, E.M. (1991a). Staging. In E.M. Myers (Ed.), *Head and neck oncology: Diagnosis, treatment, and rehabilitation* (pp. 105–125). Boston: Little, Brown and Company.

Myers, E.M. (1991b). Planning. In E.M. Myers (Ed.), *Head and neck oncology: Diagnosis, treatment, and rehabilitation* (pp. 129–148). Boston: Little, Brown and Company.

Myers, E.M. (1991c). Neck dissection. In E.M. Myers (Ed.), *Head and neck oncology: Diagnosis, treatment, and rehabilitation* (pp. 311–327). Boston: Little, Brown and Company.

Myers, E.M., & Ogura, J.H. (1979). Completion laryngectomy. *Annals of Otology, Rhinology, and Laryngology, 88*, 172–177.

Negus, V.E. (1949). The second stage of swallowing. *Acta Otolaryngologica* (Stockholm), 76–81.

Neel, H.B., & DeSanto, L.W. (1986). Factors in the choice of treatment of patients with laryngeal cancer. In R.L. Keith & F.L. Darley (Eds.), *Laryngectomee rehabilitation* (pp. 291–293). San Diego: College-Hill Press.

Neel, H.B., Devine, K.D., & DeSanto, L.W. (1980). Laryngofissure and cordectomy for early cordal carcinoma: Outcome in 182 patients. *Otolaryngology—Head and Neck Surgery, 88*, 79–84.

Nichols, A.C. (1976). Confusions in recognizing phonemes spoken by esophageal speakers: I. initial consonants and clusters. *Journal of Communication Disorders, 9*, 27–41.

Nichols, A.C. (1977). Confusions in recognizing phonemes spoken by esophageal speakers: III. terminal consonants and clusters. *Journal of Communication Disorders, 10*, 285–299.

Norante, J.D., & Rubin, P. (1978). Head and neck tumors. In P. Rubin & R. Bakemeire (Eds.), *Clinical oncology for medical students and physicians: A multidisciplinary approach* (5th). New York: American Cancer Society.

Nordman, E., Joensuu, H., Kellokumpu-Lehtinen, P., Minn, H., & Mantyla, M. (1990). It it possible to predict the outcome of radiation therapy of head and neck cancer? *Acta Oncologica, 29*, 521–524.

Ogura, J.H. (1955). Surgical pathology of cancer of the larynx. *Laryngoscope, 65*, 867–926.

Ogura, J.H., & Biller, H.F. (1969). Glottic reconstruction following extended fronto-lateral hemilaryngectomy. *Laryngoscope, 79*, 2181–2184.

Olofsson, J., & van Nostrand, A.W.P. (1973). Growth and spread of laryngeal and hypopharyngeal carcinoma with reflections on the effect of preoperative irradiation: 139 cases studied by whole organ serial sectioning. *Acta Otolaryngologica* (Suppl.), *308*, 28–29.

Oppenheimer, R., & Leader, B. (1990). Device for testing the Singer-Blom prosthesis. *Laryngoscope, 100*, 556–557.

Ossoff, R.H., Sisson, G.A., & Shapshay, S.M. (1985). Endoscopic management of selected early vocal cord carcinoma. *Annals of Otology, Rhinology, and Laryngology, 94*, 560–564.

O'Young, J., & McPeek, B. (1987). Quality of life variables in surgical trials. *Journal of Chronic Diseases, 40*, 513–522.

Palmer, E.D. (1976). Disorders of the cricopharyngeus muscle: A review. *Progress in Gastroenterology, 71*, 510–519.

Palmer, J.M. (1970). Clinical expectations in esophageal speech. *Journal of Speech and Hearing Disorders, 35*, 160–169.

Pearson, B.W. (1981). Subtotal laryngectomy. *Laryngoscope, 91*, 1904–1912.

Pearson, B.W. (1986). Office examination of the laryngectomee. In R.L. Keith & F.L. Darley (Eds.), *Laryngectomy rehabilitation*, (pp. 253–262). San Diego: College-Hill Press.

Pearson, B.W., Woods, R.D., & Hartman, D.E. (1980). Extended hemilaryngectomy for T3 glottic carcinoma with preservation of speech and swallowing. *Laryngoscope, 90*, 1950–1961.

Pellitteri, P.K., Kennedy, T.L., Vrabec, D.P., Beller, D., & Hellstrom, M. (1991). Radiotherapy, the mainstay in the treatment of early glottic carcinoma. *Archives of Otolaryngology and Head and Neck Surgery, 117*, 297–301.

Perez, C.A., Holtz, S., Ogura, J.H., Dedo, H.H., & Powers, W.E. (1968). Radiation therapy of early carcinoma of the true vocal cords. *Cancer, 21*, 764–771.

Perez, C.A., & Marks, J.E. (1985). Radiation therapy for carcinoma of the larynx. In B.J. Bailey & H.F. Biller (Eds.), *Surgery of the larynx* (pp. 417–433). Philadelphia: W.B. Saunders.

Pillsbury, H.R.C., & Kirchner, J.A. (1979). Clinical versus histopathologic staging in laryngeal cancer. *Archives of Otolaryngology, 105*, 157–159.

Pressman, J.J. (1954). Cancer of the larynx: Laryngoplasty to avoid laryngectomy. *Archives of Otolaryngology, 59*, 395–412.

Pressman, J.J. (1956). Submucosal compartmentalization of the larynx. *Annals of*

Otology, Rhinology, and Laryngology, 65, 766–673.

Pressman, J., Dowdy, A., & Libby, R. (1956). Further studies upon the submucosal compartments and lymphatics of the larynx by injection of dyes and radioisotopes. *Annals of Otology, Rhinology, and Laryngology, 65,* 963–971.

Pressman, J., Simon, M., & Monell, C. (1960). Anatomical studies related to the dissemination of cancer of the larynx. *Transactions of the American Academy of Ophthalmology and Otolaryngology, 64,* 628–625.

Prutting, C.A. (1982). Pragmatics as social competence. *Journal of Speech and Hearing Disorders, 47,* 123–134.

Public Health Service—National Institutes of Health (1984). *Cancer incidence and mortality in the United States: SEER program.* Bethesda, MD: NIH Publication #85-1837.

Putney, F.J. (1958). Rehabilitation of the post-laryngectomized patient: specific discussion of failures, advanced and difficult technical problems. *Annals of Otology, Rhinology, and Laryngology, 67,* 544–549.

Quigley, K.M. (1989). The adult cancer survivor: psychosocial consequences of cure. *Seminars in Oncology Nursing, 5,* 63–69.

Rabuzzi, D.D., Chung, C.T., & Sagerman, R.H. (1980). Prophylactic neck irradiation. *Archives of Otolaryngology, 106,* 454–455.

Ranney, J.L. (1975). Rehabilitation through employment. *Laryngoscope, 85,* 674–676.

Records, N.L., Tomblin, J.B., & Freese, P.R. (1992). The quality of life of young adults with histories of specific language impairment. *American Journal of Speech-Language Pathology, 1,* 44–53.

Reed, C.G. (1983a). Surgical-prosthetic techniques for alaryngeal speech. *Communicative Disorders, 8,* 109–124.

Reed, C.G. (May, 1983b). *Alaryngeal speech: What are the speech options for the laryngectomee?* Paper presented at the 1983 ASHA Western Regional Conference, Honolulu, HI.

Reed, G.F., Mueller, W., & Snow, J.B. (1959). Radical neck dissection: A clinicopathological study of 200 cases. *Laryngoscope, 69,* 702–743.

Report of Surgeon General. (1986). *The health consequences of involuntary smoking.* Rockville, MD. United States Department of Health and Human Services: Office on Smoking and Health.

Rizer, F.M., Schecter, G.L., & Coleman, R.F. (1984). Voice quality and intelligibility characteristics of the reconstructed larynx and pseudolarynx. *Otolaryngology—Head and Neck Surgery, 92,* 635–638.

Robe, E.Y., Moore, P., Andrews, A.H., & Holinger, P.H. (1956). A study of the role of certain factors in the development of speech after laryngectomy: Site of psuedoglottis. *Laryngoscope, 66,* 382–401.

Robbins, J. (1984). Acoustic differentiation of laryngeal, esophageal, and tracheoesophageal speech. *Journal of Speech and Hearing Research, 27,* 577–585.

Robbins, J., Fisher, H.B., Blom, E.D., & Singer, M.L. (1984). A comparative acoustic study of normal, esophageal, and tracheoesophageal speech production. *Journal of Speech and Hearing Disorders, 49,* 202–210.

Robbins, J.A., Christensen, J.C., & Kempster, G. (1986). Characteristics of speech production after tracheoesophageal puncture: Voice onset time and vowel duration. *Journal of Speech and Hearing Research, 29,* 499–504.

Robbins, K.T., Medina, J.E., Wolfe, G.T., Levine, P.A., Sessions, R.B., & Pruet, C.W. (1991). Standardizing neck dissection terminology. *Archives of Otolaryngology—Head and Neck Surgery, 117,* 601–605.

Robin, P.E., Powell, J., Holme, G.M., Waterhouse, J.A.H., McConkey, C.C., & Robertson, J.E. (1989). *Cancer of the larynx: Clinical cancer monograph, Volume 2.* London: MacMillan Press Ltd.

Rollin, W.J. (1987). *The psychology of communication disorders in individuals and their families.* Englewood Cliffs, NJ: Prentice-Hall.

Rothfield, R.E., Johnson, J.T., Myers, E.N., & Wagner, R.L. (1989). The role of hemilaryngectomy in the management of T1 vocal cord cancer. *Archives of Otolaryngology—Head and Neck Surgery, 115,* 667–680.

Rothfield, R.E., Johnson, J.T., Myers, E.N., & Wagner, R.L. (1990). Hemilaryngectomy for salvage of radiation therapy failures. *Otolaryngology—Head and Neck Surgery, 103,* 792–794.

Rothman, H.B. (1978). Analyzing artificial electronic larynx speech. In S.J. Salmon & L.P. Goldstein (Eds.) *The artificial larynx handbook* (pp. 87–111). New York: Grune & Stratton.

Rothman, H.B. (1982). Acoustic analysis of artificial laryngeal speech. In A. Sekey (Ed.),

Electroacoustic analysis and enhancement of alaryngeal speech (pp. 95–118). Springfield, IL: Charles C. Thomas.

Ryan, W., Gates, G.W., Cantu, E., & Hearne, E. (1982). Current status of laryngectomee rehabilitation: III. Understanding esophageal speech. *American Journal of Otolaryngology, 3,* 91–96.

Sacco, P.R., Mann, M.B., & Schultz, M.C. (1967). Perceptual confusions among selected phonemes in esophageal speech. *Journal of the Indiana Speech and Hearing Association, 26,* 19–33.

Salmon, S.J. (1978a). Patients talk back. In S.J. Salmon & L.P. Goldstein (Eds.), *The artificial larynx handbook* (pp. 43–53). New York: Grune & Stratton.

Salmon, S.J. (1978b). Looking ahead. In S.J. Salmon & L.P. Goldstein (Eds.), *The artificial larynx handbook* (pp. 145–147). New York: Grune & Stratton.

Salmon, S.J. (1979). Pre- and postoperative conferences with laryngectomized and their spouses. In R.L. Keith & F.L. Darley (Eds.), *Laryngectomee rehabilitation* (pp. 379–402). San Diego: College-Hill Press.

Salmon, S.J. (1986a). Pre- and postoperative conferences with the laryngectomized and their spouses. In R.L. Keith & F.L. Darley (Eds.), *Laryngectomy rehabilitation* (pp. 277–290). San Diego, CA: College-Hill Press.

Salmon, S.J. (1986b). Adjusting to laryngectomy. *Seminars in Speech and Language, 7,* 67–94.

Salmon, S.J. (1986c). Laryngectomee visitations. In R.L. Keith & F.L. Darley (Eds.), *Laryngectomy rehabilitation* (pp. 351–369). San Diego: College-Hill Press.

Salmon, S.J. (1986d). Methods of air intake for esophageal speech and their associated problems. In R.L. Keith & F.L. Darley (Eds.), *Laryngectomy rehabilitation* (pp. 55–69). San Diego: College-Hill Press.

Salmon, S.J. (1986e). Factors that may interfere with acquiring esophageal speech. In R.L. Keith, & F.L. Darley (Eds.), *Laryngectomy rehabilitation* (pp. 357–363). San Diego: College-Hill Press.

Salmon, S. (1989). Using an artificial larynx. In E. Lauder (Ed.), *Self-help for the laryngectomee* (pp. 62–65). San Antonio, TX: Lauder Publishing.

Salmon, S.J. (1990). The efficacy of speech-language pathology intervention: laryngectomy. *Seminars in Speech and Language, 11,* 256–272.

Salmon, S.J., & Goldstein, L.P. (1978). *The artificial larynx handbook.* New York: Grune & Stratton.

Sanchez-Salazar, V., & Stark, A. (1972). The use of crisis intervention in the rehabilitation of laryngectomees. *Journal of Speech and Hearing Disorders, 37,* 323–328.

Sandberg, N. (1970). Motility of the pharynx and esophagus after laryngectomy. *Acta Otolaryngology, 263,* 124–127.

Sands, H. (1865). Case of cancer of the larynx successfully removed by laryngectomy. *New York Academy Medical Journal, 1,* 110–126.

Sasaki, C.T. (1983). Horizontal supraglottic laryngectomy. In B.W. Jafek & C.T. Sasaki (Eds.) *The atlas of head and neck surgery* (pp. 333–338). New York: Grune & Stratton.

Scarpino, J., & Weinberg, B. (1981). Junctural contrasts in esophageal and normal speech. *Journal of Speech and Hearing Research, 46,* 120–126.

Schaefer, S., & Johns, D.F. (1982). Attaining function esophageal speech. *Archives of Otolaryngology, 108,* 647–650.

Schechter, G.L. (1986). Conservation surgery of the larynx. In C.W. Cummings (Ed.), *Otolaryngology—Head and neck surgery.* St. Louis, MO: C.V. Mosby.

Schechter, G.L., & El-Mahdi, A.M. (1984). Conservation surgery of the larynx—when? *Otolaryngologic Clinics of North America, 17,* 215–225.

Schleper, J.R. (1989). Prevention, detection, and diagnosis of head and neck cancers. *Seminars in Oncologic Nursing, 5,* 139–149.

Schottenfeld, D., Gantt, R.C., & Wynder, E.L. (1974). The role of alcohol and tobacco in multiple primary cancers of the upper digestive system, larynx, and lung: A prospective study. *Preventive Medicine, 3,* 277–293.

Schutt, A.H. (1986). Physical and occupational therapy for the patient with laryngectomy: Why and what for? In R.L. Keith & F.L. Darley (Eds.), *Laryngectomy rehabilitation,* (pp. 295–308). San Diego: College-Hill Press.

Scripture, E.W. (1916). Speech without using the larynx. *Journal of Physiology, 50,* 397–403.

Sedory, S.E., Hamlet, S.L., & O'Connor, N.P. (1989). Comparisons of perceptual and acoustic characteristics of tracheoesophageal and excellent esophageal speech.

Journal of Speech and Hearing Disorders, 54, 209–214.

Sessions, D.G. (1976). Surgical pathology of the larynx and hypopharynx. *Laryngoscope, 86,* 814–839.

Sessions, D.G. (1980). Extended partial laryngectomy. *Annals of Otology, Rhinology, and Laryngology, 89,* 556–557.

Sessions, D.G., Maness, G.M., & McSwain, B. (1965). Laryngofissure in the treatment of carcinoma of the vocal cord: A report of forty cases and a review of the the literature. *Laryngoscope, 75,* 490–502.

Shames, G.H., Font, J., & Matthews, J. (1963). Factors related to speech proficiency of the laryngectomized. *Journal of Speech and Hearing Disorders, 28,* 273–287.

Shanks, J.C. (1979). Essentials for alaryngeal speech: psychology and physiology. In R.L. Keith & F.L. Darley (Eds.), *Laryngectomee rehabilitation* (pp. 469–489). San Diego, CA: College-Hill.

Shanks, J.C. (1986a). Evoking esophageal voice. *Seminars in Speech and Language, 7,* 1–11.

Shanks, J.C. (1986b). Development of the feminine voice and refinement of esophageal voice. In R.L. Keith & F.L. Darley (Eds.), *Laryngectomy rehabilitation* (pp. 269–276). San Diego: College-Hill Press.

Shanks, J.C. (1986c). Essentials for alaryngeal speech: Psychology and physiology. In R.L. Keith & F.L. Darley (Eds.), *Laryngectomy rehabilitation* (pp. 337–349). San Diego, CA: College-Hill Press.

Shapiro, M.J., & Ramanathan, V.R. (1982). Trachea stoma vent voice prosthesis. *Laryngoscope, 92,* 1126–1129.

Shapshay, S.M., Hybels, R.L., & Bohigian, R.K. (1990). Laser excision of early vocal cord carcinoma: Indications, limitations, and precautions. *Annals of Otology, Rhinology, and Laryngology, 99,* 46–50.

Shedd, D., Schaaf, D., & Weinberg, B. (1976). Technical aspects of reed fistula speech rehabilitation following pharyngolaryngectomy. *Journal of Surgical Oncology, 8,* 305–310.

Shiffman, S., Cassileth, B.R., Black, B.L., Buxbaum, J., Celentano, D.D., Corcoran, R.D., Gritz, E.R., Laszlo, J., Lichtenstein, E., Pechacek, T.F., Prochaska, J., & Scholefield, P.G. (1991). Needs and recommendations for behavior research in the prevention and early detection of cancer. *Cancer, 67,* 800–804.

Shipp, T. (1967). Frequency, duration, and perceptual measures in relation to judgment of alaryngeal speech acceptability. *Journal of Speech and Hearing Research, 10,* 417–427.

Shipp, T. (1970). EMG of pharygoesophageal musculature during alaryngeal voice production. *Journal of Speech and Hearing Research, 13,* 184–192.

Shipp, T., Deatsch, H.H., & Robertson, K. (1970). Pharyngoesophageal muscle activity during swallowing in man. *Laryngoscope, 80,* 1–16.

Shook, R. (1983). *Survivors: Living with cancer.* New York: Harper & Row.

Sigler, B.A. (1989). Nursing care of patients with laryngeal cancer. *Seminars in Oncology Nursing, 5,* 160–165.

Silver, C.E. (1981). *Surgery for cancer of the larynx and related structures.* New York: Churchill-Livingstone.

Silver, F.M., Gluckman, T.L., & Donegan, J.O. (1985). Operative complications of tracheoesophageal puncture. *Laryngoscope, 95,* 1360–1362.

Silverberg, E. (1980). *Cancer statistics: 1980.* New York: American Cancer Society.

Silverberg, E. (1983). *Cancer statistics: 1983.* New York: American Cancer Society.

Silverberg, E. (1984). *Cancer statistics: 1984.* New York: American Cancer Society.

Silverberg, E., & Lubera, J.A. (1989). Cancer statistics, 1989. *CA, 39,* 12.

Simpson, I.C., Smith, J.C.S., & Gordon, M.T. (1972). Laryngectomy: The influence of muscle reconstruction on the mechanism of esophageal voice production. *Journal of Laryngology and Otology, 86,* 961–989.

Singer, M.I. (1983). Tracheoesophageal speech: Vocal rehabilitation following total laryngectomy. *Laryngoscope, 93,* 1454–1465.

Singer, M.I. (1988). The upper esophageal sphincter: Role in alaryngeal speech acquisition. *Head and Neck Surgery,* (Suppl.II), S118–S123.

Singer, M.I. & Blom, E.D. (1980). An endoscopic technique for restoration of voice after laryngectomy. *Annals of Otology, Rhinology and Laryngology, 89,* 529–533.

Singer, M.I., & Blom, E.D. (1981). Selective myotomy for voice restoration after total laryngectomy. *Archives of Otolaryngology, 107,* 670–673.

Singer, M.I., & Blom,. E.D. (1985). Voice rehabilitation with prosthetic devices. In B.J. Bailey & H.F. Biller (Eds.), *Surgery of the larynx* (pp. 367–384). Philadelphia: W.B. Saunders.

Singer, M.I., Blom, E.D., & Hamaker, R.C. (1981). Further experiences with voice restoration after total laryngectomy. *Annals of Otology, Rhinology and Laryngology, 90,* 498–502.

Singer, M.I., Blom, E.D., & Hamaker, R.C. (1983). Voice rehabilitation after total laryngectomy. *Journal of Otolaryngology, 12,* 329–334.

Singer, M.I., Blom, E.D., & Hamaker, R.C. (1984). Surgical restoration of voice after laryngectomy. In G.T. Wolf (Ed.), *Head and neck oncology.* Boston: Martinus Nijhoff.

Singer, A.I., Blom, E.D., & Hamaker, R.C. (1986). Pharyngeal plexus neurectomy for alaryngeal speech rehabilitation. *Laryngoscope, 96,* 50–54.

Singer, M.I., Blom, E.D., & Hamaker, R.C. (1988). *Voice restoration following total laryngectomy,* Instructional videotape. Santa Barbara, CA: InHealth Technologies and Hansa Medical Products.

Singer, M.I., Hamaker, R.C., & Blom, E.D. (1989). Revision procedure for the tracheoesophageal puncture. *Laryngoscope, 99,* 761–763.

Sisson, G.A., McConnel, F., Logemann, J., & Yeh, S. (1975). Voice rehabilitation after laryngectomy: Results with the use of a hypopharyngeal prosthesis. *Archives of Otolaryngology, 101,* 178–181.

Skolnik, E.M., Yee, K.F., Wheatley, M.A., & Martin, L.O. (1975). Carcinoma of the laryngeal glottis: Therapy and end results. *Laryngoscope, 85,* 1453–1465.

Smith, D. (1981). *Survival of illness.* New York: Springer.

Smith, B.E., Riesberg, D.J., Hill, J.H., & Maddox, C.M. (1985). A preoperative counseling aid for tracheoesophageal puncture. *Otolaryngology—Head and Neck Surgery, 93,* 686–687.

Smith, B.E., Weinberg, B., Feth, L.L., & Horii, Y. (1978). Vocal roughness and jitter characteristics of vowels produced by esophageal speakers. *Journal of Speech and Hearing Research, 21,* 240–249.

Smith, K., & Lesko, L. (1988). Psychosocial problems in cancer survivors. *Oncology, 2,* 33–40.

Snidecor, J.C. (1975). Some scientific foundations for voice restoration. *Laryngoscope, 85,* 640–648.

Snidecor, J.C. (1978a). Speech therapy for those with total laryngectomy. In J.C. Snidecor (Ed.), *Speech rehabilitation of the laryngectomized* (2nd ed., pp. 180–193). Springfield, IL: Charles C. Thomas.

Snidecor, J.C. (1978b). The artificial larynx. In J.C. Snidecor (Ed.), *Speech rehabilitation of the laryngectomized* (2nd ed., pp. 199–208). Springfield, IL: Charles C. Thomas.

Snidecor, J.C. & Curry, E.T. (1959). Temporal and pitch aspects of superior esophageal speech. *Annals of Otology, Rhinology and Laryngology, 68,* 1–14.

Snidecor, J.C., & Curry, E.T. (1960). How effectively can the laryngectomee expect to speak? *Laryngoscope, 70,* 62–67.

Snidecor, J.C., & Isshiki, N. (1965). Air volume and air flow relationships of six esophageal speakers. *Journal of Speech and Hearing Disorders, 30,* 205–216.

Som, P.M. (1987). Lymph nodes of the neck. *Radiology, 165,* 593–600.

Som, M.L., & Silver, C.E. (1968). The anterior commissure technique of partial laryngectomy. *Archives of Otolaryngology, 87,* 42–49.

Somerville, S.M., Rona, R.J., & Chinn, S. (1988). Passive smoking and respiratory conditions in primary school children. *Journal of Epidemiology and Community Health, 42,* 105–110.

Sontag, S. (1978). *Illness as metaphor.* New York: Farrar, Straus, and Giroux.

Spofford, B., Jafek, B., & Barcz, D. (1984). An improved method for creating tracheoesophageal fistulas for Blom-Singer or Panje voice prostheses. *Laryngoscope, 94,* 257–258.

Square, P.A. (1986a). The role of the rehabilitation team in counseling the family and friends of the laryngectomy. In R.L. Keith & F.L. Darley (Eds.), *Laryngectomy rehabilitation* (pp. 129–133). San Diego: College-Hill Press.

Square, P.A. (1986b). Death and dying. In R.L. Keith & F.L. Darley (Eds.), *Laryngectomy rehabilitation* (pp. 173–176). San Diego: College-Hill Press.

Stack, F. (1986). The feminine viewpoint on being a laryngectomee. In R.L. Keith & F.L. Darley (Eds.), *Laryngectomy rehabilitation* (2nd ed., pp. 263–268). San Diego, CA: College-Hill Press.

Stalker, J.L., Hawk, A.M., & Smaldino, J.J. (1982). The intelligibility and acceptability of speech produced by five different electronic artificial laryngeal devices. *Journal of Communication Disorders, 15,* 299–307.

Stewart, I.A., & Sherwen, P.J. (1987). Tracheoesophageal puncture simplified. *Laryngoscope, 97,* 639–640.

Stewart, J.G., Brown, J.R., Palmer, M.K., Cooper, A. (1975). The management of glottic carcinoma by primary irradiation with surgery in reserve. *Laryngoscope, 85,* 1477–1485.

Stiernberg, C.M., Bailey, B.J., Calhoun, K.H., & Perez, D.G. (1987). Primary tracheoesophageal fistula procedure for voice restoration: The University of Texas Medical Branch experience. *Laryngoscope, 97,* 820–824.

Stoicheff, M.L. (1975). Voice following radiotherapy. *Laryngoscope, 85,* 608–618.

Stoicheff, M.L., Ciampi, A., Passi, J.E., & Fredrickson, J.M. (1983). Irradiated larynx and voice. *Journal of Speech and Hearing Research, 26,* 482–485.

Stoll, B. (1958). Psychological factors determining the success or failure of the rehabilitation program of laryngectomized patients. *Annals of Otology, Rhinology, and Laryngology, 67,* 550–557.

Strong, M.S. (1975). Laser excision of carcinoma of the larynx. *Laryngoscope, 85,* 1286–1290.

Strong, E.W. (1976). Operative management of carcinoma of the larynx. In J.S. Najarian & J.P. Delaney (Eds.), *Advances in cancer surgery* (pp. 211–220). New York: Stratton.

Subtelny, J.D., Worth, J.H., & Sakuda, M. (1966). Intraoral pressure and rate of flow during speech. *Journal of Speech and Hearing Research, 9,* 498–518.

Tait, N., & Aisner, J. (1989). Nutritional concerns in cancer patients. *Seminars in Oncology Nursing, 5,* 58–62.

Tanner, D.C. (1980). Loss and grief: Implications for the speech-language pathologist and audiologist. *Asha, 22,* 916–928.

Tardy-Mitzell, S., Andrews, M.L., & Bowman, S.A. (1985). Acceptability and intelligibility of tracheoesophageal speech. *Archives of Otolaryngology, 111,* 213–215.

Taub, S. (1980). Air bypass voice prosthesis: An 8-year experience. In D.P. Shedd & B. Weinberg (Eds.), *Surgical and prosthetic approaches to speech rehabilitation* (pp. 17–26). Boston: G.K. Hall.

Taub, S., & Bergner, L.H. (1973). Air bypass voice prosthesis for vocal rehabilitation of laryngectomees. *American Journal of Surgery, 125,* 748–756.

Taub, S., & Spiro, R.H. (1972). Vocal rehabilitation of laryngectomees: preliminary report of a new techic. *American Journal of Surgery, 124,* 87–90.

Taylor, S.G. (1989). Chemotherapy in the combined modality treatment of head and neck cancer. In A.R. Kagan & J. Miles (Eds.) *Head and neck oncology: Clinical management* (pp. 166–170). New York: Pergamon.

Thomas, L. (1983). *The youngest science: Notes of a medicine watcher.* New York: Viking.

Tikofsky, R.S. (1965). A comparison of the intelligibility of esophageal and normal speakers. *Folia Phoniatrica, 17,* 19–32.

Till, J.A., England, K.E., & Law-Till, C.B. (1987). Effects of auditory feedback and phonetic context on stomal noise in laryngectomized speakers. *Journal of Speech and Hearing Disorders, 52,* 243–250.

Titze, I.R. (1980). Comments on the myoelastic-aerodynamic theory of phonation. *Journal of Speech and Hearing Research, 23,* 495–510.

Torgerson, J.K., & Martin, D.E. (1976). Acquisition of esophageal speech subsequent to learning pharyngeal speech: An unusual case study. *Journal of Speech and Hearing Disorders, 41,* 233–237.

Trudeau, M.D. (1987). A comparison of the speech acceptability of good and excellent esophageal and tracheoesophageal speakers. *Journal of Communication Disorders, 20,* 41–49.

Trudeau, M.D., Hirsch, S.M., & Schuller, D.E. (1986). Vocal restorative surgery: Why wait? *Laryngoscope, 96,* 975–977.

Tucker, G.F. (1961). A histological method for the study of the spread of carcinoma within the larynx. *Annals of Otology, Rhinology, and Laryngology, 70,* 910–924.

Tucker, G., Alonso, W.A., & Speiden, L.M. (1971). Comparative application of revised (1971 "T") classification, pathological findings and five-year end results in surgically treated cancer of the larynx. *Laryngoscope, 81,* 1512–1521.

Union Internationale Contre le Cancer (UICC). (1980). *Guidelines for developing a comprehensive cancer centre* (2nd ed.), UICC Technical Report Series—Volume 53. Geneva.

Union Internationale Contre le Cancer (UICC). (1987). *Manual of clinical oncology*. Berlin: Springer-Verlag.

United States Department of Health and Human Services (1984). *Cancer incidence and mortality in the United States—1973–81*. Bethesda, MD. Public Health Service and National Institutes of Health Publication.

van den Berg, J., & Moolenaar-Bijl, A.J. (1959). Cricopharyngeal sphincter, pitch, intensity, and fluency in esophageal speech. *Practical Otorhinolaryngology, 21*, 298–315.

van den Berg, J., Moolenaar-Bijl, A.J., & Damste, P.H. (1958). Oesophageal speech. *Folia Phoniatrica, 10*, 65–84.

van Nostrand, A.W.P., & Brodarec, I. (1982). Laryngeal carcinoma—modifications in surgical technique based on an understanding of tumor growth characteristics. *Journal of Otolaryngology, 11*, 186–190.

Van Riper, C. (1978). *Speech correction: Principles and methods*. Englewood Cliffs, NJ: Prentice-Hall.

Verdolini, K., Skinner, M.W., Patton, T., & Walker, P.A. (1985). Effect of amplification on the intelligibility of speech produced with an electrolarynx. *Laryngoscope, 95*, 720–726.

Vermund, H. (1970). Role of radiotherapy in cancer of the larynx as related to the TMN system of staging. *Cancer, 25*, 485–504.

Viani, L., Stell, P.M., & Dalby, J.E. (1991). Recurrence after radiotherapy for glottic carcinoma. *Cancer, 67*, 577–584.

Vrticka, K., & Svoboda, M. (1961). A clinical and x-ray study of 100 laryngectomized speakers. *Folia Phoniatrica, 13*, 174–186.

Wagenfield, R.L., & Bryce, D.P. (1979). Some aspects of the management of laryngeal cancer. *Journal of Otolaryngology, 8*, 274–283.

Wang, C. (1983). Carcinoma of the hypopharynx/carinoma of the larynx. In *Radiation therapy for head and neck neoplasms* (pp. 155–199). Boston: PSG

Ward, P.H. (1988). Complications of laryngeal surgery: etiology and prevention. *Laryngoscope, 98*, 54–57.

Ward, P.H. (1989). Informed consent in the patient with advanced cancer of the aerodigestive tract. In A.R. Kagan & J. Miles (Eds.), *Head and neck oncology: Clinical management*. New York: Pergammon

Ward, P.H., Berci, G., & Calcaterra, T.C. (1977). New insights into the causes of postoperative aspiration following conservation surgery of the larynx. *Annals of Otology, Rhinology, and Laryngology, 86*, 724–736.

Ward, P.H., Hanafee, W.N., Mancuso, A.A., Shall, J., & Berci, J. (1979). Evaluation of computerized tomography, cinelaryngoscopy, and laryngography in determining the extent of laryngeal disease. *Annals of Otology, Rhinology, and Laryngology, 88*, 454–456.

Ward, P.H., & Hanson, D.G. (1988). Reflux as an etiological factor of carcinoma of the laryngopharynx. *Laryngoscope, 98*, 1195–1199.

Warr, D., McKinney, S., & Tannock, I. (1984). Influence of measurement error on assessment of response to anti-cancer chemotherapy and a proposal for a new criteria of tumor response. *Journal of Clinical Oncology, 2*, 1040–1041.

Warren, D.W. (1982). Aerodynamics of speech. In N. Lass, L. McReynolds, J. Northern, & D. Yoder (Eds.), *Speech, language, and hearing, Vol. I*. Philadelphia: W.B. Saunders.

Watts, R.F. (1975). Total rehabilitation of laryngectomees. *Laryngoscope, 85*, 671–673.

Weinberg, B. (1982). Speech after laryngectomy: An overview and review of acoustic and temporal characteristics of esophageal speech. In A. Sekey (Ed.), *Electroacoustic analysis and enhancement of alaryngeal speech* (pp. 5–48). Springfield, IL: Charles C. Thomas.

Weinberg, B. (1983a). Voice and speech restoration following total laryngectomy. In W.H. Perkins (Ed.), *Voice disorders* (pp. 109–125). New York: Thieme-Stratton.

Weinberg, B. (1983b). Evaluation of treatment effectiveness: voice disorders In W.H. Perkins (Ed.), *Voice disorders* (pp. 147–153). New York: Thieme-Stratton.

Weinberg, B. (1985). Speech rehabilitation of the laryngectomized patient: Advances and issues. In J.M. Costello (Ed.), *Speech disorders in adults* (pp. 113–126). San Diego: College-Hill Press.

Weinberg, B., & Bennett, S. (1971). A study of talker sex recognition of esophageal voices. *Journal of Speech and Hearing Research, 14*, 391–395.

Weinberg, B. & Bennett, S. (1972). Selected acoustic characteristics of esophageal speech produced by female laryngectomees. *Journal of Speech and Hearing Research, 15*, 211–216.

Weinberg, B., & Bosma, J.F. (1970). Similarities between glossopharyngeal breathing and injection methods of air intake for esophageal speech. *Journal of Speech and Hearing Disorders, 35,* 25–32.

Weinberg, B., Horii, Y., Blom, E.D., & Singer, M.I. (1982). Airway resistance during esophageal phonation. *Journal of Speech and Hearing Disorders, 47,* 194–199.

Weinberg, B., Horii, Y., & Smith, B.E. (1980). Long time spectral and intensity characteristics of esophageal speech. *Journal of the Acoustical Society of America, 67,* 1781–1784.

Weinberg, B., & Riekena, A. (1973). Speech produced with the Tokyo artificial larynx. *Journal of Speech and Hearing Disorders, 38,* 383–389.

Weinberg, B., Shedd, D.P., & Horii, Y. (1978). Reed-fistula speech following pharyngolaryngectomy. *Journal of Speech and Hearing Disorders, 43,* 401–403.

Weinberg, B., & Westerhouse, J. (1971). A study of buccal speech. *Journal of Speech and Hearing Research, 14,* 652–658.

Weinberg, B., & Westerhouse, J. (1973). A study of pharyngeal speech. *Journal of Speech and Hearing Disorders, 38,* 111–118.

Weisberger, E.C. (1991). Laryngology. In E.C. Weisberger (Ed.), *Lasers in head and neck surgery* (pp. 197–220). New York: Igaku-Shoin.

Weisler, M.C., Weigle, M.T., Rosenman, J.G., & Silver, J.R. (1989). Treatment of the clinically negative neck in advanced cancer of the head and neck. *Archives of Otolaryngology—Head and Neck Surgery, 115,* 691–694.

Weismann, A., & Worden, J. (1975). Psychosocial analysis of cancer deaths. *OMEGA, 6,* 61–75.

Weiss, M.S., & Basili, A.G. (1985). Electrolaryngeal speech produced by laryngectomized subjects: perceptual characteristics. *Journal of Speech and Hearing Research, 28,* 294–300.

Weiss, M.S., Yemi-Komshian, G.H., & Heinz, J.M. (1979). Acoustical and perceptual characteristics of speech produced with an artificial larynx. *Journal of the Acoustical Society of America, 65,* 1298–1308.

Welch, R.W., Gates, G.A., Luckmann, K.F., Ricks, P.M., & Drake, S.T. (1979). Change in the force-summed pressure measurements of the upper esophageal sphincter prelaryngectomy and postlaryngectomy. *Annals of Otolaryngology, 88,* 804–808.

Welch, R.W., Luckmann, K.F., Ricks, P.M., Drake, S.T., & Gates, G.A. (1979). Manometry of the normal upper esophageal sphincter and its alterations in laryngectomy. *Journal of Clinical Investigation, 63,* 1036–1041.

Welch-McCaffrey, D., Hoffman, B., Leigh, S.A., Loescher, L.J., & Meyskens, F.L. (1989). Surviving adult cancers. Part 2: Psychosocial implications. *Annals of Internal Medicine, 111,* 517–523.

Wellisch, D.K. (1984). Work, social, recreational, family, and physical states. *Cancer, 53,* 2290–2302.

Wenig, B.L., & Applebaum, E.L. (1991). The submandibular triangle in squamous cell carcinoma of the larynx and hypopharynx. *Laryngoscope, 101,* 516–518.

Wenig, B.R., Mullooly, V., Levy, J., & Abramson, A.L. (1989). Voice restoration following laryngectomy: The role of primary versus secondary tracheoesophageal puncture. *Annals of Otology, Rhinology, and Laryngology, 98,* 70–73.

Wetmore, S.J., Johns, M.E., & Baker, S.R. (1981). The Singer-Blom voice restoration procedure. *Archives of Otolaryngology, 107,* 674–676.

Wetmore, S.J., Krueger, K., & Wesson, K. (1981). The Singer-Blom speech rehabilitation procedure. *Laryngoscope, 91,* 1109–1116.

White, R.M. (1991). Chemotherapy. In E.M. Myers (Ed.), *Head and neck oncology: Diagnosis, treatment, and rehabilitation* (pp. 149–160). Boston: Little, Brown and Company.

Williams, N.H. (1961). Speech rehabilitation of the laryngectomized patient. *CA, 11,* 126–130.

Williams, S., & Watson, J.B (1985). Differences in speaking proficiencies in three laryngectomy groups. *Archives of Otolaryngology, 111,* 216–219.

Winans, C.D. (1972). The pharyngoesophageal closure mechanism: A manometric study. *Gastroenterology, 63,* 768–777.

Winans, C.S., Reichback, E.J., & Waldrop, W.F. (1974). Esophageal determinants of alaryngeal speech. *Archives of Otolaryngology, 99,* 10–14.

Wolfe, R.D., Olson, J.E., & Goldenberg, D.B. (1971). Rehabilitation of the laryngectomee: The role of the distal esophageal sphincter. *Laryngosope, 81,* 1971–1978.

Wood, B.G., Rusnov, M.G., & Tucker, H.M. (1981). Tracheoesophageal puncture for laryngectomy voice restoration. *Annals of*

Otology, Rhinology and Laryngology, 90, 492–494.

Wynder, E. (1975). Toward the prevention of laryngeal cancer. *Laryngoscope, 85,* 1190.

Wynder, E.L., Bross, I.J., & Day, E. (1956). Epidemiological approach to the etiology of cancer of the larynx. *Journal of the American Medical Association, 160,* 1384–1391.

Wynder, E.L., Covey, L.S., Marbuchi, K., Johnson, J., & Muschinsky, M. (1976). Environmental factors in cancer of the larynx, a second look. *Cancer, 38,* 1591–1601.

Wynder, E.L., Fijita, Y., Harris, R.E., Hirayama, T., & Hiyama, T. (1991). Comparative epidemiology of cancer between the United States and Japan. *Cancer, 67,* 746–763.

Wynder, E.L., & Stellman, S.D. (1977). Comparative epidemiology of tobacco-related cancers. *Cancer Research, 37,* 4608–4622.

Yoshida, G.Y., Hamaker, R.C., Singer, M.I., Blom, E.D., & Charles, G.A. (1989). Primary voice restoration at laryngectomy: 1989 update. *Laryngoscope, 99,* 1093–1095.

Zaino, C., Jacobson, H., Lepow, H., & Ozturk, C. (1967). The pharyngo-esophageal sphincter. *Radiology, 89,* 639–645.

Zemlin, W.R. (1988). *Speech and hearing science: Anatomy and physiology* (2nd ed.). Englewood Cliffs, NJ: Prentice Hall.

Zwitman, D.H. (1986). The effect of the laryngectomy on pseudoglottis function: Is there a need for surgical improvement? In R.L. Keith & F.L. Darley (Eds.), *Laryngectomy rehabilitation* (pp. 225–236). San Diego: College-Hill Press.

Zwitman, D.H., & Disinger, J.L. (1975). Experimental modification of the Western Electric #5 electrolarynx to a mouth-type instrument. *Journal of Speech and Hearing Disorders, 40,* 35–39.

Zwitman, D.H., Knorr, S.G., & Sonderman, J.C. (1978). Development and testing of an intraoral electrolarynx for laryngectomy patients. *Journal of Speech and Hearing Disorders, 43,* 263–269.

Index